WOMEN IN NURSING
IN ISLAMIC SOCIETIES

WOMEN IN NURSING
IN ISLAMIC SOCIETIES

Edited by
NANCY H. BRYANT

OXFORD
UNIVERSITY PRESS

OXFORD

UNIVERSITY PRESS

Great Clarendon Street, Oxford OX2 6DP

Oxford University Press is a department of the University of Oxford.
It furthers the University's objective of excellence in research, scholarship,
and education by publishing worldwide in

Oxford New York

Auckland Bangkok Buenos Aires Cape Town Chennai
Dar es Salaam Delhi Hong Kong Istanbul Karachi Kolkata
Kuala Lumpur Madrid Melbourne Mexico City Mumbai Nairobi
São Paulo Shanghai Taipei Tokyo Toronto

Oxford is a registered trade mark of Oxford University Press
in the UK and in certain other countries

ISBN 0 19 579888 0

Typeset in Times
Printed in Pakistan by
New Sketch Graphics, Karachi.
Published by
Ameena Saiyid, Oxford University Press
5-Bangalore Town, Sharae Faisal
PO Box 13033, Karachi-75350, Pakistan.

For all the nurses
working to improve and enhance the
profession in Islamic societies.

Contents

Preface

When I initially thought of writing a book about women in nursing in Islamic societies, I had already completed eight years of professional work at the Aga Khan University School of Nursing in Karachi, Pakistan. My husband and I had 'retired' to our home in the woods of Vermont to enjoy a pleasant, somewhat remote life, but with continued connections to the rest of the world which has always been an essential part of our lives.

Then, in the Spring of 1997 we were both asked to return to AKU for a year while the university recruited replacements for our positions. I arranged to work part time as Director of the BSc Nursing programme in order to begin work on this book.

At first, I considered researching and writing the book myself. Within a short time, I realized that many of the topics could be written better by national nurses who lived and worked in South Asian and Middle Eastern countries and by others who were experts in the fields of labour relations, girls'/women's education and nursing standards, regulations, and employment issues. I decided to go forward with an edited book.

It was not hard to find topics that should be included. Many colleagues gave excellent suggestions for possible chapter titles. My problems began when I considered which topics to include and whom to ask to write them. As in all professions, nursing leaders and academics are overly busy, highly committed, and stretched thin with work and outside responsibilities.

I used the academic year 1997-1998 to develop a general outline of the book and to begin contacting possible contributing authors. At the same time I contacted Oxford University Press, Karachi to determine their interest in publishing the book. OUP gave me a favourable response and so did several authors I contacted. I used my year in Karachi to travel to nearby countries in the Middle East to meet nurses at conferences and to visit Dr Enaam Abou Youssef, then Nursing Adviser for the Eastern Mediterranean Region of the World Health Organization in Alexandria, Egypt.

After the summer of 1998, I began the process of getting authors committed to writing their chapters, setting and extending deadlines, and adding new chapters when exciting issues and remarkable events occurred over the next three years. Examples of these later additions are the chapters on violence against nurses in the workplace, the American nurse's experiences in the troubled times of Lebanon, and the current situation of nursing in Afghanistan. Although this process delayed publication, I believe these additions have strengthened the overall content.

Mention must be made here about the marvels of computers and e-mail. There is no question that this book would not have been completed if I had not been able to receive chapters as attachments to e-mails, download and edit them and send them on to OUP in Karachi without relying on surface or air mail. In fact, in May of this year, while visiting with my husband in Kenya, I received a long overdue chapter at the cybercafe in Kisumu, on the shores of Lake Victoria, printed it, edited it and sent the edited version on to Karachi within two days.

I wish to sincerely thank the contributing authors who so generously donated their time, effort and expertise in writing these chapters. For some it meant much extra research and commitment to obtain up-to-date data, assemble new tables, and refine their writing. For others it meant trying to complete a chapter within an impossibly busy schedule. Still others, whose chapters met my first deadline, began to wonder if this book would ever be published as we waited for the last of the chapter proofs to be returned.

Friends, colleagues and family members deserve praise for their assistance with advice, recommendations, editing suggestions as well as encouragement and support. My friends and colleagues Dr Lucie Kelly and Dr Mary Norton provided thoughtful guidance along the way. Nursing leaders at WHO, Dr Naeema Al-Gasseer and Dr Abou Youssef, and Judith Oulton of the International Council of Nurses made excellent suggestions for possible chapter authors and issues to be covered in the book.

In addition, I am extremely grateful for the help of my family, especially my sister Ruth Landini, for her substantial help and skills in editing and providing a non-health professional sounding board for ideas and concepts. I have her husband, Tony, to thank for the transmission of scanned images from the US to Karachi to be used on the book cover. My other sister Elizabeth Myhre cheered on her husband, Trygve, while he solved almost every computer problem I encountered (and there were many) and helped with data and tables. Finally, my husband, Jack, deserves my eternal gratitude for his constant encouragement and enthusiasm for this project. His contribution of time, ideas, suggestions and frequent flyer miles made this book possible.

I am also indebted to my friend and colleague, Dr Paula Herberg, who not only produced a late arriving chapter on nursing in Afghanistan, but also helped in conceptualizing and ordering of the chapter material.

Lastly, I want to thank my editor, Daleara Jamasji-Hirjikaka, for her patience and help in seeing this book to fruition and to OUP for their willingness to encourage and support me in this once in a lifetime effort.

Nancy Halsted Bryant
Moscow, Vermont
August, 2002

Foreword

I was very pleased to be asked to contribute to this important and timely publication. In addressing current issues in Muslim societies it tackles education, violence, working conditions, nursing regulations and women's roles. It presents a realistic picture of conditions and what must be done to improve upon them. Throughout the book we face the burden of the low status and image of nurses, and the lack of skilled national nurses. These are indeed not peculiar to Islamic countries, but are global issues.

Today the shortage of nurses is reaching crisis proportions in many parts of the world. Nurses are working double shifts or days off in industrialized and developing countries, and often still find themselves understaffed. Stress and burn out are common. Working conditions are far from optimal and workplace violence is a reality in every nation. Often remuneration lags behind other workers in the same or equivalent sectors.

We hear stories from countries in Africa, South America, Eastern Europe and Asia of nurses going without pay for weeks and sometimes months. There is a tremendous brain drain from poor to wealthier countries. In many instances this disrupts family life as nurses leave families behind in order to find better paying work and better working conditions. And, as nurses leave, others are recruited to fill their place. Sometimes nurses from other cultures arrive to fill gaps. And often less skilled workers are introduced and given broad skills. Without some attention to human resources planning and the underlying infrastructure issues, this quick fix has long-term implications for the ability to deliver quality care.

An underlying problem worldwide is the lack of a strong policy voice for nursing. It reflects the lack of strong nursing leadership and political skills, as well as the weak nursing voice in governments and parliaments. Nursing regulation is frequently a government role and governments are the primary employer.

The majority of nurses in Islamic countries find themselves in this situation today, a condition that is not new to them. However, in recent years, the problem has been exacerbated by a focus on building hospitals and on developing medical specialization. As a result community-based care is limited and few resources are available for primary health care in countries where most health problems could be tackled by good community-based primary health care services.

The situation is compounded by cultural and traditional practices that discourage young women from entering nursing or from remaining in the profession once married. This problem is more severe in rural areas than cities. It is being partially remedied by the growing number of men in nursing. Their presence should bring greater prestige to the profession, better pay and better care, provided: 1) they have selected nursing as their first choice of profession; 2) they are not all fast tracked into management and teaching positions; and 3) the government monitors numbers so that there is a sufficient gender balance to provide care (since women may find it difficult to receive care from men, and men may object to being nursed by females.)

Addressing human resource and infrastructure issues is critical if citizens are to have access to safe care, particularly in rural and underserved areas where there is often no nurse or physician. Moreover, the reliance on an expatriate workforce, particularly in urban areas, means that those who are clinically competent but are unfamiliar with the language, culture and the health system may provide care.

A long-term strategy will be needed to address issues of the image of nursing, remuneration, access to continuing education, public and physician attitudes, and leadership roles for women and nurses. The Gulf area and other wealthier Islamic countries are already making excellent strides in education, working conditions, regulation and leadership. In the poorer countries the challenge is much greater. Nurses have little access to continuing education, have few career and promotion opportunities, and find themselves lacking clinical competence and motivation.

This picture is bleak but by no means is it all downhill. There is an increasing recognition of the need to address nursing issues such as education, regulation and national planning. There is a growing nursing momentum and a developing leadership base. Skilled nurse leaders in the regional World Health Organization (WHO) offices are helping build strength at national levels. National plans have been developed (though not yet fully funded) aimed at strengthening nursing and midwifery. And nursing education is increasingly being strengthened though telecommunications technology has yet to be well exploited.

There are large numbers of university-prepared nurses in several countries and nursing research is adding evidence to support change. Nurses are organizing in national associations and unions and are more aware of their advocacy roles. WHO Collaborating Centres, donors, nursing strategic alliances, NGOs and government and inter-country hospital twinning initiatives are adding expertise and resources. There is growing support for nursing development. For example in Jordan, Princess Muna, mother of King Abdullah II, is playing an active role in the development of a nursing council. And in Lebanon the Nurses Association has been successful in having a Nurses Act passed to regulate nursing. New associations are in various stages of development, with leadership available from the more established ones.

The International Council of Nurses (ICN) has been involved in nursing and health issues in Islamic countries for many years, assisting with professional issues and helping establish standards and strengthen nursing leadership. Working in cooperation with WHO regional offices and national governments we are currently helping selected nurse leaders at senior and middle levels of the health services acquire requisite knowledge and skills for effective management of nursing services, as well as enhancing their contribution to national health development. It is expected that they will:

- influence policy and health system improvements;
- develop quality, cost-effective models of delivering nursing services in hospital settings;
- be effective contributors to the broader health care team;
- contribute to ongoing leadership/management development programmes for others; and
- influence changes in nursing and midwifery curricula and other training programmes.

The programme, which will run in a number of Islamic countries over the next few years, uses action learning in all programme components including workshop activities, other activities undertaken by participants between workshops, and the development and implementation of team projects. The approach has been successfully offered in over fifty countries and our early observations from both Myanmar and Bangladesh are very encouraging. Through their team projects they are changing approaches in hospitals and schools of nursing. One surgical unit has negotiated a change in admission policy which has already reduced length of stay and addressed overcrowding and excess visitors. Another group—implementing improved aseptic techniques to reduce hospital-acquired infection—is proving successful and is showing a gradual reduction in post-operative stay in hospitals. Interest in the projects and their replication is spreading to other parts of some hospitals, and outside.

There are reasons to be optimistic in the long-term. Even with the rising wave of conservativism globally, there is a growing cadre of committed women and world leaders that should prevent a backlash. However, to reach the goal of healthier Islamic nations we will need continued advocacy for the education of girls, for easier access for women to the working world, and for better education, working conditions and career prospects for nurses. Above all we need politicians, policy makers, the public and other professionals to understand that quality nursing services are essential to better health, and only by strengthening nursing can this happen.

This book is a welcome contribution to nursing globally, and to health care in Islamic countries in particular. It will appeal to all segments of nursing and should be read by students as well as practitioners.

Judith A. Oulton
Chief Executive Officer
International Council of Nurses
Geneva, Switzerland

1

Introduction

Nancy H. Bryant

There is a story that needs to be told about the role of women in modern nursing in Muslim countries. In-depth or even cursory documentation of their status has long been neglected. It is a subject of great concern, affecting the extent and quality of health care delivery in many Islamic societies, and it deserves increased attention from not only medical and nursing professionals, but also from governments and the public as well. The purpose of this compilation of pertinent papers is to heighten awareness of the status of these women nurses and to encourage action for positive and effective change—by health professionals, government officials, educators and laymen alike.

My interest in the subject of women in nursing began when I joined the faculty of The Aga Khan University School of Nursing (AKUSON), Karachi, Pakistan in early 1985. Some nine years of working there with Pakistani female nursing faculty and nursing students, followed by several years of research and study tours to other developing countries, provided an incentive to take a comprehensive look at the issues of modern nursing in Islamic societies. The choice of countries included mostly those within the Eastern Mediterranean Region (EMR) of the World Health Organization (WHO) and a few from South Asia.

I use the term 'modern' nursing to define the time period and educational requirements of the professional nurse that we know today. This is not to say that midwifery service and care of the sick, poor and disabled have not been part of Middle East societies since ancient times. In fact, both medicine and nursing had their early beginnings in this same geographic region prior to Islam and before shifting westward into Europe and beyond.

In ancient Egypt, physicians had developed treatments for numerous illnesses and had established public hygiene and sanitation to a remarkable scale. A concise summary of the contributions of Arabian medicine and the most important physicians of the time is found in Jamieson, Sewall, and Suhrie. They state:

> To this Islamic interest in learning, medicine owes a great deal. Physiology and hygiene were studied and an extensive materia medica developed. Although Moslem belief in the uncleanliness of the dead forbade dissection, surgeons practiced and learned to use hyoscyamus, cannabis indica and opium as anesthetics.... With advancing knowledge of medicine, great hospitals were built and those of Bagdad and Cordova became famous. We hear of women working in them, but instruction seems not to have gone beyond bedmaking.[1]

From ancient times women have assumed the role of nursing the sick, whether it was within the family, during epidemics or when caring for battlefield casualties. Since the history of modern nursing has evolved from the work of women in the early Christian Church, it is necessary to briefly examine the role of these women and note how it has changed over time.

Deaconesses were the earliest orders of women workers in the Church and the ones especially concerned with nursing. They were generally considered to be the first 'visiting nurses,' since their responsibilities included distribution of food and medicines, caring for the sick in their homes and in prisons, as well as performing clerical duties. Phoebe (AD 60), a friend of Saint Paul, was the first deaconess. She had a high social standing and wealth of her own. The order of deaconesses spread over Asia Minor into Syria and throughout Italy into Spain, Gaul and Ireland. It was especially active in the Eastern Church, where Olympia, the young widow of the Roman prefect of Constantinople, organized and guided the work of forty deaconesses.

The order of deaconesses died out early in Rome because the Western Church (Rome) opposed the role they played in conducting churchly functions. 'The female diaconate lasted in the East as an institution until the eighth century, but Schafer says that from the end of the fourth it steadily declined in importance. It was deprived of its clerical character by the decrees passed by the Gallic councils of the fifth and sixth century.'[2]

This action seems to be an early example of power and status being taken from women who were performing 'nursing' and charity roles. The church leaders did not want them on an equal footing with the clergy, and resented their ordination and their freedom of mobility and lifestyle. The women workers of the church who were tolerated and brought into the formal structure were widows and virgins. These women became nuns, joined orders and lived in convents under the rule of male clergy.

Another group of women who distinguished themselves in the field of nursing were noble Roman matrons. 'These were women of wealth, intelligence and social leadership who, having been converted to Christianity, founded hospitals and convents and worked for the good of others.'[3] The best known of these matrons were St. Helena (AD 250–330), Empress Flacilla (AD 346–395), St. Marcella (AD 340–420), St. Fabiola (AD 390) and St. Paula (AD 347–404).

During the early medieval period three famous hospitals were built outside monastery walls; they are still in existence today. They are the Hotel Dieu in Lyons, established in AD 542, where nursing was carried out mainly by repentant women and by widows called sisters and male nurses called brothers; the Hotel Dieu in Paris, founded in AD 650, where the nursing staff was composed of Augustine sisters; and the Santo Spirito Hospital in Rome, founded in AD 717, mainly to care for the sick rather than serving solely as an almshouse.[3] The pattern of nursing that developed during the Middle Ages continued well into the nineteenth century. This is the situation that largely prevailed when Florence Nightingale took up the torch in the mid-1800s.

Although very little information is recorded in Western books about the early role of Islamic women in nursing, several publications from the East include reports of nursing activities carried out by females during the time of the Prophet Muhammad (PBUH). Shaikh and Abbasi report that women nursed wounded soldiers and provided water and food to needy persons.[4] One woman, Umme Atiya, claimed that she participated in seven battles along with the Holy Prophet, prepared food and attended the sick and wounded. The authors give the names of many other Muslim women who at that time carried out similar duties on the battlefields and helped establish tent hospitals.

An interesting account by Hussein about Rufida, the 'First Nurse In Islam,' was published in the Bulletin of Islamic Medicine as part of the Proceedings of The First International Conference on Islamic Medicine in January 1981. Rufida learned healing and nursing skills from her father, Saad al-Aslamy, a prominent healer in Yethreb, Arabia. Hussein claims that Rufida started the first nursing school in Islam when she organized a team of Muslim women and young girls and taught them the art of nursing the wounded and sick. Rufida continued her work in the development and improvement of nursing, even after the battles were over, until her death. According to the author, 'She laid down the first code of Nursing Rules and Ethics in the world. This was fourteen centuries ago and she is still a symbol of noble deeds and self-denial. Twelve centuries later came Florence Nightingale who followed her footsteps.'[5]

After these early reports, however, there are few recordings of progress in nursing among Muslim women until Western missionaries reintroduced these activities in the 1880s.

There has always been an urgent need for women doctors and nurses in Islamic countries. Cultural and traditional practices, as well as the institution of *purdah* in some societies, make it difficult for women to receive care from men. Although this situation is changing somewhat, in the more traditional and conservative societies of the Middle East and South Asia, women are still reluctant to be seen by male health workers.

There are numerous factors that restrict young Muslim women from entering the profession of nursing: the general level of education of girls/women; their status in society; resistance from family members; and cultural and traditional constraints.

In addition, the low status and image of nursing, low pay, poor working conditions and security concerns are major barriers for young women (and their parents) when making a career choice. This situation contributes to a severe shortage of nurses throughout the region.

This book begins with an overview of the global and regional issues of nursing and midwifery, including some of the specific obstacles facing the nursing profession in the Eastern Mediterranean Region. The work of international organizations, such as the International Council of Nurses and the World Health Organization, are viewed as they pertain to nursing in the above region. These chapters are followed by an analysis of the place of girls'/women's education in Islam and its current status; the past and present status and role of women in many Muslim societies; and various aspects of the modern nursing profession in the Middle East and South Asian regions.

Authors in the last portion describe nursing in a selection of countries, ranging from Bangladesh to wartorn Lebanon and Afghanistan. The book concludes with a look at the future direction of nursing in the regions.

Dr Gillian Biscoe, in her analysis of global trends of nursing and midwifery, first examines the key global health trends that are affecting all countries, but at differing times and magnitudes, and then discusses the challenges presented by changes such as evolving medical technology, migration of health care workers and health care management reform.

Her examples include health system reform and development (HSRD) undertaken by widely differing countries such as Thailand, Nepal, New Zealand, Viet Nam, China, etc.

She points out, 'For nurses and midwives, they need to understand HSRD and ensure that proposed changes address values and attitudes, as well as the skills, competencies and organizational cultures needed to support appropriate change in health policy and the health system.' She notes, however, that in making these reforms, both developed and developing countries often fail to recognize that 'capable and motivated staff are the lifeblood of an effective state.' Biscoe also cites the Magnet Hospital Study conducted by the USA which found that nurses and midwives were attracted to organizations where the organization's culture placed value on them, where there was respect between health professionals and workers and the focus was on excellence in care.

The conclusions of this study appear to be self evident, but many countries and organizations have not made appropriate changes in their organizations to reflect these findings and recommendations. The author also places some blame on nurses and midwives (and other health professionals) who do not understand the complexities of the health care system, and have not prepared themselves for decision-making roles in policy and management issues and are, therefore, not included in the process.

It is heartening to learn what can be accomplished when a country such as New Zealand makes the effort to prepare nurses, midwives and others to qualify for senior roles in the health care system. Biscoe is an example of a nurse who took this opportunity and served in high Ministry of Health positions in both New Zealand and Australia. It must be noted that the role and status of women in a country also helps determine the emphasis that that country will place on nurses and midwives in senior administrative and policy positions. Biscoe uses case studies to illustrate various efforts that have been made in Eastern Mediterranean Region countries, China and elsewhere to address challenges for raising the educational level, status and image of nursing and midwifery, while at the same time making the health care systems more efficient and effective. Many but not all of these efforts have been successful.

Concerning nursing and midwifery leadership, Biscoe stresses the need for working in conjunction with government and health ministries to develop and implement long-term goals that will strengthen and upgrade the professions. This is especially true in a time of reduced budgets and high profile health challenges. In addressing the global and international issues related to nurses and midwives, the author also includes lessons from non-health organizations that can be useful for affecting change. Finally, she looks at what the future holds for nurse and midwifery graduates of the year 2005 and makes some assumptions about what changes must occur for them to fulfill a role of leadership and management.

One person who has provided guidance and support to all the countries in the regions under consideration in this book, is Fadwa Affara. In fact, as a consultant in Nursing and Health Policy for the International Council of Nurses (ICN), she provided these services to all countries whose national nursing associations are members of ICN. Her chapter, 'Issues of Control: The Role of Nursing in the Regulation of the Profession,' examines the role that standards and regulations play in empowering the nursing profession.

Affara states that for ICN, regulation is conceptualized in its broadest sense, whereby order, consistency, identity and control are brought to the profession. She points out that in each country, numerous agencies, organizations, institutions, etc. have a part in regulating and setting standards for the nursing profession. Of particular interest are the issues which deal with the question 'Who controls nursing?' and how nursing is regulated in Islamic countries. We learn about the problems these countries face in trying to establish standards of practice and educational qualifications when there is a lack of consensus as to the proper functions of nursing. The author also discusses the problems facing nursing associations and how these problems may weaken the role of the individual nurse and the associations within the health care system, and in the eyes of the public.

Education of girls and women is known throughout the world as a major issue in the Islamic social context. Dr Nagat El-Sanabary has conducted an in-depth analysis of the educational status of girls/women in many Muslim countries. She has researched educational and gender issues in the Middle East and North Africa for over twenty-five years. Her chapter, 'Educating Girls and Women in Islamic Countries: What is the Problem?' is a comprehensive comparison of the progress made and obstacles still existing in the development of girls' and boys' education since the early 1970s by various countries within the region. Her central theme is that all Muslims, whether male or female, are instructed to search for knowledge. Parents want both their sons and daughters to be educated, but many circumstances and obstacles have prevented this from happening. Although the number of girls being educated at all levels—primary, secondary and higher education—has increased substantially in nine selected countries, the author is careful to point out the problems that still persist after thirty years of government, donor agency and private efforts.

It is no surprise that poorer countries of the regions have not done as well as the oil-rich Gulf States. What is interesting is the vast disparity between girls' educational levels in urban and rural areas within the same country, and the reasons for this disparity. Another pertinent observation is the impact of population growth. Although countries such as Bangladesh, Pakistan and Egypt have substantially increased the total number of girls receiving all three levels of schooling, the rates of illiteracy are either unchanged or are higher than in the 1970s. Much of this can be attributed to high population growth rates. El-Sanabary recognizes that unless governments undertake some drastic measures to provide education for all children, along with increased resources from private organizations and donor agencies, these countries will fall hopelessly behind their neighbours and the rest of the world in the twenty-first century.

One issue that remains a long-standing problem in a country's effort to provide education for girls is the severe lack of female teachers. This was the case when Woodsmall wrote about it in 1930 and it is the case today. She writes, 'Throughout the Near East, the Middle East and India, the one profession which has long been accepted for women is teaching. Certainly from Egypt to India, marriage and teaching have been, and still are, the only unquestioned avenues for a woman's activity.'[6] However, it becomes a vicious circle when there are not enough girls educated to become the future teachers. Gradually, more and more young women have entered the teaching profession.

'The development of teaching as a professionally acceptable position for women helped nursing in two ways. First, it provided the opportunity for girls to receive an education, without which they would not be prepared for any professional job, and second, once women were allowed to enter one profession, the opportunity to choose others was bound to follow. This is exactly what happened, but not at the same speed in each country.'[7]

Of broad interest to health planners, Ministries of Health, financial officers, and nursing leaders, educators and employee organizations in many developing countries, is Hedva Sarfati's chapter on 'Remuneration of Nurses in Islamic Countries: An Economic Factor in a Social Context.' As a former Branch Chief at the International Labor Organization (ILO), she brings the knowledge and background of an organization that has studied working conditions of health professionals around the world for many years.

Her chapter presents an in-depth summary of the past and current health care labour needs and trends in the Middle East and South Asian countries. In comparing the public expenditures on health as a percentage of GNP in 1960 and 1990, Sarfati notes that expenditures have grown significantly in most countries of the regions, but are still low when compared with public expenditures for health in industrialized countries. Health policy makers, therefore, must take into account indicators such as demographic trends, income and health levels, access to health services, trends in public health expenditures, distribution of physicians and nurses, and gender gaps in education when planning for the future with limited resources.

Using figures from the UNDP Human Development Report, World Bank Reports, WHO publications and various ILO reports, Sarfati compares income and health indicators, numbers of physicians and nurses per population, women's share of the labour force and so forth in selected Middle East and North African (MENA) and South Asian countries. In addition, she deals specifically with the difficulty of trying to compare remuneration of nurses between and within countries when factors such as merit increments, seniority, special bonuses, and cash and non-cash allowances are taken into account. Added to the above are the issues of the gender factor, personnel shortages, leadership, status, need for primary care providers, migration and working conditions as they pertain to the nursing profession.

Sarfati points out that there is a lack of basic data on the health sector and particularly for nursing personnel, and urgently recommends the establishment of a reliable database with up-to-date statistics on employment, pay and conditions of work in health services in general, and for nursing personnel in particular in order to plan health care services.

A common issue raised in chapters by Amarsi and Sarfati and demonstrated in the Lebanon situation by Mouro, has to do with the concern about security in the workplace for nurses and nursing students. This concern is more closely analyzed by Dr Mireille Kingma in her chapter on 'Violence Against Nurses: Violation of Human Rights.'

For many years Kingma has researched the field of employment conditions for nurses as a consultant for the International Council of Nurses in Geneva, Switzerland. The startling and disturbing facts and figures presented by the author may be familiar to some persons working in the fields of violence and abuse, but will likely come as a shock to most readers. Kingma points out that since most incidents of violence worldwide are against women, it is understandable that a mostly female profession such as nursing would reflect what is, unfortunately, often a cultural norm.

In fact, the situation is much worse than expected. Here is a sample of some statistics she presents:

- Health care staff is at greater risk from work-related violence than the general population.
- The *Health and Safety Executive* has identified nursing as the most hazardous occupation in the United Kingdom.
- In the US...Nurses are more likely to suffer nonfatal injuries while at work than are members of any other profession.
- In Nova Scotia (Canada), 80 per cent of nurse respondents reported experiencing some form of violence in their nursing careers.
- In Turkey, 75 per cent of nurse respondents reported having been sexually harassed during their nursing practice.
- Male physicians were identified as the major perpetrators of sexual harassment in a study undertaken in Pakistan.
- Recent cases of abuse against nurses are not isolated incidents, but form a long history of violence that has been associated with the nursing profession in Pakistan.

Kingma summarizes: 'Violence against nurses is world-wide and appears to be increasing although the degree of underreporting continues to be high. Of great concern is the widespread practice of colleagues, co-workers and administrators of blaming the victim of violence for provoking the incident. Societal values, the treatment of women and the status of nursing as a profession determine the framework or context within which nursing is practiced. In addition, they influence the level of work-related violence experienced by nurses.'

The author then analyzes the issues of health sector risk factors, the consequences of nurse abuse, impact on health services and nurse response to violence. To address these problems, she includes six factors that need to be considered when planning for a secure workplace, including: social structure, legal context, clinical issues, organizational climate, physical environment and staff competence.

As a sociologist, contributing author Kausar S. Khan, has wide knowledge and experience concerning the status of women in Pakistan and other Islamic societies. Her chapter, 'Women in Pakistan: Trapped but Struggling,' uncovers the discouraging facts of oppression, suppression and in some cases, extreme violence against women. Over time, these affronts have been exposed by the press, human rights groups, concerned women's organizations, etc. We are led to believe that conditions are improving, but as she maintains, positive actions by the government to protect women and prosecute the perpetrators fall short of what is required.

Educating young women to the level where they can enter modern nursing programmes has been an ongoing problem in many countries of the world and has been especially troublesome in the Middle East and South Asia. Several factors and influences have been working against one another to cause the situation described in Dr Fariba Al-Darazi's chapter on nursing and nursing education in the Eastern Mediterranean Region (EMR) of WHO, which includes twenty-two countries extending from North Africa, across the the Middle East and into Pakistan.

Most of modern nursing in the region was begun by colonial governments, missionary groups or individual doctors and nurses, and was usually patterned after nursing in their home countries. Early on, there were very few young women with the necessary educational backgrounds to enter Western style nursing programmes. Instead, short courses to produce nursing aides, auxiliaries and midwives to serve mostly in hospitals were begun and later expanded into the usual three-year diploma programme. These programmes varied in content and quality from country to country and even within countries.

As more foreign aid donors provided resources for female nursing education, students often went abroad to study, obtain higher degrees and return to help upgrade their institutions. Foreign advisers and returning nationals with higher education were welcomed, but they also created some problems, such as developing modern nursing curricula based on Western style medicine and health care delivery systems; and making decisions about which medium of language to use—local or foreign—and how many levels of nursing education are required, to name a few.

The WHO Advisory Panel on Nursing for EMRO addressed these many issues at its meeting in 1995. In Al-Darazi's report of this meeting she describes the many programmes of basic nursing education within the twenty-two EMR countries—their varied lengths, educational entrance requirements, curriculum content and capabilities of the graduates. The same troubling issues are reviewed for post-basic nursing education programmes. The panel discussed the need for developing regional standards for basic nursing education, levels of practice and standard-setting for the profession, and priorities for nursing specialization that would be appropriate for the EMR. The recommendations from the advisery panel meeting have been further developed into *A Strategy for Nursing and Midwifery Development in the EMR*, which was published by WHO in 1997.

Some of the uncertainty about the capabilities of nurses in the EMR is reflected in the manner in which nursing human resources are addressed in many of the countries of the region. This is especially true in Pakistan, which serves as an example for Dr Yasmin Amarsi in her chapter, 'Nursing Health Human Resources in Pakistan.' In interviews with federal and provincial government officials, nurse leaders and nursing personnel, Amarsi found numerous shortcomings and differing opinions about planning, production and management of nursing human resource development (NHRD). Using Hall's expanded COHHRD (coordinated health human resource development) model, Amarsi found that in Pakistan planning was hierarchical, with a top-down approach, and was ineffective. The production of nursing personnel did not appear to be coordinated with the planning of nursing personnel for health services. Further, the management of nursing human resources was characterized by a poor working environment, job dissatisfaction, and inadequate salary and benefits for nursing personnel.

It is important to note that Pakistan is not the only country facing problems with NHRD; therefore, the author's summary implication and recommendations will be valuable for health planners, ministries of health, financial officers, and nursing leaders and educators in many developing countries as they seek to raise the quality and adequacy of their nursing services.

Several authors portray nursing in a selection of countries in the Middle East (Saudi Arabia, Iraq, and Lebanon), and South Asia (Afghanistan and Bangladesh) along with one country, Malaysia, from South East Asia. All of the countries in this section have a large if not majority Muslim population, but nurses and the profession of nursing function somewhat differently in each. We can easily compare their similarities and differences.

Reflecting on the chapters in the book as a whole, there are numerous positive signs of change underway that will benefit nursing, including the increase in female education and women being accepted in non-agricultural areas of employment. Leaders in the nursing profession, as through WHO, ICN and national nurses associations, are working hard to upgrade educational programmes and standardize the competencies and roles of nurses in order that international norms can be established to guide the training and employment of nurses.

The future of nursing is strongly dependent on the value that governments, health care systems, the corporate sector and universities place on the profession. It will take positive action from enlightened parties to define the roles and improve the status and image of the modern nurse.

While women play strong and important roles in Muslim family life everywhere, in the more modernized societies of some countries they play increasingly influential roles outside the home. It is from these changing and enlightened societies that more young women will be drawn into the nursing profession. To be sure, however, the needs of the health care systems require that nurses come from all levels of society and from rural as well as urban areas. At the same time, we are constantly reminded that the image and status of nursing must be changed and improved before parents and young women will consider nursing as a career for their daughters or themselves.

The concluding chapter reviews the problems that nursing has faced in the West and East since very early times in its efforts to become a respected profession. While the obstacles have been and still are substantial, particularly in the East, progress is apparent. There is reasonable evidence that continued effort to advance the cause of nursing will result in important gains for the profession and for those who will benefit from the committed and devoted service of nurses around the world.

NOTES

1. Elizabeth M. Jamieson, Mary F. Sewall, and Eleanor B. Suhrie, *Trends in Nursing History: Their Social, International and Ethical Relationships* (6th ed.), Philadelphia: W.B. Saunders, 1966, pp. 89-90.

2. Adelaide Nutting and Lavinia L. Dock, *A History of Nursing*, Vol. 1, New York: G. P. Putnam's Sons, 1935, p. 114.

3. Josephine A. Dolan, *Nursing in Society: A Historical Perspective*, (14th ed.), Philadelphia: W.B. Saunders, p. 45.

4. N.M. Shaikh and S.M. Madni Abbasi, *Women in Muslim Society*, Karachi: International Islamic Publishers, 1981.

5. Suad Hussein, 'Rufida Al-Asalmia: First Nurse in Islam,' Proceedings of the First International Conference on Islamic Medicine, *Bulletin of Islamic Medicine* 1: (2), pp. 261-2.

6. Ruth F. Woodsmall, *Women in the Changing Islamic System*, New York: The Round Table Press, 1936, p. 241.

7. Nancy H. Bryant, 'Progress and Constraints of Nursing and Nursing Education in Islamic Societies,' in *Global Perspectives on Health Care*, Eugene B. Gallagher and Janardan Subedi (eds.), Englewood Cliffs, N.J.: Prentice Hall, 1995, p. 51.

2

Nursing and Midwifery: The Global Context

Gillian Biscoe

This chapter focuses on nursing and midwifery within its global context.[1] Why? Because interdependency between countries and regions is increasing, from finance, to trade, to politics, as new knowledge is shared and embraced. This increasing interdependency affects countries' social and economic development, and together with the rapid global sharing of new knowledge, the development of their health systems and the development of nursing and midwifery. Thus, while detailed issues in nursing and midwifery remain unique to each country, common global themes are emerging. Globally, regionally and nationally, the complexity of health systems is being increasingly understood, with efforts being made in many countries to improve or 'reform' their health systems. These changes, fuelled by rising costs, increasing technology, changing community expectations and knowledge, have placed health higher on countries' government agendas. The pace of system change in the health sector is accelerating in many countries. Where it is not, the pressures for change are increasing.

Nurses and midwives need to understand, keep pace with, and influence these changes, to ensure ongoing relevant and appropriate clinical practice, and to deal with and successfully manage the changing context of their work. Serious global issues in nursing and midwifery include: in many countries a reduction in younger people choosing to become nurses and midwives as a greater range of career opportunities open up for women; a disparity between countries on the education, role and utilisation of nurses and midwives; while, paradoxically, global interdependency is resulting in recruitment of nurses and midwives from one country to the other.

For example, England has a shortage of nurses and midwives. To overcome this shortage England is recruiting from countries as differing as South Africa, Australia, the Philippines and the People's Republic of China. South Africa, as a consequence, is now experiencing a shortage of nurses and midwives, a matter raised between the two countries at the highest political level. In Kuwait, nursing is not always seen as a desirable profession for young Kuwaiti women. Consequently Kuwait's health system is heavily reliant on recruitment of nurses and midwives from abroad, including India.

A generation ago, it was perhaps sufficient to educate neophyte nurses and midwives in their professions' clinical practice only. This is no longer sufficient as nurses and midwives continue in their careers in a rapidly changing global environment. In 1993, the South East Asian Region of the World Health Organization held a five-day strategic planning workshop for senior nurses and midwives. The aim was to develop a Regional ten year plan for nursing and midwifery development. In this it was successful. However, the words of one senior participant encapsulate the statement above: 'We must become "citizens of the world" in our understanding of the influences on us, on our health policies, our health systems, on our professions. If we do not understand these, then how can we influence change, and, as importantly, how can we successfully manage the changes which seem often to be imposed on us.'

Understanding the Global Context

The usual points on global trends need to be presented. However, this is done with some caution. The danger always is that because a label or concept is familiar, there is an assumption that there is shared understanding of the real issues and potential implications. If environmental scanning and rigorous analysis is not repeated regularly within organizations, is it safe to use concepts and labels learned five or eight or ten years ago and assume a shared understanding? There is a need to apply ongoing intellectual rigour to understand new or potential implications, when times continue to change apace.

Globalisation is seen by some to have detrimental affects within countries. Concerns are many and varied but include potential global homogeneity of societal values, exploitation of workers in economically weaker countries, and the accumulation of profit by multinationals with little or no economic return to the host country. Thus, with caution, some key global trends are presented below. The question is, for all of us, what do they actually mean in terms of their potential impact and influence, over time? And importantly, if these are global trends, implying that 'sooner or later' they will happen in most countries, then what are the most effective strategies to adapt and manage these trends successfully within individual countries and organizations? Some key global trends are:

• Economic globalisation and integration.
• Technology and its impact.
• Structural adjustment and privatisation.
• Ensuring sustainable development.
• Emerging new work systems.
• The shift from personnel administration to strategically focused HR efforts.
• Changes in leadership style from bureaucracy to entrepreneurship.[2]
• Changes in organizational culture from risk averse bureaucracies to innovative and effective organizations.

Added to these are the increasing global challenges of keeping abreast with new health knowledge and its implications, from the explosion of knowledge in the genetic field to communicable and non-communicable diseases. While sophisticated technological advances continue, we are faced with the paradox of growing resistance of infectious diseases to antibiotics and the potential for uncontrollable epidemics. For this and other global health challenges, globalisation provides a platform for solutions, given that the magnitude of many of the challenges is greater than the capacity of one nation to successfully address.

Globalisation is defined, for the purpose of this Chapter, as 'the process whereby nations increase their interrelatedness and interdependency through the spread of democracy, the dominance of market forces, the integration of economies in a world-wide market, the transformation of production systems and labour forces, the spread of technological change and...the media revolution.'[3]

In this new world of global competitiveness, perhaps the ideal scenario is a dynamic equilibrium between wealth creation and social cohesiveness, with governments balancing the need for local, social, value-added policies (e.g. health policies) against the need for developing a comparative advantage for their country to actively participate in the global integration of the value chain. Local, social, value-added policies are seen by some to be relatively market and cost-inefficient. However, they are essential for social development. There seems little point in a country being wealthy while civil society crumbles around the pot of gold, leading inexorably to poverty and despair.

The policy issues that governments, and thus society, grapple with are how to finance these social policies, whether privatisation and 'free' market forces will reduce the cost burden, and how to manage the social cost of increased efficiency (e.g. unemployment). Even where governments have sound social policies, globalisation is resulting increasingly in the internationalisation of previous domestic markets such as supermarkets and hospital chains, with some authors saying that this diminishes the direct power and control of government in the domestic market.[4]

We see some countries with health workforce policies focused on both the global and domestic markets, for example the Philippines' overproduction of doctors and nurses, stimulating their 'export'. Overseas-earned income is thus provided to the Philippines because of strong family ties and money being sent home. In other countries, there are barriers protecting domestic markets for example in Australia registration for Australian-resident foreign trained doctors has traditionally been achieved with some difficulty, while there are now some changes in progress.

The migration overseas of 50 per cent of new medical graduates from Thailand in 1965 resulted in the government implementing a three-year compulsory contract for public sector services for all new medical graduates. In 1997, as privatised, competitive health services reached their peak in Thailand, giving choice of employer to medical graduates, 22 per cent of new medical graduates resigned from the public sector to join the private sector, even though the financial penalty for breaking their three-year contract was $US10,000 to US$15,000 in fines. The reasons for resignation included mismanagement of human resources.[5]

In other countries, for example Fiji, increased outward migration of the health workforce has resulted from internal political changes placing strain on the capacity of the health system. In South Africa, as mentioned earlier, an acute shortage of registered nurses is being exacerbated by a similar shortage in the United Kingdom, with the latter recruiting from the former. In both Fiji and South Africa, nurses and midwives have sound education programmes and are therefore 'in demand'.

From time to time, suggestions are made that reducing the quality of nurses and midwives (and other health professionals), making a country unattractive as a source of recruitment, would overcome this problem. This approach raises many complex philosophical issues, but at its simplest level, would reduce the quality of the health system in the home country. Instead, the core reasons why well-trained health professionals want to leave a country should be addressed. As well, health professionals gaining international experience, particularly in their early years of practice, has long been a tradition in developed countries, and gives an additional return-on-investment to the home country, through the additional experience gained when the health professional returns. The ratio of those leaving to work overseas and those returning is the statistic that needs studying. And different countries will be looking for different results (e.g. South Africa vs. the Philippines).

Understanding the Health System

First, within health systems there are competing and conflicting goals. Three of these are society's desire for equitable distribution of health care irrespective of socio-economic status; clinical freedom of medical doctor providers to organize health care as they see fit, and economic freedom to charge prices they deem appropriate or to be paid a salary reflecting their own perceived value; and economic and budgetary controls, with health benefits at the margins justified by costs, and households, insurance agencies and governments being able to budget for the coming year and beyond.[6]

Second, there is knowledge, values and attitude dissymmetry between different categories of health providers, between providers and consumers, and between providers and governments,[7,8] which skew equality and rationality of communication and information exchange and subsequent policy development, including for nursing and midwifery. This dissymmetry creates a market that is unlike other markets, with public sector production failure,[9] and health systems consequently sometimes responding atypically to some management and human resource strategies that are effective in non-health markets.

Third, the goals of a country's health system are, or should be, good health, responsiveness to people's expectations, and fairness of contribution to financing the health system. And that to achieve these goals, a country needs to have effective service provision, resource generation, financing and stewardship.[10]

Fourth, attraction and retention of people to nursing and midwifery, is more than simply education and training, pay, working conditions, and performance and career development. Increasingly the multidimensional nature of organizations is being understood. This multidimensional nature involves interdependency between an individual and the organizational culture, policies and structures, and requires enabling strategic capacity for linkages between a myriad of issues such as information, ethics, awareness, motivation and behaviour.[11]

Fifth, basic knowledge is becoming obsolete at an unprecedented rate, requiring ongoing learning, updating and adaptation as new working styles and labour markets develop.[12] In the author's experience this complexity is ill-understood in the management of health systems, with effective leadership and management too often weak as a result and that, while health sector reform is 'sweeping the developing world, its wider implications for human resources have been largely ignored'.[13]

And finally, the competing and conflicting goals, dissymmetry, and sociohistorical values that underpin each country's health system, create health systems that are inherently resistant to system change. Leadership, management and human resource development strategies are a key vehicle to achieve system change, with maximum effect obtained when strategically linked to health policy and financing strategies. The development of nursing and midwifery needs to be seen by governments as an effective vehicle to assist in achieving stronger health systems, it needs to be linked to health policy and financing strategies, and needs to be seen by governments and other key stakeholders, including the community, as an opportunity to be supported.

Understanding Health System Reform and Development (HSRD)

Health systems are thus complex. They are also neither immune nor divorced from the impact of the new global order. Attempts are being made in most countries of the world to adapt or transform health finance and service delivery structures accordingly.

There have been many lessons learned over the last decade in HSRD. Paradoxically there is little information in the literature on how nursing and midwifery policies and strategies relate to government and health sector reforms. Perhaps the one thing that is clear is that, as with computer systems, a turn-key solution, that is, one country's approach to nursing and midwifery, unilaterally applied to another country, is not the answer, both because of historical, sociopolitical, religious, economic and cultural differences and because of differing national internal capacity and capability. However, global best practice principles can be incorporated in country thinking with adapted specific strategies developed.

Precise definitions of HSRD are not internationally agreed. HSRD can incorporate both health management reforms and health market reforms and it is useful to distinguish the differences (although some countries, for example New Zealand and the UK, undertook both concurrently in the late 1980s), as each has a different impact on the health system and thus the health workforce.

Health management reforms generally include structural changes (e.g. decentralization), health financing reforms (e.g. health insurance), policy process improvements, and strengthened management accountability through financial and human resource (HR) delegations (e.g. to hospitals from the health ministry or central government agencies). Health market reforms, on the other hand, are aimed at creating market forces in the health system, through internal markets of limited or more open competition. Thailand is currently pulling back from a perceived over-competitive health system and developing instead health management reform approaches, as is New Zealand, while the specifics in each country differ. Nepal, on the other hand, is encouraging the further development of largely unrestricted internal markets as it pursues health market reforms. Viet Nam is currently seeking the policy and regulation balance between private sector market forces in health and health management reforms.

Sophisticated HR development strategies are a key component for successful health management reforms, and this includes for nursing and midwifery.

The general global pattern over the last fifteen years has been health management reforms followed by health market reforms. In those countries where the latter precedes the former, for example Nepal, the proliferation of the private sector in the absence of the elements of health management reforms, creates inequities, quality and cost dilemmas, and policy and management dilemmas, because of inadequate capacity and capability.

The starting point for HSRD is often un-planned, and results from *ad hoc* influence for change. At macro-policy level and institutional policy level, this leads to a diversity of non-harmonized policies, policy gaps and capacity and capability challenges. Developing countries have the additional burden of embracing medical and other technological advances in a restricted economic environment, while most health professionals would say their country's health systems were under-resourced. However, this is indeed a relative concept.

In Viet Nam, for example, the amount of money spent per capita on health by the government is US$4. The amount spent per capita directly in the private sector, is US$6. On current trends, both figures are expected to double in ten years. Current government policy approaches aim to redress this. A recent study in China found that 40 per cent of the rural population reporting as seriously ill did not contact a professional health care provider due to the high costs. Again, the government is taking rigorous steps to overcome this.[14] In developed countries, the very policies that led to success, for example Japan, may turn into liabilities as priorities change and institutional inertia prevents people adapting to the new requirements (e.g. Japan's care of the elderly and pursuit of higher quality).

During the 1990s the circular influence of poor health reducing income and generating poverty and poverty-related diseases became more widely understood. The circular influence of high medical expenses forcing sick people in need of professional health services into poverty is only recently receiving wider policy attention.[15]

Globally, the shift from public to private funding of health care services typically resulted from economic crises, often as part of IMF/World Bank structural adjustment programmes, with these privatisation approaches translated into health sector reform. This approach is under increasing criticism by some for its negative social affects. However, predominantly private sector health systems have traditionally existed in some countries. The United States of America spends 14-15 per cent of GNP on health care with around 45 million people uninsured and many more people underinsured. In West Europe, 8-9 per cent of GNP is spent on publicly funded health services. There appears to be no difference in the quality of health care provided. In West European health systems, a person being driven into poverty by high health care expenses is a marginal problem. In the USA, high health expenses cause 25 per cent of all private bankruptcies.[16]

To respond to the impact of global trends, HSRD needs to be comprehensive and address priority setting, public/private mix, organizational design, research, values, information systems, productivity, performance and incentives. For nurses and midwives, they need to understand HSRD and ensure proposed changes address values and attitudes, as well as the skills, competencies and organizational cultures needed, to support appropriate changes in health policy and the health system. HSRD needs to be responsive to societal needs, and the long-term effects of change need to be known and predicted.

The Health Workforce

As countries face the challenges of structural adjustment and transition to market economies, countries and regions are competing with each other to expand or maintain economic capacity. The International Labor Organization (ILO), recognizing that the efficiency of the public service is a key variable to success and that the general image of public service personnel has been on the decline for many years, included human resource development in its 1998-99 programme of sectoral meetings.

The basis of ILO's deliberations included the reality that there has been weak analysis of how the various factors contributing to successful HSRD are linked and interact. 'Public service personnel' is defined by the ILO as those employed in ministries and other public administration agencies and also those working in services in the public or general interest, including health services. The ILO concluded 'without qualified, committed and motivated staff, the State cannot play the role assigned to it in a rapidly changing and globalised economy.'

In 1996 the OECD concluded, on the basis of country surveys, that more effective management of people would lead to more efficient and effective public service administration.[17] In 1997 the World Bank stated the issue succinctly: '...whether making policy, delivering services or administering contracts, capable and motivated staff are the lifeblood of an effective state.'[18] This is not always recognized in health systems in developed or developing countries. Even where it is, where overall stewardship is weak, the public service culture may not be conducive to its achievement.

This is a major issue for nursing and midwifery. In the early 1980s the USA government commissioned the national 'Magnet Hospital Study'. Why were some hospitals able to attract and retain nursing and midwifery staff, in a time of acute national shortage, and others not? Essentially, the study found that nurses and midwives were attracted to organizations because of the organization's culture: how the organization was led and managed and how this translated into the environment in which they worked, the emphasis placed on valuing nurses and midwives, the respect and complementarity between them and other health professionals and workers, the focus on excellence in care.

While this has been known for nearly twenty years, and intuitively understood for years before, change has been slow in coming to many countries and organizations.

In the author's experience, nurses and midwives (and many other health professionals) frequently do not clearly understand the core health policies, the health system's complexities and ideosyncracies, or the complexities of the various sub-cultures within health. Where this is the case, nurses and midwives are not in a strong position to develop, argue for, and implement the sort of strategic approaches needed to facilitate systemic strengthening of stewardship, service provision, financing and resource generation, ultimately leading to a health system satisfactory to the community and to those who work in it.

Where nurses and midwives are perceived by decision-makers as lacking these capacities, their strategic consultation on system change issues is not usually part of that health systems' culture. This fuels feelings of being under-valued and disempowered, which in many systems has become a chronic and festering source of discontent within nursing and midwifery. This becomes circular in its impact: where nurses and midwives are either not usually consulted as the norm, and/or are not active participants at the 'right' decision-making tables, exposure to new and different thinking is limited, and if and when consulted, their useful input is limited, and consultation and inclusion remains *ad hoc* and minimal.

However, when nurses and midwives have sound basic education as well as ongoing and appropriate development opportunities (e.g. the International Council of Nurses' global leadership and management development programme), then some remarkable change can happen in knowledge and understanding, in how nurses and midwives perceive themselves, how others perceive them, and in what influence they achieve.

In New Zealand's first wave of health system reforms, from around 1988, there was considerable government investment in experiential, multidisciplinary leadership and management development,[19] seen as a key foundation to achieve, and sustain, health strategy change. These programmes were multidisciplinary and their impact is still being seen. Among other programmes (e.g. for existing CEO's, middle managers, younger people with potential) there was a Transitions Programme for senior clinicians (medical, nursing/midwifery and other health professions), who wanted to make the change from a clinical role to a middle or senior management role. The New Zealand government recognised that the health system is complex and that its effective leadership and management is complex. Having clinical qualifications alone does not equip anyone to lead and manage these complexities.

And yet still, in many countries, a medical qualification is seen as the background needed for senior appointments. In these countries, nurses and midwives cannot be appointed to senior health positions, only to nursing or midwifery specific positions. Does this matter? Yes, it does. The health system needs a variety of perspectives and backgrounds at decision-making level for sound policy and management decisions. As well, nurses and midwives should have the same career opportunities in health as others, where competence is equal. In New Zealand, for example, nurses and midwives compete equally for senior executive positions, and are highly respected and successful in these roles. However, the point is stressed that having a clinical background alone is insufficient to take senior leadership, management and policy roles. This requires additional and broader experience and development.

Given the predominance of women in nursing and midwifery, the local societal view of women cannot be disentangled from the status and respect given to nursing and midwifery.

In New Zealand, women arguably enjoy greater equality than the majority of other countries. The last two New Zealand prime ministers have been women. The current Director-General of Health is a woman.[20] Many women hold such very senior positions in New Zealand.

In Australia, there has never been a woman prime minister, and around 98 per cent of permanent secretaries (or director-generals) are men, as are around the same proportion or higher of Chairman and CEOs of major businesses. One (female) nurse/midwife has been a Permanent Secretary for Health in Australia, and others now hold senior policy, planning and hospital CEO positions.[21] They did not achieve these positions only on their clinical qualifications and experience. They studied further, took risks, challenged the status quo, and achieved change.

In many other countries, however, this is not the case. Change becomes more challenging where there is a duality of predominating forces: the political and civil service culture predominately values men, and the role of women and the status of nursing and midwifery is low. Such countries may be poor or rich. This is not the key variable. The variables arise from complex socio-historical forces, often including religion.

The philosophical questions are many. Globalisation has had an impact on the equality of women. Some countries see this trend as a threat to their socio-historical and religious context, the country's culture, and there is strong community and even government resistance to improving the status of women. Similarly, if nursing and midwifery has historically been an under-educated profession, low in status and self confidence, where is the line to be drawn, in the view of some countries, between improving health services and perceptions of 'going too far' in changing a country's culture, changing traditional roles, traditional approaches to 'how we do things here'.

There are sometimes extreme differences in knowledge and competency between nurses and midwives in different countries, while common titles are usually used ('nurse', 'midwife'). Nursing and midwifery has the same need to keep abreast of new knowledge as any other health profession. The challenge in countries where nursing is at a low base is first to persuade governments that nursing and midwifery needs strengthening; second, to determine the speed of change needed and third, in which direction should this change go. The USA model? The UK model? The Egyptian model? Indian?

A new model? If the last, from which countries will elements be taken, who will design the country-specific innovations, how will teachers be prepared to teach the new curriculum, how will practising nurses be prepared to support students and graduates etc.?

And ultimately, what is the problem the country is trying to solve and will this strategy help solve it?

While to some nurses and midwives it sounds harsh, the basic premise in any workforce planning and development is: what is the least cost necessary in inputs to achieve the desired outputs of appropriate quality. Thus competencies, skills, attitudes, behaviour, flexibility, capacity to embrace new learning all become part of the puzzle to determine what inputs will be most efficient and most effective. For example, in 2000, the World Health Organization analysed the impact of nurses and midwives as one input to health, in ten countries.

CASE HISTORY NO. 1

In the mid-1990s the World Health Assembly passed Resolution 49.1 (WHA 49.1), which effectively requested member states to improve and develop the capacity of their nursing and midwifery professions. Since that time, and prior to it, there have been remarkable efforts by nurse/midwifery leaders to systemically improve the capacity of nurses and midwives in many countries. WHO's Eastern Mediterranean Regional Office (EMRO) perhaps deserves special mention because of its key role over many years in providing leadership, mentoring and wise advice on nursing and midwifery throughout the mainly Islamic countries of EMRO.

Dr Enaam Abou Youssef's nursing and midwifery leadership at EMRO, and the capacity and commitment of nurse/midwifery leaders in countries ranging from Iran to Oman, and from Bahrain to Syria, have resulted in some developments and strategies for reforms in nursing and midwifery.

In 1991, Dr Abou Youssef convened a group of around fifteen nurse/midwifery leaders from throughout the region. The author was privileged to be the facilitator of this first meeting to develop a Strategic Plan for Nursing and Midwifery Development in EMRO, and to work closely with Dr Abou Youssef in many countries in

EMRO subsequently. This group evolved into a Regional advisory council on nursing and midwifery.

Through this council, nurses and midwives across EMRO provided input into WHO EMRO policy and strategy development, with this subsequently providing EMRO's input to WHO's Global Advisory Group on Nursing and Midwifery. National strategic plans for nursing and midwifery development were developed in many countries including Bahrain and Iran. Regional leadership and management development programmes for nurses and midwives were held, hosted by Syria. Oman now has a very successful ongoing programme of international nursing and midwifery conferences. Regional nursing and midwifery education standards were set. Iran and other countries are exploring community nursing.

WHO Fellowships provided international study opportunities to nurses and midwives.

While there is still an enourmous amount of work to do to ensure consistent standards of nursing and midwifery practice across EMRO, it is exactly this sort of strategic approach, with mid to long term time lines, that achieves system change in nursing and midwifery.

CASE HISTORY NO. 2

In 1989, the author went to the People's Republic of China for WHO to do a base-line analysis of nursing and midwifery, its current standards, status, educational preparation. In 1991, a national strategic plan for nursing development was developed. In 1995 this received four-year funding from the United Nations Development Programme. In 1999, progress was assessed. An important part of the national plan was to improve quality of care at the point of delivery. To do this pilot 'holistic nursing wards' in hospitals were implemented.[22] In 1999, more than 2000 hospitals had implemented holistic nursing wards. Patient and nurse satisfaction was measured pre and post implementation, with satisfaction exponentially improved post implementation.

From the outset, hospital chief executives and clinical doctors were kept fully informed. Their satisfaction in the perceived standards of nursing care was also measured. It had also increased greatly. Because holistic nursing care was successfully introduced, it had a system impact in the hospitals. As a result, new categories of staff were introduced (e.g. ward clerks, couriers between wards and laboratories) to enable nurses to focus on patient care.

The next step for China is the introduction of community based nursing, for which they have developed a national curriculum and begun pilot implementation. And finally, as with the Case History above on EMRO, none of this would have happened if it had not been for visionary and consistent leadership, in this case through China's Chief Nurse, Dr Quong.

Sometimes countries need external leadership and support at certain stages of their development. In China's case, several nurses and midwives have been key, two of whom need mentioning to illustrate the importance of global networks and external support to countries at critical stages of their development in nursing and midwifery. The first is Terry Miller, formerly of WHO's Western Pacific Region (and now enjoying art and university life in Tucson, Arizona, USA) who knew what was needed to support the Chinese, and found ways to overcome challenging obstacles to give them support. And the second is Dr Ruth Starke, RN, who took over from Terry Miller (and who is now one of the new historic appointments of women heading up WHO country offices, and the first nurse to ever be appointed to such a position [in Papua New Guinea]) and found funds for consultants and gave technical and personal support, to ensure the project did not falter.

CASE HISTORY NO. 3

Some countries have no national agenda of priorities to guide the development of nursing and midwifery. Why is this so? Is it the professions' lack of capacity? Governments? This varies between countries, but it is food for thought that some assert that problems in strategic and coordinated health system development, including for nursing and midwifery, is compounded by '...too many governments know(ing) far too little about what is happening in the provision of services to their people.'[23]

A case history of one developing country (an analysis done by the author in 2000) has elements similar to many other poorer developing countries. It highlights the complexity of determining both the appropriate starting point for sustainable nursing and midwifery development and the complexity of determining the relative responsibility of the health workforce, governments and the community.

In this country, there are more than 250 national and international non-government organizations (NGOs) supporting health projects. Their activities are not currently strategically coordinated. There is little private or NGO focus on the poorest areas. It is in these same areas that publicly provided services are most weak. The quality of NGO services varies and they, and the private sector, are largely unregulated.

The aim of this country's health system is decentralization but, despite, legislative changes, actual decentralization is minimal. While, structurally, fairly even access to health services across the country appears assured, the reality differs. There is weak capacity for strategic planning, policy development, leadership and management, finance and other resource disbursement, analysis and decision-making at all levels. The geographical location of health facilities is not always ideal to meet population health needs. Staff availability, including for nursing and midwifery, is inconsistent and absenteeism is high.

Centralized management continues. Personnel administration, including staff deployment and transfer, is centralized. Family, economic, social and security disadvantages of working in rural and remote areas make staffing problematic. Problems in drug and other supplies, transport and financial disbursements, together with low or absent staff, compromise services including outreach services.

There are over forty health worker cadres in (country); the majority of them have limited training. Nurse training ranges from one year to three years. Bachelor and masters programmes are available, and have been for a decade or more.

There is a shortage of absolute numbers of nurses and midwives. There is an over-supply of doctors with increasing production of both doctors and nurses and midwives in the pipeline through private medical colleges. There are perceptions that standards of new medical, nursing and other health worker graduates are uneven. There is no overall health workforce planning to facilitate the balance between supply and demand.

There is geographical maldistribution of all health workers in favour of urban areas. Staffing levels are further compromised by poor motivation and widespread absenteeism because of poor wages in the public sector, higher wages and incentives in the private and NGO sectors, and staff not taking up positions when transferred to rural and remote areas with which they are not familiar. This is especially true for nurses and midwives who are expected to live and work in remote areas, as young single women, sometimes many days walk from other towns, roads and transport. Their personal security is a concern for them and their families, with rape and molestation cited as 'common'.

Most health workers in urban areas, and in some rural areas, supplement their incomes in the private sector. For nurses, this often means dual employment. For doctors, it often means public sector employment and private practice, even where some private health organizations in which they are employed provide financial incentives for them not to concurrently run a private practice.

Donors emphasize training. This translates into a myriad of discrete and non-integrated training courses, usually directed at the less-educated health cadres who frequently must leave their health centre unattended and travel long distances, including on foot, to attend them. The narrowly focused training programmes for nurses and midwives and others, means opportunities are lost to develop capacity for integrated care, holistic care.

The higher wages paid by NGOs and the proliferating and unregulated private hospital sector attract the talented and able away from the public health system, compromising the latter's capacity.

Finances are a major constraint in improving health services. Because of the weak administrative and management capacity, strategies to strengthen aspects of the health system follow an *ad hoc* pattern.

Staff reluctance to serve in remote areas far from home and families, where there are no financial incentives to do so, usually no accommodation (provided for doctors but not for other health workers), and security fears, means that health facilities may have no staff or *ad hoc* staffing patterns, constraining access. Illiteracy and poverty in a user-pays system further constrains access. Travel distance and the terrain, and perhaps no staff, no drugs and no other supplies when the patient arrives, complete the access constraints.

For staff, their low wages have recently been increased to a minimum living wage. This has yet to be paid. Despite the low wages, there are more applicants to study medicine and nursing than there are student positions. It is very attractive to staff to attend donor-supplied training courses, and to be paid for them, whether or not they are a priority or perceived to be relevant to their day-to-day work.

The Ministry of Health's absorptive capacity for its donor funding is low. The 1999 data indicates that around two-thirds of external development resources allocated were released and about 60 per cent utilized, and about 20-40 per cent of the Ministry of Health (MOH) development budget has not been utilized. The MOH budget is heavily reliant upon donor funding including for recurrent costs, with no strategies apparent to reverse this situation.[24]

A nurse and midwife registration board has recently been established. Its first priority has been to register nurses and midwives, regardless of educational background or competency. Its next priority is to attempt to develop standards, based on continuing education, on which future practise certification will be based. The basic nurse curriculum has not been revised for nearly twenty years.

Senior nurses in management have traditionally led the national nursing association. The younger generation of nurses and midwives are impatient with the status quo and the perception that these senior nurses are satisfied with their senior status, and thus reluctant to challenge the status quo. Medical doctors (all men) hold all senior MOH and hospital management positions. Nursing and midwifery is predominantly female. The younger generation (in this culture, those approaching their 40s) are developing strategies to challenge low pay, lack of career opportunities for nurses and midwives including to senior health management positions, security fears etc. These strategies include strikes and refusal to do some aspects of work.

Clearly, to continue with *ad hoc* and uncoordinated approaches for a better health system, better health care and improved health status in this country, will mean much effort will be expended for unsatisfactory gain. However, where nurse/midwifery leadership is weak, as in this country, little influence can be exerted at decision-making levels to develop a coordinated approach to health system reform, and within this, nursing and midwifery development.

NURSING AND MIDWIFERY LEADERSHIP

Leadership has been described as the ability to envision and remove barriers, enabling people and organizations to maximize their effectiveness to achieve a common goal.[25] Where it is clear that stewardship needs strengthening, either at the political or public service level, or both, then stronger leadership should be exercised by nursing and midwifery to develop strategic alliances needed to support strengthening the government's and health ministry's stewardship.

Research shows that nursing and midwifery development achieves much greater return on investment when conducted within a clear strategic plan endorsed by government, where priorities are determined, and where there is active management of the plan's implementation within realistic time lines.[26]

Where nursing and midwifery leadership is generally weak, the myriad of lower-level efforts will not achieve sustainable, or perhaps even desirable, results in the absence of higher government-level activity. Higher-level nursing and midwifery activity needs to focus on national policies that address priority public service system weaknesses, health system needs and the nursing and midwifery profile needed to address these needs. Lessons learned in many countries is that nursing and midwifery development is more problematic where national ministries of health are weak, and where there is insufficient focus on strengthening health service delivery.[27] In many environments, ministries of health have little flexibility to respond to and embrace needed new approaches in the health workforce. The MOHs exist in a bureaucratic environment of 'administering the rules' when 'managing innovation' is needed for health systems to be successful.[28]

The bureaucratic demarcations that characterize national public service structures are often repeated at international level. Strengthened strategic alliances and partnerships are needed between nursing and midwifery organizations and between them and non-nursing and midwifery organizations, to conduct joint situational analyses and a coherent strategic approach to health sector reform and health workforce change.

In a climate of tightening health budgets, it can be difficult to persuade governments to spend money on health system strengthening, such as through strengthening nursing and midwifery, when there are high profile health challenges to which to respond for example malaria, TB, HIV/AIDS, maternal and infant mortality. In the same way as other technical experts in health often have little understanding of nursing and midwifery and its importance, so too with governments. This is particularly prevalent where nursing and midwifery is weak, and so there is no observable evidence of its potential effectiveness. There needs to be strengthened national, regional and global political understanding of the potential return on investment, social and economic, of a strong, well educated, and well performing nursing and midwifery workforce.

NURSING AND MIDWIFERY AND OTHER SECTORS

The health system is not renowned for actively engaging with other industries to share stories and lessons learned for mutual benefit. And the reverse is true. While there are some changes at international level, cross-sector collaboration at national level is not the norm. While the health 'market' may be atypical to other markets, there are many best practice organizational and human resource management practices and principles that are generalisable. Some of these are present in some health systems. However, as most health systems tend to work in isolation from others sectors, and they from health, it is not surprising to note their relative absence. There are lessons learned from non-health sectors that can be used by nurses and midwives to influence change.

These lessons learned include the central premise that developing the workforce has a positive economic impact by improving the economic condition of the individual, as well as his/her family and community. Other lessons learned include:

• Understanding that transparency and accountability play a key role in building public trust, equity, access and the social partnerships required among stakeholders for workforce development;
• The importance of experiential learning in contrast to the Taylorist-like principle of knowledge and training being presented in discrete bits to be assembled together at a later date (e.g. New Zealand's former Health Services Management Development Unit, see above);
• Developing systems thinking in ways that allow stakeholders to learn from one another and connecting systems and strategies at points that promise highest leverage for mutual benefit (e.g. Australia and New Zealand's Learning Sets);[29]
• Understanding the basic concept of customer-oriented learning and helping people to learn skills they want to learn because they can see the potential benefits (e.g. micro-financing for poor women in Ahmedabad, India; the military retraining programme in the Ukraine);

- Ensuring HR strategies are demand-driven, tied into local, regional, national and/or international need and being able to minimize gaps between the demand and supply of skills;
- Ensuring transparent criteria for access to education and other workforce development strategies; seeking out groups who have not previously participated (e.g. more women in medicine; more men in nursing; those disabled being recruited into the health workforce etc.);
- Basing workforce development strategies on improving competencies rather than on length of training;
- Creating multiple entry points for education programmes instead of the usual one-entry-point more usual in most health professional training, including nursing and midwifery;
- Ensuring portability of skills: local, regional or international geographic portability and portability across occupations (e.g. *Schluesselqualifikionen* in Germany);
- Developing generic skills for portability across occupations include learning how to learn, plan, effectively communicate in a variety of media, budget, problem solve and generate alternatives with traits such as leadership, flexibility, curiosity and 'coachability' being even more portable, traits that seem difficult for many nurse and midwifery education programmes to instil, and which seem even more difficult for health delivery service environments to nurture and encourage; and finally,
- Exploring public-private partnerships and the linking of multiple stakeholders, key for workforce or human resource development.[30]

There is little evidence that these principles are widely understood by international organizations and governments across many sectors, including health generally and nursing and midwifery specifically. Where health experts have accountability and responsibility for leadership and management of health issues in-country, the absence of HR knowledge and workforce development issues is apparent.[31]

Two among many case histories support the premise that there is a lack of general HR knowledge and expertise. In Guinea, maldistribution of health workers and low staff morale are the critical HR issues. The HR strategies in Guinea, however, are focused on in-service training when it is organization and management of the health system that needs strategic targeting. In Costa Rica, the health sector reform plan recognizes the lack of HR policies, standards and procedures but strategies are focused on worker productivity and short-term contracts, contributing to greater grievances among public sector employees.[32] However, Fiji provides a case history of a clear understanding of the strategic importance of developing a health workforce to meet changing needs, with their very successful recent introduction of nurse practitioners.

INTERNATIONAL STRATEGIC ALLIANCES: TURNING DELIBERATIONS INTO ACTION

Strategic alliances among international agencies is becoming more apparent as is the swing away from the hard edge of economic rationalism to include a greater social and people focus. For example, the World Bank and Asian Development Bank announcements in the last three years to refocus their strategies, in response to the widespread perception that development efforts had been successful only in narrowly defined terms, with often inadequate human relevance and impact, and, the Jakarta Plan of Action on Human Resources Development in the ESCAP Region.[33]

The challenge now for nursing and midwifery is to understand and read the winds of change, and assist in creating the future for their countries, their health systems, and themselves and their fellow health workers.

The International Council of Nurses, successfully reading these winds of change, convened an historic meeting of international nursing and midwifery organizations in Miami in November/December 2000, to specifically discuss global socio-political and economic issues, trends and challenges over the next five to ten years, and within this environmental context, the global issues, trends and challenges for nursing and midwifery, looking beyond the status quo.

It was agreed that the global goal of nursing and midwifery is global health based on cooperative nursing and midwifery leadership and partnership, evidence and ethics, in three fields: policy, workforce and education.

Globally, the three key messages are:

Policy
Nurses and midwives engage in essential, effective policy development and implementation.

Workforce
Quality of care demands a well prepared, well compensated and valued nursing and midwifery workforce.

Education
Changing environments and roles require skills and knowledge to provide quality health care to individuals, families and communities.

Where there is relative marginalization from decision-making, leadership and broader competencies in these three areas are key to changing both perception and reality.

Licensing

Licensing of nurses and midwives is a critical factor in maintaining and strengthening standards and capacity, and protecting the public. Many countries have licensing provision for nurses and midwives, but many do not. In some countries the Ministry of Health is the licensing authority (e.g. Jordan for medical doctors; Myanmar for nurses and midwives). In other countries, autonomous or relatively autonomous councils have the responsibility (e.g. South Africa's Interim Medical and Dental Council; Australia's state-based nurse and midwifery registration boards).

The International Council of Nurses has had a sustained and strategic approach over many years, supporting countries to develop nurse licensing regulation and procedures.

With globalisation a new concept has been raised. In September 2000, at a nursing conference of members of the Asian Productivity Organization, one speaker proposed a phased approach from early to mid-twenty-first century, for global licensing, discipline and nursing education requirements.[34]

Leadership and management

Those countries which responded early to the impact of global trends, in the late 1980s, focused strongly on multidisciplinary best practice leadership and management development strategies for their most senior managers and for health professionals (e.g. the UK and

New Zealand). The positive impacts of these strategies are still being felt more than a decade later. In South Africa, the Oliver Tambo Leadership Development Programme aims similarly to strengthen leadership and management capacity and capability. The International Council of Nurses, initially funded by the W.K. Kellogg Foundation, has a global initiative and conducts leadership and management development programmes for current and 'next generation' nurse and midwifery leaders across the world. WHO is developing leadership and management development programmes which will initially commence in Egypt, with the medical profession taking the lead in its design.

The increased awareness of the importance of sound leadership and management is heartening. However, the design and execution of leadership and management programmes is critical. Process is as important as content if participants are to genuinely, and sustainably, move beyond the status quo and achieve change. Key at a certain stage of a country's nursing and midwifery development, is that programmes are multidisciplinary and that current and potential leaders are the participants. One group of participants in a 'health leadership programme' made a study tour to another country. The question of the host country was: 'Why do you have people on such programmes who do not have now, and clearly will never have, the capacity or capability to be leaders?'.[35]

The magnitude of the leadership and management task in health, and in nursing and midwifery, is high. The interest in, and understanding of, best practice leadership and management development to ensure real expertise in senior and middle level managers in the health sector, is uneven globally.

As well, discrete and disparate leadership and management development programmes may assist individual capacity building but do not necessarily strengthen organizational or health stewardship capacity or capability. Organizational development (OD) strategies are as ill-understood by many health leaders as HSRD, notwithstanding the plethora of available OD literature. At the end of the day it is improved system capacity and capability that should be the aim, and OD provides the framework to achieve this.

Maintaining the relative capacity and capability of a health system is critical as the global pace of change continues.

THE FUTURE

What does the future hold for nursing and midwifery? For the person graduating as a nurse or midwife in 2005, and assuming they continue to work for twenty-five years at least, what changes will they need to lead, anticipate and/or manage?

A first assumption is that targeting nursing and midwifery development in isolation from health system reform and development reduces chances of sustainable success. Strong strategic alliances are therefore needed between nurses and midwives and other key stakeholders.

A second assumption is that where nursing and midwifery leadership is weak, credibility is absent, political leadership is unpersuaded, and the required linkages between nursing and midwifery development and health policy and planning is weak or absent. Strong, informed, wise and competent leadership is a key to the future and its development needs to be supported.

The third assumption is that basic and continuing education for nurses and midwives needs to facilitate their capacity for life-long learning, for clinical practice and to anticipate, understand, contribute to, and manage their environment's change.

The fourth assumption is that to achieve system change, requires realistic time lines, and sustained leadership and management, and a robust strategic framework, with a clear strategic intent and goals to be achieved.

The fifth assumption is that health ministries need to shift from the prevalent rigid bureaucratic approach to cultures of flexibility and innovation. Unless this happens, health system capacity to embrace new knowledge, achieve quality outcomes, and attract and retain staff, will be slow or minimal.

Given these assumptions, nursing and midwifery should anticipate and manage:

- harmonisation of international standards;
- a consistent global image based on the consistent international standards;
- greater interdependency between education and practice;
- greater multiple entry points to 'professional' nursing and midwifery with more options and flexibility in education;

- a richer nursing and midwifery workforce profile (class, gender, ethnicity);
- an expanded role, where, using today's terms, the first level nurse's training and knowledge base will be at nurse/midwife practitioner level, with a clear focus on holistic care and competencies and skills, soundly based on knowledge, with 2nd level nurses and midwives carefully educated as complementary support workers;
- legal, ethical and financial requirements for evidence-based practice fuelling research as the norm;
- increased diversification, career choices and specialisation;
- increasing numbers of nurse and midwife entrepreneurs;
- blurring of boundaries between professions leading to rapid change in roles and functions, team work and interdependency.[36]

And finally, globally, in any country, the nursing and midwifery culture will be characterised by measurable effectiveness and efficiency; caring and supportive attitudes and behaviour; values and curiosity leading to life-long learning and research for the continuous improvement of clinical practice; and well-rewarded trust and respect from society, including within the health sector.

NOTES

1. Some parts of this Chapter were first prepared as a paper for the WHO December 2000 meeting in Annecy, France on global human resource issues.
2. J. Prokopenko, *Globalization, alliances and networking: A strategy for competitiveness and productivity*. Enterprise and Management Development Working Paper EMD/21/E. International Labour Organization, 2000. (Internet communication, 27 September 2000 at http://www.ilo.org/public/english/employment/ent/papers/emd21.html)
3. M. Gonzalez Block, *Comparative research and analysis methods for shared learning from health system reforms*. (Internet communication, 17 February 1999 at http://www.insp.mx/ichsri/ch/index.html
4. J. Prokopenko, 2000, op. cit.
5. P. Wongwatcharapaiboon et al., 'The 1997 massive resignation of contracted new medical graduates from the Thai Ministry of Public Health: What reasons behind?' *Human Resources for Health Development Journal (HRDJ)* Vol. 3, No. 2, May-August 1999.
6. D. Dunlop et al. (eds.), *An International Assessment of Health Care Financing*. Economic Development Institute Seminar Series. The World Bank. 1995.

7. P. Degeling et al., 'A comparison of the impact of hospital reform on medical subcultures in some Australian and New Zealand hospitals.' *Australian Health Review*, Vol 22, No. 4, 1999, pp. 173-188.

8. H. Kahssay et al. (eds.), *Community involvement in health development: a review of the concept and practice.* Public Health Action 5. World Health Organization. 1999.

9. A. Preker et al., *Market mechanisms and the health sector in Central and Eastern Europe.* Technical Paper Series No. 293. World Bank. 1996 (Translations in English, Russian, Hungarian, Polish, Romanian and Czech.).

10. *Health System: Improving Performance.* The World Health Report 2000. World Health Organization. Geneva, 2000.

11. *Human resource development in the public service in the context of structural adjustment and transition.* Report for discussion at the Joint Meeting on Human Resource Development in the Public Service in the Context of Structural Adjustment and Transition. International Labour Office. Geneva, 1998.

12. M. Bargellini, *Libraries: A key role in lifelong learning.* (Internet communication at http://www.jrc.es/pages/iptsreport/vol41/english/ICT2E416.htm).

13. R. Kolehmainen-Aitken, *Defining human resource responsibilities in the era of health sector reform.* APHA conference. 2000. In-press. (Internet communication at http://apha.confex.com/apha/128am/techprogramme/paper_2922.htm).

14. Wei Fu et al., *Health Care for China's Rural Poor, International Health Policy Programme.* Occasional paper. Washington. April 1999.

15. G. Dahlgren, *The Medical Poverty Trap.* Unpublished. 2001.

16. Ibid.

17. *Integrating people management into public service reform.* OECD. Paris, 1996.

18. *World Development Report 1997: The State in a Changing World.* World Bank, 1997, in *Human resource development in the public service in the context of structural adjustment and transition.* International Labour Office. Geneva, 1998, op. cit.

19. The New Zealand Government established the Health Services Management Development Unit (HSMDU), at arms length from Government to enable it to have greater flexibility. They recruited globally, with Bob Dearden of the UK and Brian Lewis of Australia, establishing HSMDU and leading the design and delivery of programmes.

20. Dr Karen Poutasi is the Director-General of Health in New Zealand.

21. For example, Gillian Biscoe was appointed Secretary, Department of Health, Canberra, ACT in 1991 and Secretary, Department of Community and Health Services, Tasmania in 1993. Geri Taylor was appointed to the Senior Executive Service in the Queensland Department of Health in 1991.

22. The work of Eric Chan of Hong Kong is acknowledged. He was a key consultant to China in introducing the Holistic Model Wards and lent great support and expertise over several years to their success.

23. *Health System: Improving Performance.* The World Health Report 2000. World Health Organization. Geneva, 2000.

24. G. Biscoe, Analysis of country 'x'. 2000.

25. R. Dearden, *The interconnectedness of system change.* Paper presented to senior executives of the Tasmanian Department of Community and Health Services, Australia, 1996. Unpublished.

26. WHO analysis of WHA49.1. Unpublished. 2000.
27. Op. cit.
28. B. Lewis, Managing Change. Paper prepared for 1998 Health Exchange, Canberra, Australia. Unpublished.
29. The Australian and New Zealand Learning Sets began in 1999, through Management Consortium Ptd. Ltd., and Brian Lewis and Kevin Hardy specifically. They are an extension of the original Australian Learning Sets, funded by the Australian Federal Department of Health, through the interest and vision of the then Deputy Secretary, Alan Bansemer, now Commissioner for Health, Western Australia Health Commission.
30. Compass to Workforce Development: 'What Works'. (Internet communication, 27 September 2000 at http://www.edc.org/CWD/s_works.htm).
31. G. Biscoe, Analyis of thirty-six WHO consultancy reports from 1989-2000 and ten donor project designs from 1997-2000 for preparing this paper.
32. D. Egger et al., Issues in health services delivery. Discussion paper No. 2. Human resources for health. Achieving the right balance: The role of policy-making processes in managing resources for health problems. World Health Organization. 2000.
33. Background of the Jakarta Plan of Action. United Nations ESCAP. 1997-2000.
34. R. Harrifan et al., International Cooperative Workforce Projection Model. Community Initiative of Nursing of Hawaii. Asian Productivity Organization Conference. Unpublished. 2000.
35. Personal communication. 2000. (It seems appropriate not to mention either country by name).
36. These elements reflect the author's thinking and that of health leaders at two meetings: (1) ICN's global strategic planning meeting in Miami in December 2000; and (2) WHO's meeting on Long Term Home Based Care in Jerusalem, 1999.

3

Issues of Control: The Role of Nursing in the Regulation of the Profession

Fadwa A. Affara

INTRODUCTION

To survive and maintain their integrity, professions have to establish some form of control over their members and their practice. The major part of forces that control nursing and nurses are exerted through regulatory systems. The International Council of Nurses (ICN), as the body representing nursing and nurses world wide, has a long history of studying the issues and processes that are involved in professional regulation.[1] For ICN, regulation is conceptualised in its broadest sense and has been defined as all of those legitimate and appropriate means—governmental, professional and private—whereby order, consistency, identity and control are brought to the profession. The profession and its members are defined; the scope of practice is determined; standards of education and of ethical and competent practice are set; and systems of accountability are established through these means.[2] At the heart of this process lies a framework of educational, practice and ethical standards to which the profession ascribes.

This paper elaborates on various aspects of that framework. It begins with examples of how regulation is carried out in the real world, and then proceeds to the issue of who controls nursing, and examines tasks, limitations and strength of arrangements for ensuring the quality of nursing in various settings. Against that background, the paper proceeds onto the important terrain of nursing regulation in Islamic countries, focusing on a series of features that point to the uncertain control nursing has over its profession and practice in many countries in the Islamic world. The paper concludes with a set of key factors that are necessary for nursing to control its own destiny.

REGULATION IN THE REAL WORLD

It is helpful to use examples to illustrate how these processes of control that bring order and consistency to the profession may be operationalised.

Nursing schools accept students with certain qualifications, provide an educational programme to meet prescribed standards, and are recognized by an external authority (e.g., a nursing board or council appointed by the government) as institutions approved or accredited to prepare nurses for professional practice.

Nurses are licensed or registered through a set of procedures and the application of various criteria. The requirements for licensure or registration are usually stated in a law and thus give nurses the legal right to practice nursing, to offer their services to the public for compensation and to use a particular title. Unlicensed or unregistered persons may not use the title stated in the law and may not practice nursing for hire.

Nurses may go on to become specialists through advanced education and experience. They are certified by an authority as having met certain standards that qualify them as specialists prepared for additional responsibilities and authorized to use a specialist title.

Nurses are bound by a code of ethical conduct. Such codes may be sanctioned by law and/or by professional associations of nurse peers. A professional or regulatory body may discipline nurses who violate the code or laws and regulations governing nursing by practising in an unsafe or unethical manner.

Nursing practice is defined within certain boundaries or limits. This 'scope of practice' may be reflected in nursing practice or other health-related laws, governmental rules and regulations, in the curricula of educational programmes preparing nurses, and in officially recognized job descriptions, role definitions and responsibilities of qualified nurses.

Health care agencies, through the process of approval or accreditation, meet standards set by an external authority such as the Ministry of Health or a voluntary accreditation body assigned to protect the public interest. Among the standards are those concerned with the numbers, qualifications and use of health care personnel, including nurses. For example, only qualified nurses may fulfill designated roles and responsibilities and supervise lesser-prepared auxiliaries.

Governments set general health care and civil service policies, ranging from health care priorities, health care financing and health care systems to the qualifications, rights, responsibilities, promotion systems, working conditions and compensation of health professionals.[3]

Nursing practice, nursing education and nurses are regulated or governed by some or all of the above mechanisms. Such mechanisms define, set standards, and identify limits and exert control of the practice, education and worklife of nurses. In doing so they work at two levels. The first level strives to assure that nurses provide services that are in the public interest. Within this intent, processes of regulation aim to make nursing care competent, effective and appropriate.[4] At the second level, regulatory systems function in a highly positive sense, for through regulation, its standard setting functions and other mechanisms, professional growth can be encouraged and advanced. Furthermore, regulatory systems should allow nurses, as individuals and members of their professional organizations, every opportunity to influence events and contribute to policy debates and decision making that affect nursing education and practice as well as the environment of practice.[5] Therefore, the significance of regulatory systems in determining nursing's potential to provide a decent level of nursing care, and to contribute to the improvement of health care in general is of paramount importance.

WHO CONTROLS NURSING?

ICN takes the position that systems that regulate professions should recognize and properly incorporate the legitimate roles and responsibilities of interested parties—the public, profession, government, employers, and other professions—in aspects of standard setting and administration.[6] In this partnership, nursing, through its professional organizations and individual nurses, plays a broad and critical part not only by monitoring the effectiveness of the system, but also through taking a leading role in its professional governance by:

- securing full participation of nurses in statutory regulatory processes and the associated administrative aspects;
- recommending standards for nursing and nurses in the form of definitions, ethical codes, educational and practice requirements;
- taking primary responsibility for the development of the knowledge and skill base for all nursing; and
- fostering post-basic specialist preparation and advanced practice.

ICN, through its worldwide study on nursing regulation involving over eighty countries concluded that certain characteristics exist when nursing's ability to make decisions for the profession is limited. These characteristics include:

- tolerance of poor educational standards for nursing;
- unclear or non-existing definitions of role, function and scope of practice;
- poor professional representation on bodies that determine standards, role, functions and scope of practice for the profession;
- if a nursing board, or council exists, its authority to establish standards is weak and its ability to enforce standards limited;
- relegation to a dependent role with respect to other health professions, especially medicine; and
- little or no evidence of activities directed to advancing theoretical knowledge and the practice base of the profession.

Conversely, when nursing exercises a legitimate level of control over the way its profession is regulated, it will demonstrate the following:

- a balance between the role of government and the profession as agents of regulation, involving the public and other professions in an appropriate way in these affairs;
- a clear structure for nursing, that defines the accountability of nurses for their practice, and delineates a scope of practice of nursing that is appropriate and capable of meeting changing practice and new health care needs;
- a parity with other professions in standards of education and autonomy of practice; and
- nurses prepared for and active in all aspects of delivery of health care services, planning of services, and health policy formulation.

NURSING AND REGULATION IN ISLAMIC COUNTRIES

Nursing, being primarily a woman's profession, will often take on the features ascribed to the status and position of women in society. It is simplistic to attribute the low status and powerlessness of women in Islamic countries to any single factor in society such as the dominant religious faith. Indeed, the Prophet Muhammad (PBUH) was a reformer in his time when it came to women's rights. He abolished such discriminatory practices as female infanticide and introduced innovations that guaranteed women the right to inherit and bequeath property, and the right to exercise full control over their wealth. It is society that fails to honour these Islamic precepts.[7]

Status and power attributed to members of a society are the result of a complex interaction of culture, social organization, economy systems, history and politics. As the 1993 report to the Regional Committee for the Eastern Mediterranean on women's role in Health For All noted, 'a large gap persists in many countries between the legal declaration of the rights of women and the full realisation of these rights in daily life, owing to cultural traditions inherent in a patriarchal society, weakness of law enforcement, cultural and national discriminatory practices, and the lack of awareness by most women of their full legal rights'.[8] This observation can also be applied to women in many non-Islamic countries.

However, a gender perspective does not fully explain all the forces acting to maintain nurses in a subordinate and passive role. For example, Morocco boasts a large percentage of men in the nursing work force, yet there the profession also struggles to exert the same level of control over its own affairs as that accorded to other health professionals in the country. Indeed, we may find that the pervasive image of a nurse, male or female, as doctor's helpmates with no control over the health service rendered[9] is a dominant perception that continues to keep nurses in a dependent and powerless role.

Several features point to the uncertain control nursing has over its profession and its practice in many of the countries within the Islamic world:

1. Nursing has no universal meaning within these countries and the word 'nurse' embraces a potpourri of students, auxiliaries, technicians and professionals.

The Eastern Mediterranean Region of the World Health Organization (EMRO), a region embracing a large number of the Islamic countries, reports 22 levels of nurses and midwives. Even more telling is that the title 'nurse' is applied to a heterogeneous range of nursing personnel. Within these categories one can find those requiring only six years of general education prior to entry into a nursing education programme, to nurses who have graduated from a university level programme. For example, Egypt has three categories of nursing personnel with the word 'nurse' attached to the title, yet their education may range from a three year programme after nine years of general education to a four year university degree.

However, the situation is changing. Nurses in the Eastern Mediterranean area, under the auspices of WHO, have articulated a clear vision and strategy for nursing in the region. Included is the declaration that nursing must move to *one level of professionally qualified practitioners*.[10] They have identified a number of regional standards, including a requirement of twelve years of general education before admission to a basic nursing programme.[11] The Nursing Technical Committee of the Gulf Cooperation Council, which covers Bahrain, Kuwait, Oman, Qatar, Saudi Arabia and the United Arab Emirates, has adopted EMRO standards for the Gulf region and has reached consensus for standards for nurse specialisation.

2. Statutory regulation of the nursing profession (regulation established by law) is lacking or, if present, is weak in its authority to set standards, and in its implementing, monitoring and enforcement processes.

Across the Eastern Mediterranean and South East Asia regions, there is wide variability in regulatory policies and practices. Bangladesh, Malaysia and Pakistan have had Nursing Councils and Nursing Acts for some time. But their focus is primarily to prescribe the qualifications of nurses and the criteria for the recognition of nursing education institutions and to maintain various types of registers.[12,13] Scope of practice issues, definition of nursing roles and setting of practice standards are largely outside the purview of these councils.

However, as the Registrar of the Bangladesh Nursing Council points out, they have learned the lesson that authority without resources and expertise to carry out functions makes the Council ineffective and powerless.[14] This leaves one to wonder how effectively these councils are able to protect the public from unsafe practitioners, to monitor and enforce educational standards, and to promote the professional growth of individual nurses.

Many countries in these regions have some form of licensing system, but it is often Civil Service based and bureaucratic.[15] Controlling and advancing the standards of nursing care and promoting professional development are low priority concerns in many of such systems. For example, while all nurses and midwives in Indonesia must report to the Provincial Health Office before taking up employment, there is in essence no licensing for nurses. There is a form of licensing for doctors, dentists, pharmacists, nutritionists and midwives and it is necessary for them to obtain a license for work in the private sector.[16] In Jordan, the professional association is charged with registering nurses, but has little authority to set, monitor and enforce standards. Egypt has made provision for health professional licensing. A unit of the Ministry of Health carries it out and the license is issued for a lifetime. In the case of nursing, nurses have little involvement in administering or monitoring this process.

Nurses in Bahrain are regulated under an umbrella law that licenses all allied health professions. It is interesting to note that physicians are treated differently and have their own law. Nevertheless, nurses and midwives have been able to obtain a ministerial order setting up a nursing committee to review license applications.[17] Through this committee, nurses began to exert some control over who can practice. In this way nurses start to acquire a more direct involvement in the processes that determine educational and other standards for entry into nursing practice.

A similar system exists in the United Arab Emirates,[18] and Oman, and other countries in the Arabian Gulf region are working towards establishing comparable mechanisms.[19] This suggests that having a major responsibility in the licensing process is one way to move towards achieving a greater degree of self-regulation.

But licensure or registration in itself is only one small aspect of regulation—a fact often not appreciated by the profession and government authorities. By itself, and in the absence of the other components of regulation as defined earlier, it is insufficient to promote improvement in standards and enhancement of professional development. Mechanisms that promote, implement, monitor, enforce and evaluate standards for nursing education, practice and the nursing services are a critical part of any system that sets out to ensure that practitioners are safe and competent.

The concept of 'self-regulation' of the profession, that is, nurses and nursing governed by nurses in the public interest, does seem to be taking root in these regions as nurses become better educated and are more directly involved in planning, policy development and management of nursing and other health services. For example, in 1996 the United Arab Emirates began formulating a nursing practice law and in 2001, Lebanese nurses succeeded in creating an order to regulate the profession and Oman has established a nursing and midwifery council. Bahrain has recently expressed its intention to move in a similar direction, while recently nurses in Egypt have taken the first steps towards acquiring a nursing practice act.

The role of properly developed systems of regulation in improving the quality of nursing care has been consistently recognised in documents from WHO's offices in the Eastern Mediterranean (EMR) and South Eastern Asia (SEAR). The EMR strategy for nursing and midwifery development identified the regulation of practice and education, at both the basic and post-basic levels, and the establishment of a legislative body (e.g. nursing council) to monitor and enforce regulation as necessary elements for proper nursing development.[20] As well as the countries already mentioned, Iran, Morocco, Jordan and Kuwait have taken initiatives to review their regulatory status. In Pakistan, a country with a nursing council, the approach adopted is to strengthen the infrastructure and functional capacity of the council.[21] In the SEAR, nurses from the region and a number of experts developed guidelines to assist countries with formulating appropriate systems for professional regulation. In addition, ICN reports an increasing number of requests for assistance in establishing new or better regulatory frameworks.

3. Nursing enjoys no universal definition of function. The scope of nursing practice as defined by law or job descriptions and other similar instruments is more restrictive than the public needs for their services.

Reports from WHO and ICN indicate that few countries under consideration in this book have reached a clear consensus as to the proper function of nursing. Lack of role definition, either through job descriptions or a legal definition of function, is often accompanied by a considerable overlap of function among the different levels of personnel in practice settings. If there is agreement on nursing's role, it is often limited to the curative and institutional settings. Nursing is usually restricted to activities concerned with providing physical care and assisting or executing the physicians' orders. The EMR reports that some member states view nursing as a technical service consisting of a series of nursing procedures and activities prescribed by a medical or administrative hierarchy of the curative health services.[22] This puts nursing at the service of the physician or health care administrator rather than of the individual, family or community requiring nursing services.

The lack of a clear focus for nursing practice is further reflected in the high percentage of time nurses may spend in 'non-nursing' jobs such as clerical work and porterage or duties with no patient contact in laboratories, X-ray, departments or pharmacies. Neglect of the 'caring' part of the nurse's role and the limited range of interventions in the prevention and health promotion fields means that nursing action is restricted in the very areas where nurses could have expertise and where needs exist.

But nurses in the Eastern Mediterranean region are challenging this concept of their work and contribution to health care. They have a vision of nurses who...

...will offer efficient practice of the highest possible standard and safety, founded on up-to-date research and knowledge. They will meet the present and future health care needs of the people as members of the health team in a cost-effective manner in a variety of settings, with the ultimate goal of contributing to the maintenance and/or improvement of quality of life.[23]

4. Educational standards are generally inadequate to meet the demands of increasingly complex health care problems and systems. No universal standards of education exist within a country.

Lack of commonly accepted standards of education for the profession are evident when multiple basic nursing programmes with different standards exist and are tolerated within a country, a situation frequently reported by WHO[24,25] and in the country reports received at ICN. This is aggravated by nursing's limited access to resources and lack of power to act to improve the quality of education in many situations.

Other conditions contribute to keeping standards at a level inadequate for society's needs. Nursing has to battle constantly with poor classroom, library and study facilities; unsuitable clinical learning settings; inadequate equipment, and limited access to up-to-date educational materials, especially in the language of the country. The number of teachers is often insufficient and many are ill-prepared, unable to make effective use of current educational methodologies. For example in Egypt, only four of the eleven Higher Institutes of Nursing that provide the country with its university-prepared nurses are headed by a nurse. There is a penury of expertise in curriculum development and educational policy development. Even where systems for monitoring standards and for approving nursing schools are present they, too often, are poorly resourced and may have little real power to enforce standards, even at the lowest level. All these factors make it difficult to establish and apply higher educational standards nationally with consistency.

Health care systems are continually evolving and becoming more complex, demanding that health professionals acquire new knowledge and competencies. However, nursing education standards in too many countries remain static, or may even fall further below the minimum required of today's health care systems. One of the largest countries in the EMR still recruits 95 per cent of its nurses from programmes requiring only nine years of general schooling. Even where standards of education are higher, it is questionable whether the education acquired really prepares nurses for the complexity and diversity of practice. ICN staff making country visits and publications of WHO have often noted the lack of access for nurses to specialty preparation, continuing education and the other educational experiences that are required to maintain continuing competency and meet new and emerging nursing needs. As noted by an EMR report, many continuing education programmes have been directed to re-education of staff rather than the development of new skills and knowledge to support changes in practice.[26]

5. The role of the profession, through the national nurses' association, other nursing organizations and individual nurses, in the processes of regulation, governance and standard setting for the profession and its members is uncertain or undeveloped in the country.

ICN firmly believes it is the responsibility of the profession to take the leading role in its governance. The profession's role includes establishing and recommending the standards in the form of definitions, ethical codes, education and service requirements and a range of related issues. Further to this, the profession must bear the primary responsibility for knowledge development and for advancing nursing through fostering relevant post-basic specialist preparation and advanced nursing practice.[27]

Strong professional organizations exist where the profession has a clear identity, is publicly recognised as a leader in nursing development and in improving the status of nurses, and is granted the same degree of control over its affairs that is given to the other professions in the country. However, nursing faces many constraints in establishing strong professional organizations in Islamic countries, as is often the case elsewhere in the world. The political system, for example, may inhibit the establishment of strong professional interest groups. Other restraints are a consequence of the very features that limit nursing's control over its affairs. They include:

• Lack of a clear identity that is often accompanied by the absence of legal recognition. This means that nursing is not taken seriously as a profession with its own knowledge base, range of expertise, standards for ethical behaviour, and capability for deciding its own future.

• Weak professional and public leadership inhibits nursing growth and limits its ability to contribute to improving health care. Skillful leadership is needed to develop an effective organization with the capacity to advance nursing and with it, the capability of demonstrating professional authority and knowledge to the public and policy makers.

• Poor participation by nurses in general is widespread in this largely female profession where multiple roles and family obligations leave little time for activities outside work and home. In addition, effective models for collective professional action, especially for female-dominated occupational groups, are hard to find in many of these countries. The potential impact of collective action in advancing nursing, both professionally and in the socio-economic field, is underestimated and poorly understood.

• Low participation from well-educated nurses in professional organizations is often the case. Several reasons may underlie this reluctance to become involved. The better educated nurses may be out numbered by a mass of lesser-qualified nurses. Consequently, they may experience difficulties in reaching leadership positions within the organization. In countries where nursing has a poor image, nurses may prefer to join better regarded organizations that have been made accessible to them as a result of their higher educational qualifications. Finally, some countries have so few well-prepared nurses that they become over committed and have to attend to other pressing nursing needs. Association strengthening takes low priority.

- The poor financial state of nursing associations limits their ability to strengthen organizational structures, communication and services to their members as nurses' low pay prevents many associations from charging realistic dues. Moreover, nursing finds it difficult to attract sponsors to support its activities. Nurses are not seen as attractive sources of revenue for commercial and other groups who will generously sponsor physicians, pharmacists and dentists. Finally, the association may have neither the contacts and the 'know how' to seek other sources of revenue, and it may lack the financial and organizational skills required to manage finances and other assets.

CONCLUSION

Regulatory systems that support good practice and prevent poor and unacceptable care are the key to keeping nursing alive and fit to meet the expectations of society for quality health care. Regulation lies at the heart of many of the issues that are discussed in other chapters in this book. It is instrumental in deciding who is a nurse, who will be accepted into a nursing programme, to what standards a nurse will be educated, to whose standards the nurse will practice, and at what level the nurse will be rewarded and recognised. As Affara and Styles[28] concluded, nursing will be able to say that it is in control of its own destiny when it can demonstrate that:

- nursing is recognised as being at the forefront of health care;
- the world, in pursuit of health for all, has full access to the best of nursing—access to its values, knowledge, skills and commitment;
- the word 'nurse' has a singular, positive meaning, and the image of nursing is sharp and distinct in the eyes of the public; and
- nursing speaks with authority and with a strong and united voice.

NOTES

1. International Council of Nurses. 'Report on the Regulation of Nursing: A Report on the Present, a Position for the Future.' Geneva, ICN, 1986, p. 7.
2. M.M. Styles and F.A. Affara, 'ICN On Regulation: Towards 21st Century Models.' Geneva, ICN, 1998, p. 2.
3. F. Affara and M.M. Styles, *Nursing Regulation Guide Book: From Principle to Power.* Geneva, International Council of Nurses, 1993, p. 1.
4. M.M. Styles and F.A. Affara, ibid., p. 18.
5. M.M. Styles and F.A. Affara, ibid., p. 23.
6. M.M. Styles and F.A. Affara, ibid., p. 22.
7. J. Godwin, *Price of Honour.* London: Warner Books, 1994.
8. World Health Organization, Regional Office for the Eastern Mediterranean. 'The Role of Women in Support of Health For All.' Document presented to the 40th session of the Regional Committee held in Alexandria, Egypt, 1993.
9. World Health Organization. 'Nursing Practice Around the World.' Geneva, World Health Organization, 1997, p. 62.
10. World Health Organization. Eastern Mediterranean Region. 'A Strategy for Nursing and Midwifery.' EMRO Technical Publications, Series 25, Alexandria, EMRO, 1997, p. 24.
11. World Health Organization, Regional Office for the Eastern Mediterranean. Report on the Third Meeting of the Regional Advisory Panel on Nursing. Tunis, 25-28 September, Alexandria, EMRO, 1996, p. 14.
12. N.I. Durrani, L. Tinevez, 'A Management System for the Pakistan Nursing Council.' Paper given at the first conference of the Global Network of WHO Collaborating Centres for Nursing/Midwifery Development, Nursing and Midwifery: Making a Difference in Health For All, Bahrain, 1996.
13. Z.S. Nessa, Brief History of the Bangladesh Nursing Council. NESP Newsletter. *Focus on Nursing,* Vol. 2:2, April 1997, p. 6.
14. Z.S. Nessa, ibid., p. 6.
15. World Health Organization. Eastern Mediterranean Region, op. cit., 1997, p. 13.
16. Personal communication with Elizabeth Percival, after her consultancy period with the Government of Indonesia, on strengthening professional association and licensing of health personnel in Indonesia.
17. State of Bahrain. Establishing a Nursing and Midwifery Licensing and Registration Committee. Ministry of Health Ministerial Order No. (19), 1992.
18. F. Rifai, 'Nursing Management Information System (NMIS)-UAE Experience.' Paper given at the first conference of the Global Network of WHO Collaborating Centres for Nursing/Midwifery Development. Nursing and Midwifery: Making a Difference in Health For All, Bahrain, 1996.
19. Third International Conference on the Regulation of Nursing Regulation, 'Across Borders: Enhancing Public Service Through International Collaboration.' Proceedings, Vancouver, Canada, p. 7.
20. World Health Organization, Regional Office for the Eastern Mediterranean, op. cit., 1997, p. 13.
21. I. Durani and L. Tinevez, 'A Management System for the Pakistan Nursing Council.' Paper given at the first conference of the Global Network of WHO

Collaborating Centres for Nursing/Midwifery Development, Nursing and Midwifery: Making a Difference in Health For All, Bahrain, 1996.
22. World Health Organization, op. cit., 1997, p. 57.
23. World Health Organization. Eastern Mediterranean Region, op. cit., 1997, p. 9.
24. Eastern Mediterranean Region of the World Health Organization. 'The Need for National Planning for Nursing and Midwifery in the EMR.' Report to the Regional Committee for the Eastern Mediterranean, EM/RC41/11, May 1994.
25. World Health Organization, op. cit., 1997, pp. 58-59.
26. World Health Organization, ibid., p. 62.
27. M.M. Styles and F.A. Affara, op. cit., 1998, p. 23.
28. F. Affara and M.M. Styles, op. cit., 1993, p. 183.

4

Educating Girls and Women in Islamic Countries: What is the Problem?

Nagat El-Sanabary

INTRODUCTION

'The Search for Knowledge is the duty of every Muslim,' (Saying of the Prophet Muhammad [PBUH]).

This saying confirms a view (injunction) unknown to many people in the Muslim world and outside it. Islam, a religion based on the book, the Holy Quran, does not distinguish between women and men in their obligation to acquire knowledge. Several Quranic verses address knowledge and its importance for Muslims and their community.[1] Hence, the high rates of illiteracy in Islamic countries, especially among women, cannot be blamed on Islam. The culprit has to be found elsewhere.

Many Western scholars and practitioners miss the point when they attribute illiteracy and the observed lag in female education in Islamic countries to Islam. There are more than one billion Muslims, roughly one-fifth of the world's population. They share a common religious creed and adhere to many similar religious practices. However, they constitute a mosaic of various ethnic, racial, cultural and economic backgrounds. This mosaic of cultural traditions, which blends variably with Islamic values, has had a major influence on the development of education generally and women's education in particular. There is neither a monolithic Muslim world nor a uniform system of education of Muslim women. The various cultural, historic, economic, demographic and political events constitute a complex web of factors that have affected and continue to affect the level and pattern of female education among and within the various states.

In this study, I show how Muslim women's education reflects the socio-economic and political context in each country. I begin with a historical overview which shows the effects of early educational development in Islamic countries, the level of exposure to Western influences including colonization, trade relations, missionary activities, and more recently, international forums and conventions on the rights of women and children, and donor support. The study focuses on nine selected Islamic countries, Arab and non-Arab. These countries differ considerably in population size, culture, economic wealth or poverty, general level of human resource development and other development indicators. I will show how these differences have affected educational development among girls and women. I highlight the major progress achieved and the persistent problems still faced in expanding educational opportunities for girls and women and reducing gender disparities in education. I focus on key issues—the high illiteracy in some countries, the challenge of achieving universal access to basic education and some of the key quality issues. Specifically, I address the problem of curriculum bias, gender role stereotypes in textbooks, the reproduction of gender divisions in the schools and school to work issues. The study is based on data from official government documents, international sources, the findings of field-based research, the burgeoning literature of international development agencies, and my own observations, study and field experience in education and gender issues in several Islamic countries. At some points the analysis focuses on the Arab countries, about which I am more knowledgeable.

Table 1 provides basic economic and demographic data for the nine countries: Indonesia, Pakistan, Bangladesh and Turkey are non-Arab, while Egypt, Saudi Arabia, Jordan, Lebanon and Kuwait are Arab countries. Most have a population of over 90 per cent Muslim except Lebanon, where Christians are close to 30 per cent. The estimated total population of these countries in the year 2000 was 662 million. They vary considerably in population size. Indonesia, Pakistan and Bangladesh alone have a combined population of about 500 million while Jordan, Lebanon and Kuwait have a combined population of just ten million. In most of them, over 30 per cent of the population is below 14 years of age. Ironically, the large-population countries have the least resources to harness for educating their sizable school-age population. Those with the smallest populations, such as Kuwait, are the wealthiest and have abundant resources for education. Although Lebanon and Jordan are not as wealthy as Kuwait, their small size population makes the educational effort more manageable than in the more populous countries. Of the countries discussed in this paper, Kuwait has the largest gross domestic product (GDP) per capita— $22,700—which is about eight times the GDP of Indonesia, Pakistan and Egypt individually. Bangladesh has the lowest GDP/capita of $1,380, or roughly 6 per cent of Kuwait's. It is no surprise that educational opportunities, especially for females, are much more advanced in Kuwait than in either Bangladesh or Pakistan. The urbanized states such as Kuwait and Turkey have better educational opportunities for females than the predominantly rural ones such as Bangladesh and Pakistan.

Table 1
GDP/capita, Total Population, Population Growth rate, and Percentage age 14 and under 1999/2000

Country	GDP/Capita 1999 est. (US$)	Population 2000 est. (millions)	Population Growth Rate	Percentage Age 14 and Under
Indonesia	2,830	224.8	1.6	31
Pakistan	2,000	141.6	2.2	41
Bangladesh	1,380	129.2	1.6	36
Turkey	6,600	65.7	1.2	29
Egypt	2,850	68.4	1.7	35
Saudi Arabia	9,000	22.0	3.8	43
Jordan	3,500	5.0	3.1	38
Lebanon	4,500	3.6	1.4	28
Kuwait	22,700	1.9	3.4	29
Total		662.2		

Sources: Population Data from the Fact Books for the Various Countries, CIA, USA, and the United Nations Demographic Yearbook 1999.

HISTORICAL OVERVIEW OF WOMEN'S EDUCATION IN ISLAMIC COUNTRIES

In the early Islamic period, from the seventh to the eleventh centuries, education was extremely informal and flourished in a variety of institutions including mosques, literary circles, bookshops, and the homes of learned men. Most children acquired basic religious teachings and life skills from their parents or other adult family members. A small proportion of boys attended religious schools called '*kuttabs*' or '*Maktabs*' for formal education in religion, reading, writing and mathematics. Girls and women were educated in the privacy of their homes where they learned homemaking skills from their mothers and the rudiments of religion from their fathers. Some families hired women readers of the Quran, called *Sheikhas*, to teach the Quran to young girls in their homes. There were no special *kuttabs* for girls; a few attended the boys' *kuttabs*, an indication of the existence of a limited form of co-education at that time.[2] Those from upper-class families received advanced education in religion, philosophy, poetry and oratory from their parents or private tutors. Some of these women became poets, orators and theologians.

The secondary-level schools (*madrasahs*)[3] established in Islamic countries during the eleventh century had a strong sectarian orientation designed for future religious leaders and government officials.[4] They had little to offer girls and women who had no role in public affairs in those days. The *kuttabs* and home study remained the main vehicles for educating Muslim girls for several centuries.

Women contributed to education and culture in many ways. Some women from ruling and prominent families contributed financial support to the *madrasahs*; mainly through endowments, which they managed themselves. Some women who received their education through the informal system had major influence in academic and literary circles. Some are reported to have taught men in some of the major mosques and had given *Ijazas* (graduation certificates) to learned men. Early Islamic education and learning resulted in major achievements by Islamic scholars in the various fields of knowledge. What came to be known as the Golden Age of Islam, when Muslims made major contributions to the sciences, humanities and art, ended with the crusade wars, the Mongol invasion, national strife in the Islamic countries and elsewhere in the world. During the Ottoman Empire and its control over much of the Muslim world, there was little support for the traditional Islamic schools and *madrasah*'s in non-Turkish speaking countries. Education in the Arab countries, for instance, became stagnant mainly because of loss of financial support. Educational reform began in the nineteenth century and accelerated in the twentieth. Women and men benefited from this reform, especially in the second half of the twentieth century, as I will show later in this chapter.

In the early decades of the nineteenth century, Western Christian missionaries introduced the first Western-type girls' schools in strategically located countries where Western traders and missionaries flocked in search of riches and religious converts. Dozens of schools were established in Egypt, Lebanon, Syria and India (that then encompassed today's Pakistan and Bangladesh). Foreign schools were established for the children of Western settlers. The missionary schools aimed to attract both native Christian and Muslim girls and boys. But Muslim parents suspected their religious intentions and proselytizing efforts. This is not surprising given the fact that Bible study was required of all students. To allay parents' fears and attract more children from modest backgrounds, these schools taught utilitarian subjects such as handicrafts and income-generating skills. To attract the upper classes they taught foreign languages, English or French— depending on the nationality of the particular mission,—Western culture and etiquette, art and music. That strategy succeeded and the numbers of both Christian and Muslim girls in these schools grew steadily. For example, by 1878 there were 3,524 girls enroled in missionary and foreign schools in Egypt, in addition to unidentified numbers who attended co-educational schools. The majority of girls in missionary schools in Egypt were non-Egyptian and non-Muslim.

Prompted by the example of missionary girls' schools, influential Muslim philanthropists began to establish their own private girls' schools and to pressure their governments to open public ones. Many of the teachers and administrators in the newly established native girls' schools in Egypt and Lebanon were graduates of missionary schools. This is an important contribution of missionary girls' schools in these countries.

Turkey was one of the first countries to open public schools for girls in the early nineteenth century. It passed a compulsory education law in 1824 during the 'Tanzeemat Period' (1780-1876), which was characterized by the introduction of Western-type institutions while maintaining traditional cultural and religious values. By 1868, 126,459 girls and 242,017 boys were enroled in 11,008 primary schools.[5] In 1895/96, there were 248,737 Muslim females enroled in Ottoman primary schools under the Ottoman Empire, mostly in Turkey. There were also 118,890 non-Muslim females in private schools.[6] Egypt opened a public girls' school in Cairo in the 1840s, but it was short-lived for lack of demand. Female public education became a reality in Egypt in 1873 with the establishment of the Saniyyah School in Cairo under the sponsorship of the Khedive's wife.[7] Around the turn of the twentieth century, prominent men and women fought tenaciously to improve the status of women. Education was on top of the list of their demands for enhancing women's status and improving standards of living among the masses. Calls for women's education echoed from India to Turkey and Egypt. Women who were educated at home, in foreign or national schools became actively involved in the nationalist liberation and feminist movements. They championed the cause of girls' education and became role models for new generations of women.

The colonial governments that extended their rule over much of the Muslim world during the late nineteenth and early twentieth centuries paid little attention to girls' and women's education, assuming that girls' education was against Islamic teachings.[8,9] Thus, under colonialism, girls' education progressed minimally or even declined. In Egypt, for instance,[10] girls' enrolment in primary schools declined during the ten years following the British occupation of Egypt. In 1884 there were 225 girls enroled in public schools in Egypt, constituting 2.9 per cent of all students. By 1894, the number had fallen to 164 or 1.7 per cent of all students. By 1914, female enrolment had risen to a mere 786 or 5.5 of total primary enrolment. These developments were a direct result of the policies of a tight-fisted British minister of education who restricted public spending on education and imposed school fees. Furthermore, under British administration, education in Egypt and elsewhere focused on preparing civil servants from among the elite classes and paid little attention to mass public education.[11]

Upon achieving national independence in the early to the mid-decades of the twentieth century, nationalist governments emphasized education for nation building. Most countries passed compulsory education laws for boys and girls and made education free of charge through the secondary or even the tertiary level. Girls and women benefited considerably from these laws and the resulting educational expansion. Progress was slow in the beginning but accelerated in the second half of the twentieth century because of rising demand from educated families, and in response to numerous international conventions on education and children's and women's rights.

Some countries, especially those that escaped the stimulation and humiliation of colonialism, and were closed to Western influences, had a late start in initiating education for females. Saudi Arabia, for instance, opened its first government girls' schools in 1960. Opposition from parents in some isolated communities did not shake the government's resolve to keep the schools open. Before that date, thousands of girls attended private girls' schools in the capital of Riyadh and the port city of Jeddah. Many Saudi families sent their daughters to schools in Egypt and Lebanon where they stayed either with relatives or in boarding schools.

While some states struggled to maintain adequate levels of economic and human development, others were blessed with new found wealth. The Arab Gulf States are a prime example. The oil boom of the 1970s catapulted these states from decades of dormancy into unprecedented affluence. The resulting phenomenal economic growth transformed these societies and allowed education of men and women to flourish, despite uneven cultural change and religious rigidities in some states. These wealthy states had the resources to build schools and provide the needed human and financial resources. Comparatively, the poor states remained at the bottom rung of the development and education scales. There, traditional cultural attitudes, combined with misconceptions about the implications of Islam for girls' education and gender roles, constrained the development of girls' and women's education. Under limited resources, religion and cultural traditions become an easy excuse and rationale for the lag in girls' and women's education, and for the restrictions on women's role in public life. Consequently, girls' and women's education progressed at a phenomenal pace in the rich states but at a much slower rate in the poor ones.

The beginning of the first UN Decade for Women, in 1975, focused international attention on girls' education as a means of improving the status of women and expanding their options beyond the domestic sphere. In the two decades that followed, academicians and development professionals produced research evidence that girls' education improves all development indicators. It increases life expectancy; reduces infant, maternal and child mortality rates; increases productivity, and slows population growth. This evidence heightened commitment to girls' education as 'probably the best investment that a country can make in its development.'[12] This research confirmed earlier concern that the lag in female education has hindered the achievement of sustainable social and economic development. To remedy the situation, researchers at universities and international donor agencies tried to pinpoint the constraints on female access to education in developing countries, and to the more subtle forms of discrimination facing girls and women in education in the industrialized Western nations. Special attention began to focus on women's education in Islamic countries, which was generally lagging behind women's education in other parts of the world except sub-Saharan Africa.

Several researchers and development professionals blamed Islam for the lag of girl's education in Islamic countries, mostly on perceived parental resistance to girls' education. Without any empirical evidence, they argued that Muslim parents are reluctant to send their daughters to schools because of alleged concern for family honour and that they sequester them at home awaiting an arranged marriage. Concerned about this issue, I began in the early 1970s to examine the relationship between girls' education and its socio-economic and political context. I came to the conclusion that we need to look at the big picture, look beyond Islam to find the constraints to the supply and demand for girls' education. I suggested a careful examination of the complex macro and micro-economic determinants of this education in order to come up with better explanations of the problem and viable remedies.[13] The model that I produced in 1973, and refined in 1989, has been widely used in the study of girls' education in all developing countries. Field research over twenty-five years has resulted in a better understanding of the constraints on female educational access, achievement and persistence in education in these and other developing countries. New strategies have been effectively used in several countries to enhance female education and reduce gender gaps in education and society, as I will show later in this chapter.

CURRENT STATUS OF FEMALE EDUCATION

The Policy Environment

Generally, educational policies of the Islamic countries do not discriminate against girls and women. Most of these countries have open admission policies and compulsory education laws that guarantee the right of all children to a free primary cycle of five to six years in some and up to eight or nine years in others.[14] Many of them provide free education through the university level. Additionally, the wealthy Arab Gulf states grant scholarships to university students, male and female, and free lodging for those who need it. In most Islamic countries co-education is common at the primary and university levels, but single-sex schools are the norm at the secondary level, the period that coincides with adolescence and hence parental concern over intermingling of the sexes. But there are exceptions on both sides. While co-education is the prevailing pattern at all levels in Lebanon, it is prohibited in Saudi Arabia except in kindergartens. Saudi Arabia is the only Arab country with a gender-specific policy that requires the complete separation of male and female schools and administrative structures and determines the mode and type of education that women receive.[15] Comparatively, the Turkish educational policy affirms that 'irrespective of sex, both males and females have equal opportunities in education.' With the increasing international focus on girls' education, more and more countries are beginning to introduce gender specific policies aimed at increasing female educational access, persistence and achievement.

As signatories to international conventions that stipulate the right to education for both sexes, these countries have committed themselves to achieving gender equity in education by the year 2015, according to the declaration of 'Education for All' (Jometien, China in 1990), to the Conventions on the Rights of the Child, and the Beijing Declaration and Platform for Action (1995). Hence, their governments are under pressure to enhance educational opportunities for girls and women, and to meet their international commitments.

But equitable policies and international obligations do not guarantee equitable access or achievement. International cooperation and donor support have helped some countries expand educational opportunities for girls and women and increased awareness of the constraints facing them. Yet the challenges are great and resources are limited. Compulsory education laws do not compensate for lack of accessible schools and school places. Furthermore, equal access does not guarantee equal outcome.

PHENOMENAL GROWTH AND EXPANDING OPPORTUNITIES

Since the early 1970s, all Islamic countries have made significant progress in increasing female access to education at all levels. The magnitude of the increase is apparent by data in Table 2 showing changes in the numbers and percentages of girls and women in primary, secondary and higher education between 1980/81 and 1996/97. During that period, female primary education enrolment increased by 50 per cent. Their secondary enrolment more than tripled, and higher education enrolment quadrupled. Specifically, female primary enrolment increased from about 22 to 33 million, secondary enrolment rose from four and a half million to fifteen and a half million, and higher education enrolment increased from about half a million to more than two million. Overall enrolment in the three educational levels in the nine countries increased from about 27 million in 1980/81 to over 50 million in 1996/97. In Indonesia, the most populous state, female enrolment increased from about 13 million to about 21 million.

These data should dispel the widely held stereotype that Islam is against women's education. The enormous increase in female enrolment in all countries has resulted, not from a change in religious values but from a better understanding of the implications of Islam for girls' and women's education, increased government commitment, growing popular demand, and participation of the private sector and civil society organizations in the development of girls' education. There has also been an increased awareness of the importance and benefits of female education. Increasingly, governments and families are recognizing female education as an investment with high personal and social returns.

UNIVERSAL PRIMARY EDUCATION: STILL AN ELUSIVE GOAL FOR THE POOR STATES

As a result of the phenomenal growth in primary education enrolment, shown in Table 2, most Islamic countries are now providing primary education to the majority of school-age children as shown in Table 3. Of the nine countries included in this study, five—Indonesia, Turkey, Jordan, Lebanon and Kuwait—have achieved close to universal access for males and females. Four countries—Pakistan, Bangladesh, Egypt and Saudi Arabia—have not yet achieved this goal. Saudi Arabia has the resources to achieve universal access and has come close to it. But for the economically constrained and populous countries, notably Pakistan, Bangladesh and Egypt, universalization of primary education remains a daunting challenge.

Table 2

Changes in the Numbers of Female Students and their Percentage of Total Enrolment 1980/81–1996/97

Country*	Primary Education (1980/81)		Primary Education 1996/97		Secondary Education 1980/81		Secondary Education 1996/97		Higher Education 1980/81		Higher Education (1996/97)	
	Female Students	%	Female Students	%	Female Students	%	Female Students	%	Female Students	%	Female Students	%
Indonesia	11,786,500	46	14,129,949	48	840,534	34 (a)	5,878,900	46	62,400	25 (a)	803,577	36
Pakistan	1,782,400	33	4,771,000	31	558,000	26	1,613,300	32	30,100	24 (b)	69,868	26
Bangladesh	3,045,000	37	5,346,700	45 (c)	636,584	24	1,880,500	33	33,400	14	68,866	16
Turkey	2,568,600	45	3,013,550	47	1,030,900	35 (c)	1,900,900	40	42,800	26	504,088	35
Egypt	1,875,900	40	3,484,000	46	1,081,504	37	3,048,300	45	255,600	32	352,900	42
Saudi Arabia	360,000	39	1,081,774	48	132,368	38	707,100	46	17,300	28	127,500	47
Jordan	216,600	43	551,385	49	119,022	45	159,900	48	16,700	46	52,900	47
Lebanon	197,157	45 (a)	187,700	48	131,300	53 (d)	179,600	52	28,500	36	40,200	49
Kuwait	71,249	48	69,600	49	83,227	46	111,700	50	7,800	57	18,300	62
Total	21,903,406		32,631,658		4,613,439		15,480,200		494,600		2,038,199	

Sources: Compiled from UNESCO, Statistical Yearbook, 1999. Several Tables.

*Arranged in Descending Order by size of a country's population

(a) 1970
(b) 1975
(c) 1990
(d) 1985
(e) 1991

Female enrolment increased much faster than male enrolment, thus narrowing the gender gap in education at all levels as demonstrated by gross enrolment ratios in Tables 3 and 4. The data reveal greater democratization of educational opportunities, with greater access for more of the eligible school age children and youth, male and female, at all educational levels. Indonesia, Lebanon, Turkey, Saudi Arabia and Kuwait have achieved gender parity. Comparatively, the gender gap remains quite high in Pakistan where the enrolment ratio for males is twice that for females, 87 versus 42 per cent. Pakistan is a prime example of how poverty and traditional values towards women combine to constrain women's educational access. Although Pakistan had doubled female primary enrolment between 1970 and 1991, more than half the girls of school age were still out of school in 1996 (Table 2). International comparisons ranked Pakistan as the sixth lowest in the world (World Bank 1989) in terms of progress toward achieving universal access of females to primary education. In 1985/86, only about one third of the approximately 940,000 five-year-old girls living in rural areas were in schools, and fewer than one in six rural girls completed five years of education.[16] International donor agencies have been helping Pakistan expand educational opportunities for girls in the educationally deprived provinces of Balochistan and the North West Frontier Province. Non-governmental organizations are supplementing government efforts to expand educational opportunities for girls in Pakistan and Bangladesh. The Bangladesh Rural Advancement Committee (BRAC) and the Balochistan Community Organizations in Pakistan have achieved substantial results in increasing female access to education in their communities.

Rapid population growth, which has slowed down in recent years, has thwarted the efforts to universalize primary school access and eradicate illiteracy in the poor states. Consequently, in these and other Islamic countries, millions of children of primary school age, the majority of whom are female, are out of school. Most live in rural areas or urban slums. According to a recent World Bank study, 'Nearly five million children (male and female) aged 6-10 and another four million aged 11-15 in the Middle East and North Africa[17] were out of school in 1995.' The report estimated the numbers would rise to 7.5 and 5.6 million respectively by the year 2015.[18] Most of these out-of-school children are females. In Egypt, females constituted two-thirds of out-of-school children, estimated at 860,000 in 1998.[19]

Table 3

Gross Enrolment Ratios in Primary, Secondary and Higher Education Between 1970–1995* by Percentage

Country and Date	Primary Education Male	Primary Education Female	Secondary Education Male	Secondary Education Female	Teritary Education Male	Teritary Education Female
Indonesia						
1970	87	73	21	11	4	1
1985	120	114	47	35	n.a.	n.a.
1995	116	111	55	48	15	8
Pakistan						
1970	51	19	20	5	3	0.8
1985	56	30	24	10	4	1
1991	87	42	33	17	4	2
Bangladesh						
1970	72	35	n.a.	n.a.	3	.04
1985	72	52	27	11	8	2
1990	77	66	25	13	7	1
Turkey						
1980	102	90	44	24	8	3
1985	117	110	52	30	12	6
1996	111	104	68	48	27	15
Egypt						
1970	81	53	38	19	10	4
1985	94	76	72	50	24	11
1997	108	94	83	73	n.a.	n.a.
Saudi Arabia						
1970	61	29	19	5	3	0.3
1985	73	57	48	31	12	9
1996	77	75	65	57	17	15
Jordan						
1980	105	97	79	63	29	24
1992	94	95	n.a.	n.a.	n.a.	n.a.
Lebanon						
1970	131	112	49	33	31	10
1991	120	116	71	76	30	28
1996	113	108	78	84	n.a.	n.a.
Kuwait						
1970	100	76	70	57	4	4
1985	104	102	95	87	15	18
1996	76	75	65	65	15	24

Source: UNESCO Statistical Yearbook, 1999. Table 11.8
Data are arranged in descending order by country population size.
* Unless otherwise indicated

Table 4

Changes in the Gender Gap in Gross Enrolment Ratios in Primary,
Secondary and Higher Education between 1970–1996*

Country	Date	Primary	Secondary	Teritary
Indonesia	1970	14	10	3
	1985	6	12	n.a.
	1995	5	7	7
Pakistan	1970	32	15	2.2
	1985	26	14	3
	1991	45	16	2
Bangladesh	1970	37	n.a.	3
	1985	20	16	6
	1990	11	12	6
Turkey	1980	12	20	5
	1985	7	22	6
	1996	7	20	12
Egypt	1970	28	19	6
	1985	18	22	13
	1997	14	10	n.a.
Saudi Arabia	1970	32	14	2.7
	1985	16	17	3
	1996	2	8	2
Jordan	1980	8	16	5
	1992	-1	n.a.	n.a.
Lebanon	1970	19	16	21
	1991	4	-5	2
	1996	5	-6	n.a.
Kuwait	1970	24	13	0
	1985	2	8	-3
	1996	1	0	-9

Source: UNESCO Statistical Yearbook, 1999. Table 11.8
Data are arranged in descending order by country population size.
* The gender gap is the difference between female and male gross enrolment ratios.

Most of the poor countries, such as Pakistan and Bangladesh have had to postpone the date of universalizing primary education. For instance, Bangladesh which aimed to enrol 90 per cent of school age children by the year 2000, by instituting compulsory education (in 1989) for all children age four to ten,[20] fell short of achieving that goal. As of 1990, only 77 per cent of the boys and 66 per cent of the girls of primary school age were in schools. All low-income countries cite shortage of finances as the culprit for not achieving this goal. According to Egypt's Human Development Report 2000, shortage of government resources limits government's effort to provide universal primary education. Despite a major school construction programme, there are not enough accessible schools or school places for all children of school age. Furthermore, a report by the Egyptian Ministry of Education indicated in 1998 that almost half of the schools were not suitable, thousands of them had no bathrooms and many were in danger of disintegration and in dire need of repair or replacement.[21] These school quality issues raise parental concern about the safety and privacy of their daughters. Furthermore, resource shortages generate internal inefficiencies, crowded classrooms, and low quality education, which in turn lead to school dropout. Low enrolment rates, low levels of basic skill acquisition, and high dropout rates perpetuate high illiteracy and its corresponding ills. Thus, the vicious cycle continues

The traditional model of education has not been adequate to achieve universal access. Hence, national governments, with support from donor agencies including the United Nations Children's Fund (UNICEF), United States Agency for International Development (USAID) and the World Bank, began experimenting with new schooling models to expand educational access for girls and boys in rural and sparsely populated areas. Participatory models, such as the community and one-room schools that involve parents, religious leaders, civil society organizations and the business community, are being used successfully in several Islamic countries.[22] Scholarships and other schemes to help parents with the direct and indirect costs of education have been successful in getting girls to enrol and to remain in school until graduation.

SECONDARY EDUCATION: INCREASED ACCESS BUT PERSISTENT DISPARITIES

Not all graduates of primary education are able to enter secondary schools, but the numbers of those enroled have been rising year after year. Total female secondary enrolment in the nine countries more than tripled between 1980/81 and 1997/98, from just over four and a half to fifteen and a half million. The increase was remarkable in Pakistan, Bangladesh, Egypt and Saudi Arabia (see Table 2).

Furthermore, the proportion of eligible females enroled in secondary education doubled in Indonesia and Turkey, more than tripled in Pakistan and Egypt, and increased ten times in Saudi Arabia (see Table 3). As with primary education, the increase in secondary enrolment has been a result of increased government commitment, growing public demand and international donor support for poor countries. Measures undertaken to increase female access to secondary education included elimination of school fees and granting of scholarships. For instance, in 1989 the government of Bangladesh made secondary education free for girls and provided scholarships to encourage female participation in secondary education. Pakistan had also instituted scholarships to increase female participation in secondary education. Free public secondary education and the availability of schools have led to phenomenal increase in female secondary education in Saudi Arabia, probably the most conservative Islamic country. This shows the power of wealth in enhancing educational opportunities for women in any Islamic country.

Numbers do not tell the whole story, though. There are some serious qualitative problems that manifest themselves in the differential access of females and males to various kinds of educational programmes available at the secondary level.

TRADITIONAL ORIENTATION IN A VASTLY CHANGING WORLD

What type of education do girls receive at the secondary level and does it differ from the education provided to boys? The majority of secondary education students, from 60 to 90 per cent, enrol in academic secondary schools[23] that are theoretically open for all those who have the qualifying grades. A small proportion enters the less prestigious vocational or technical schools, while enrolment in teacher training has been dwindling steadily as elementary teacher training shifts to the college level.

Theoretically, no difference exists between the education available to females and males at the academic secondary level. The differences emerge when students are faced with a curriculum choice between a scientific or literary track in preparation for appropriate specialization in colleges and universities. A system of self-selection occurs here. It is true that thousands of girls choose the scientific track and often excel over their male counterparts. The majority, however, choose the literary track based on a commonly held stereotype that these are female-appropriate subjects suited for women's feminine and nurturing psyche and delicate physique. Economic circumstances play a part also. Furthermore, scientific and technical studies are more expensive fields of study than literature and social sciences. Working class girls often shy away from secondary school science fields because of the cost and the required length of study were they to pursue higher education. For all female students, choice of the literary track limits their educational options in higher education and career opportunities afterwards. Unknowingly, girls and women help perpetuate gender divisions in the home and marketplace.

The majority of girls are not getting adequate education in math, science and technology to prepare them for the technological revolution of the twenty-first century. Instead, many of them get a low quality education that may qualify them for higher education, but has little relevance to the world of work. These educational systems have traditionally allowed for relatively high rates of participation of girls and women in math and science, but most of them have not kept pace with the new technological revolution. Thousands graduate from high schools and college with no marketable skills and very little chance of finding employment. Nonetheless, academic secondary education remains the most viable option for girls. This is because the disparities in academic secondary education pale in comparison with those in vocational and technical education, the real class and gender marker.

VOCATIONAL EDUCATION: KEEPING WOMEN IN THEIR PLACE

Vocational secondary education is generally unpopular. Its class stigma and repute, as the dump basin for those who cannot succeed in academic secondary schools, has made it virtually out of bounds for middle class girls. Yet it remains a viable option for many working class girls seeking practical skills for gainful employment.

Traditionally, the only type of vocational education available for girls focused on home-making skills, sewing and tailoring, knitting and crochet, and nursing. It aimed to prepare women for their adult roles as homemakers, mothers and caretakers. Over the past two decades, several countries have expanded vocational education opportunities for women to allow them access to most fields of studies available to males. As the focus expanded, so did female enrolment.

Despite the progress, the proportion of girls enroled in vocational education is minimal compared to enrolment in the academic secondary schools.

Available statistics underscore the low female participation in vocational education and the major differences among the various countries. Generally, the gender-integrated economies of Turkey and Egypt promote greater access of females to vocational education than countries such as Pakistan and Saudi Arabia. In gender-segregated Saudi Arabia, the only type of vocational education available to girls is nursing education and some training in sewing and handicrafts. In 1990, the only female vocational enrolment in Saudi Arabia consisted of 2,520 girls enroled in secondary-level nursing institutes run by the Ministry of Health, and another 1,000 in tailoring schools run by the General Presidency of Girls' Education (GPGE).[24] The first prepares assistant nurses, the second homemakers.

In these countries, as in many others, vocational education is a major gender and class marker. Most girls enrol in programmes that prepare them for motherhood or for traditional female occupations. Even in countries with diversified vocational programmes for women like Turkey, domestic science schools, which enrol most female vocational education students, offer general home economic subjects, rug weaving, garment making and related 'female crafts'. For instance, in 1981/82 females constituted 100 per cent of the enrolment in domestic sciences, 39 per cent in commerce and tourism, 94 per cent in health and nursing, 10 per cent in agricultural schools, 13.4 per cent in Muslim teacher training schools and 9.6 in other vocational programmes. About six per cent of the enrolment in boys' vocational schools were females.[25] In 1990, the Turkish Ministry of National Education substantially increased female enrolment in vocational and technical education. It had 386 vocational and technical lycees enroling 50,301, of whom 47,265 were in 352 Vocational Lycées for girls, 319 in three Technical Lycées, 2,573 in 30 Anatolian Vocational Lycees and 144 in one Anatolian Technical Lycee.[26] The stated goal of these schools for girls is 'to make them productive so that they can contribute to the Turkish economy.'

Egypt has also expanded its programmes in commercial education for girls to increase their employment in clerical and sales occupations. It expanded female vocational education enrolment considerably and broadened women's curriculum choices. In 1997/98, 844,000 girls were enroled in vocational secondary schools, or 28 per cent of total enrolment. However, little is known about the effectiveness of this education in providing its graduates with marketable skills. Available evidence indicates that this education has not increased women's occupational options or earning potential. Unemployment among vocational education graduates in Egypt is extremely high, especially among females. This is because employers prefer to hire academic secondary graduates whom they consider to be better qualified than graduates of vocational schools.[27]

In the 1980s Bangladesh embarked on a major initiative focusing on strengthening vocational education and skills training for women. Training in animal husbandry, garment making, food processing and other fields was initiated in 250 training-cum-production centres, household or village-based industry development, with provision of microcredit through rural development banks to help the graduates undertake income-generating enterprises. The government allocated one third of the education budget to this vocational training education (VTE), the second largest after basic primary and secondary education. The plan faltered, though, when the government shifted its emphasis to Universal Primary Education in its development plans for 1980-2000.[28]

In Pakistan, vocational and technical education for girls remains much more limited than for males and more traditionally 'feminine' in focus. In 1991/92 the proportion of girls enroled in vocational secondary education in Pakistan was less than one per cent (11,970 out of 1,613,300). Most of them were enroled in the government's Vocational Institutes for Girls (GVIGs), which offer one- to two-year diplomas in traditional female fields such as sewing, knitting, dressmaking, leather goods, handicrafts, and more recently, typing and hairdressing. Vocational opportunities are much more limited in rural than in urban areas. Girls living in cities could enrol in one of the polytechnic institutes, which offer diplomas in commerce, radio, television, electronics and design and dress-making, or in one of the technical training centres (TTCs) under the National Vocational Training Project.[29]

It is commonly accepted that vocational education for males and females has not kept pace with social and technological change. In most countries, vocational education generally, and for women in particular, suffers from poor quality, lack of good curriculum materials, and irrelevance of the curriculum to students' lives. Education and work linkages are almost completely lacking. There is no educational or occupational guidance, no linkage with employers and no placement service. Consequently, unemployment, especially among females, is a pervasive problem among vocational education graduates. Those who enrol in this educational programme with some occupational aspirations are often frustrated by lack of jobs and negative attitudes among employers. There is a need for major reform of vocational education especially for females in order to meet individual, family and community needs. There are signs of hope. Several workforce development programmes in these countries, initiated during the past few years in collaboration with international donor agencies, have introduced measures to improve the quality of vocational education, to involve the business community, and to develop apprenticeship programmes and other school-to-work measures. It is not known to what extent these programmes take women's needs into account. Failing to do so would perpetrate the disenfranchisement of women in countries with high rates of unemployment, especially among vocational education graduates.

Teacher training in secondary schools used to be a viable option for thousands of young women seeking a career-oriented education. It has been phased out in favour of college-level teacher education in order to produce better-qualified teachers for primary education. At the same time, Egypt, Pakistan and Bangladesh provide short-term training for thousands of secondary school graduates to prepare them to teach in community schools and one-classroom schools run by the government. This new teacher training option has helped increase the supply of teachers and enhance educational opportunities for out-of-school girls and dropouts in remote villages and rural areas.

Nursing education in secondary-level nursing institutes is available in several countries, but enrolment is generally small and has its own problems which characterize all nursing education in these countries. I have discussed this in another paper.[30] Suffice it to say here that nursing education and nursing in general are stigmatized by low status, low class association, intermingling with male patients and doctors, and the risks of working night shifts. Yet the demand for qualified nurses is great and the supply continues to be limited.

HIGHER EDUCATION: FROM ELITIST TO MASS ORIENTATION

At the turn of the twentieth century, feminist voices echoed in Egypt, Lebanon, Syria and Iraq calling for greater opportunities for women in education and public life. Women had been working as schoolteachers and nurses for several decades and were then needed in other professions, especially medicine. Yet, prior to the 1920s Arab women wishing to continue their education beyond secondary level had to go abroad, if their parents had the means and the desire to let them do so. This option existed for very few women from wealthy and educated families at a time when women's mobility was very limited and international travel very difficult. The first Arab women seeking professional education abroad were Lebanese, Egyptian and Palestinian women who traveled mostly to Europe, financed by their families, to study medicine.[31]

The American University in Beirut was the first university in the Arab countries to admit women (1921/22) to professional schools of medicine, pharmacy and dentistry. Three years later the university admitted women to other fields of study. Students came not only from Lebanon but also from Egypt, Syria, Palestine and Iraq. The first woman graduated with a pharmacy degree in 1928. In 1931, two women graduated with medical degrees and two with a degree in law from that university.[32] This all occurred at a period of extreme conservatism as well as changing social attitudes toward women and their role in society following the First World War. The University of St. Joseph in Beirut also began admitting women in the 1920s.

National universities, opened in several countries during the early 1920s, began admitting women around 1924/25. By the 1950s almost all Arab countries had admitted women to higher education. The small Gulf States did not have national universities until after oil wealth. However, shortly there after they began to admit women. Saudi Arabian women were among the late comers to higher education. The first group of women entered Riyadh University as external students in 1961. Those first university entrants were graduates of private schools which existed in Jeddah and Riyadh for about a decade prior to the opening of public schools. It was not long before thousands of Saudi women were enroled in the increasing number of universities in various major cities in Saudi Arabia. This is in addition to thousands of others enroled in teacher training colleges under the auspices of the General Presidency of Girls' Education.

In all countries, female higher education enrolment increased slowly before the 1960s but has skyrocketed since the 1970s. By 1996/97 over two million women were enroled in higher education in the nine countries included in this study. Indonesia alone had more than 803,000. The most dramatic increase occurred between 1970 and 1996 in Turkey where the number of women enroled rose from 32,000 (19 per cent) in 1970 to more than half a million in 1996/97 (35 per cent). Egypt's female higher education enrolment increased dramatically between 1970 and 1980, from 61,000 in 1970, to 255,600 in 1980/81, and then to 352,900 in 1996/97, excluding female enrolment at Al-Azhar University.[33]

These countries generally follow gender-blind admission policies. Hence, women continue to edge toward parity with men in higher education, but major differences still exist among them. In 1996/97 females made up 62 per cent of total higher education enrolment in Kuwait, but only 16 per cent in Bangladesh.

Saudi Arabia illustrates the power of wealth in enhancing educational opportunities for girls and women. It expanded educational opportunities for women so rapidly that by 1995/96 this country of 20 million people had about twice the female enrolment in higher education of both Pakistan and Bangladesh, each of which has about six times the population of Saudi Arabia. This highly gender-segregated and conservative country has achieved a higher percentage of women in higher education than the much more open and liberal, but economically poor, Egypt, which has a much longer history of female higher education. Saudi Arabia educates as many of its eligible females in higher education as Turkey (15 per cent), and is exceeded only by Lebanon, Jordan and Kuwait (with rates of 28, 24 and 24 per cent respectively), as shown in Table 3.

Middle Eastern women pursue graduate studies in large numbers, mostly in national universities, but also in Western universities, notably in the US and England. Tens of thousands of Muslim women hold Masters and PhD degrees. Egypt alone claims to have 4,221 women with PhD degrees.[34] Saudi Arabia has a large number of women with Masters and PhD degrees, many of them obtained in US universities. Women also constitute a large proportion of professional staff in universities and colleges. Around 1996 there were approximately 57,000 women teaching in colleges and universities in these nine countries. Women make up from 33 per cent of the teachers in Lebanon and Turkey to about 10 per cent in Indonesia. Turkey, Lebanon, Egypt and Saudi Arabia have the highest ratio of women faculty in higher education, while Bangladesh and Indonesia have the lowest ratios. Saudi Arabia has a high ratio because of its gender-segregation policy that prohibits male faculty from teaching in female colleges and universities. Its wealth enables it to hire women faculty from other Islamic and Western countries, but predominantly from Egypt. In all these countries women hold advanced positions in colleges and universities including department chairpersons and college deans, but they have not yet broken the glass ceiling to the presidency of any university.

As for the fields of study in higher education, women in Muslim countries, like their western sisters, tend to concentrate in the traditional fields of the humanities, social sciences and education. But they have an edge over their Western sisters in their representation in medicine and some engineering and science fields. Teaching, medicine and social work have traditionally been the most acceptable fields of study for women. They serve women's need for education and health while maintaining gender segregation. As women's enrolment increased, so did their curriculum options, but major differences still remain among the various states. In some countries such as Egypt, Turkey and Jordan, women enter all fields of study if they have the qualifying grades in the national high school graduation exams. Hence, in these countries, thousands of women study nontraditional fields such as the natural sciences, engineering, mathematics, computer science and business. By contrast, Saudi Arabia's gender-specific policy bars women from engineering, earth sciences and architecture.

Medicine is the most prestigious field of study for women in all Islamic countries. It fits with religious and cultural values that favour treatment of female patients by women doctors. Consequently, female enrolment in medicine in Islamic countries is often close to 50 per cent, exceeding the numbers and percentages of women in medicine in many Western countries. Ironically, while nursing is also considered an appropriate profession for Muslim women, it has not been a popular field of study or employment in many Islamic countries. There, nursing colleges are struggling to attract women students.[35] One of the main reasons for the unpopularity of nursing is a widely held low image of the nurse as a doctor's helpmate and excessive concern in some countries about the intermingling of nurses with male doctors, patients and nurses in hospitals during night shifts.[36] By contrast, concern over intermingling of the sexes has not diminished the demand for medical education for women in these countries, because of its high status and prestige. Women continue to enter medical colleges in large numbers even though the field has become saturated and employment opportunities for women doctors have declined considerably in countries such as Egypt and Saudi Arabia. Saudi women continue to get medical degrees, even with little prospect of employment, just because of its status and the hope that job opportunities may expand.

Jordan provides a broad range of opportunities for women in higher education. In 1995/96 there were 32,343 women students in higher education, 42 per cent of total enrolment. Jordanian women outnumbered men in education (58%), humanities and religious studies (66%), social and behavioral sciences (64%), natural sciences (60%), dentistry (53%) and architecture (52%). They were also highly represented in several non-traditional fields.[37]

PERSISTENT PROBLEMS

In discussing the history and current status of female education in Islamic countries, I have highlighted the remarkable progress made in expanding educational opportunities at the various levels and some of the problems encountered. Following is a brief discussion of two persistent problems.

ILLITERACY: THE PARADOX OF DECLINING RATES AGAINST RISING NUMBERS

High illiteracy rates among adults, especially females, have been a persistent problem in most Islamic countries. Illiteracy rates among women, which stood at over 90 per cent in many Islamic countries during the 1960s, have declined substantially over the past four decades. Most countries have reduced illiteracy rates significantly through formal schooling and literacy education, as documented by the data in Table 5. Indonesia, Turkey, Lebanon, Jordan and Kuwait started the 1980s with illiteracy rates at or below 50 per cent, which they all reduced to about 20 per cent by the year 2000. Comparatively, Pakistan, Bangladesh, Egypt and Saudi Arabia had female illiteracy rates above 65 per cent in 1980. Oil rich Saudi Arabia was able to cut the illiteracy rate for females from 67 to about 33 per cent. By contrast, resource-constrained and populous Pakistan and Bangladesh still maintain a female illiteracy rate double that of Saudi Arabia (over 70%). The decline in illiteracy rates has been greater for females than for males, resulting in a substantial reduction of the gender gap in illiteracy in all countries except Pakistan where the gap actually increased from 27 to 30 per cent (see Table 5).

The declining rates in all countries obscure an insidious problem, namely a constant increase in the absolute number of illiterates. For instance, Egyptian sociologist Hamid Ammar, in a 1994 report written for the Economic and Social Commission for Western Asia (ESCWA), noted that in the Arab countries the number of female illiterates increased from 49 million in 1975, to 61 million in 1985 and to 63.7

Table 5
Changes in Illiteracy Rates and the Number of Illiterates
1980–2000*

Country	Year	Illiteracy Rates** in per cent		Number of Illiterates in thousands	
		Male	Female	M	F
Indonesia	1980	21	40	9,080	18,298
	2000	8	18	5,911	13,329
Pakistan	1980	59	86	14,799	19,419
	2000	42	72	20,079	31,592
Bangladesh	1980	59	83	14,434	19,238
	2000	48	71	20,739	28,881
Turkey	1980	19	50	2,540	6,736
	2000	6	23	1,555	5,542
Egypt	1980	46	75	6,171	9,906
	2000	33	56	7,466	12,368
Saudi Arabia	1980	33	67	999	1,552
	2000	16	33	1,187	1,764
Jordan	1980	18	46	137	330
	2000	5	16	104	292
Lebanon	1980	17	37	134	306
	2000	8	20	82	225
Kuwait	1980	27	41	137	128
	2000	16	20	109	122

Source: UNESCO Statistical Yearbook, 1999. Table 11.2
* Data for 2000 are estimates
** Rates rounded to the nearest per cent

million in 1990. He estimated the number to reach 69 million in the year 2000. The increase between 1975 and 2000 was 20 million, that is roughly the total size of the Egyptian population in 1952, the year of the Egyptian revolution. Country-specific data shown in Table 5 substantiate this serious trend in Pakistan, Bangladesh and Egypt. In Bangladesh, the number of female illiterates increased from just over 19 million in 1980 to about 29 million in 2000. The corresponding increase was from about 19 to more than 31 million in Pakistan, and from 10 to 12 million in Egypt during the same period. Official statistics in Egypt show an increase, but of somewhat lower numbers, from ten and a half million in 1986 to twelve and a half million in the year 2000.[38] While the number of illiterate women has been rising, that of illiterate men has declined except in Pakistan, Egypt and Bangladesh, where the numbers of both illiterate women and men have been rising. In these and other Islamic countries, illiteracy is a rural phenomenon caused by inadequate educational access, poor socio-economic conditions and cultural lag. For instance, one study put the literacy rates for the various Pakistani provinces in 1982 as follows: 0.8 per cent in Balochistan, 3.4 per cent in Sindh and 7.4 per cent in the Punjab, (cited in Bergsma and Chu 1989, p. 47). In Egypt, literacy rates are lowest in the rural areas of Upper Egypt.

Several factors contribute to this disturbing trend: failure of primary education to accommodate all primary-school-age children, especially girls; dropout and wastage especially among girls; poor quality education and the inadequacy of most adult literacy programmes, especially women's. The problem is compounded by a vastly growing population and the large proportion of children under 14 years of age, roughly 35 per cent in several countries. This problem has created a vicious circle. The large numbers of illiterates, especially among women, tend to perpetuate low demand for female education; high fertility; high infant, child and maternal mortality rates; and low options for women in the personal and public spheres. Illiteracy compromises the well being of women, their families, communities and countries.

EDUCATION CONTINUES TO PERPETUATE GENDER ROLE DIVISIONS

Undoubtedly, education has opened new opportunities for women and increased their power in the family and community. Analysis of data from recent Demographic Health Surveys (DHSs) indicates that education improves all development indicators. Educated women have greater decision-making power in the family, desire fewer children, have higher expectations for their daughters' education, provide better care for their children and families and help increase their children's educational and nutritional status. Education increases women's productivity in the home and marketplace, and their participation in public life and civil society organizations.

In various Islamic countries, educated women occupy leading positions in education, the economy, the political system and in civil society organizations. They are the backbone of the educational system as teachers, supervisors and administrators. Women are highly represented in the sciences and professions. Many have excelled in business as owners and managers with their own business associations. Women occupy prominent positions in the political system as appointed cabinet members, elected members of parliament, ambassadors, judges (in a few states) and airline pilots, and three have been prime ministers (in Turkey, Pakistan and Bangladesh).

But these are lands of contrast. Prominent women are shining stars in a large scale of illiteracy and poverty. Class distinction, especially for women, remains strong despite major democratization. The traditional curriculum orientation, in most educational systems, helps perpetrate gender role divisions. In schools, girls are socialized into accepting the predominant gender role divisions that exist in the family and the wider society. School textbooks continue to ignore women's multiple roles and contributions to the community and wider society. Instead, they portray women mainly in traditional roles as homemakers, mothers, daughters or grandmothers. Young girls receive virtually no educational or career guidance. Hence, females continue to be concentrated in traditional fields of education and employment such as teaching, social welfare and office clerical work. This does not ignore the thousands of women who play an active role in society. Yet most of the female and male graduates lack marketable skills and join the ranks of the unemployed or unpaid family workers. Women suffer disproportionately from unemployment, a growing problem in many Islamic countries. The problem has intensified in recent years as a result of economic reform and structural adjustment programmes undertaken in several countries. Available data from various countries consistently show higher unemployment rates for women than men graduates holding secondary and higher education degrees. For instance, Egypt and Saudi Arabia, two vastly different countries culturally and economically, suffer from a severe problem of unemployment among educated women. Even women graduates with degrees in medicine and nursing have been having difficulty finding employment either because of economic stringency in Egypt or because of strict restrictions on women's employment in Saudi Arabia. Women with nursing degrees in Saudi Arabia face numerous hurdles in their efforts to enter and continue in nursing positions.[39]

GENERAL DISCUSSION AND CONCLUSION

The preceding discussion reflects research evidence and my own thinking and research on the education of Muslim women over the past twenty-five years. Since the 1970s, I have challenged the stereotype that Islam has been an obstacle to girls' education. Islam is a religion based on the holy book, the Quran, which encourages reading and knowledge acquisition. I have argued instead, that religion has been an easy excuse used to justify limited resource allocations to girls' education, especially under constrained economic conditions.

I have argued that a country's level of economic development, rather than adherence to strict religious values, is a major determinant of educational development in general and girls' education in particular. Poor countries with a large population and a large proportion of school age children and youth have not been able to provide all the schools and the needed human, physical and educational resources needed to educate school age children and youth. Children, especially girls, cannot go to school if there are no accessible schools or school places. Compulsory education laws cannot make up for the lack of schools, teachers or textbooks. Enrolment data by rural/urban communities in all countries show a strong correlation with female enrolment and literacy rates. Furthermore, the poor condition of many schools and lack of sanitary facilities arouse parental concern about the safety and security of their children, especially girls. Lack of school textbooks, or texts that arrive late, and irrelevance of the curriculum to students' lives are factors that lead to loss of motivation for schooling. Attitudes of teachers and administrators often discourage girls from persisting in their education. These are all part of the complex web of factors that influence the supply and the demand for girls' education in these and many other developing countries.

There is no doubt that dominant cultural and social values intertwine with religious beliefs to influence public and government decisions regarding girls' and women's education. One important social and cultural value is the dominant perception about women and their role in the family and society, i.e. gender role divisions or stereotypes. Most Muslims believe that women's and men's roles are complementary rather than equal. Neither is superior to the other. Woman has a basic responsibility for home and family, man for family economic support. These notions, of course, have changed with the spread of education and the increasingly active role of women in the economy. Many families now need the income of two family members. Educational decision-makers often ignore the fact that women have shouldered and continue to shoulder heavy multiple responsibilities in the home and the workplace for which education is indispensable. International conventions and forums on the rights of women and children over the past fifty years, since the first UN Declaration of Human Rights in 1948, have heightened awareness of education as important in itself, but also as the foundation for empowering women to perform their multiple responsibilities and contribute more effectively to the well being of their families, communities and wider society.

Predominant cultural values about women and their role in society influence the supply and demand for girls' education in all countries. On the supply side, predominant values affect the policy makers' decisions about resource allocation for building schools, training teachers and providing curriculum and other school supplies. These values also influence the demand for girls' education. They affect family decisions as to whether or not to send their daughters to schools and for how long to keep them there

Concern over the free intermingling of the sexes and its potential effects on girls' and women's reputations and family honour shape parental attitudes toward and desire for their daughters' education. Therefore, most Muslims prefer single-sex to co-educational secondary schools, which coincide with adolescence. Nonetheless, many parents would send their daughters to a boys' school if that were the only school in their village. Evidence of this comes from countries as far apart as Pakistan and Egypt. Support for single-sex schools, though, has boosted the education of girls in many Muslim communities. Furthermore, most conservative Muslim parents prefer female teachers in girls' schools. Increased sensitivity to these issues has prompted international donor and development agencies to recommend single-sex schools and training of adequate numbers of female teachers. These measures are working very well. So are efforts to introduce innovative education programmes that involve parents and communities in children's education. Many countries are also developing gender-sensitive educational curricula. Education campaigns that garner parental and community support for girls' education have also helped.

Micro-economic factors, especially the socio-economic background of parents, have an important effect on the demand for girls' education. Class and family income are important. Upper- and middle-class parents have always found the means to educate their daughters, in public or private schools, at home or abroad. For instance, Egyptian and Syrian parents sent their daughters to missionary and foreign schools in Lebanon before such schools were available in their own countries. Likewise, educated Saudi Arabian fathers sent their daughters to schools in Egypt and Lebanon in the 1950s before public girls' schools were founded in Saudi Arabia in 1960. In fact, some Saudi women obtained PhD degrees in Egypt before girls' could enter a public primary school in Saudi Arabia.

By contrast, million of girls from low socio-economic backgrounds, especially those living in rural areas, continue to have no access to schooling. Survey data from various countries show that the majority of out-of-school children live in rural areas, or poor urban households. Girls from very poor families are often kept at home to help with domestic work or sent at a tender age to work as domestics or seasonal farm laborers to supplement family income. Research conducted in Egypt, Bangladesh and Pakistan found that heavy domestic and work responsibilities were a major hindrance to girls' school attendance. Another reason is family concern about a girl's safety and security on the way to and from school, especially if girls have to walk a long distance on unpaved roads or in harsh weather conditions. Family size has also been shown to affect girls' chances of entering school or continuing their education. Large families, who cannot afford to send all their children to school, usually decide in favour of the boys. In recent years, research has demonstrated that a mother's level of education has a major effect on the education of her daughters. Educated mothers desire better education for their children, especially the girls.

Efforts to address the constraints to girls' education in these countries have focused on both the supply- and demand-side of the problem. In recent decades academicians and practitioners alike, particularly those working with international development agencies, have started to address a myriad of constraints to girls' education. To address the supply-side constraints, donors have provided many countries that receive donor assistance with funding for school construction, teacher training and curriculum development. To address the demand-side constraints, donors are helping governments provide scholarships for girls from poor families to compensate them for the direct and indirect cost of educating their daughters. Some countries, with donor assistance, provide school uniforms and supplies; others provide gender awareness training and education campaigns to familiarize parents and communities with the personal and social benefits of girls' education. It has become evident that the task of educating all children is beyond the ability of many governments and that it requires the collaboration of civil society organizations, religious leaders and the private sector. Innovative programmes involving communities in girls' education have been effective in increasing girls' school attendance, achievement and persistence in countries such as Egypt, Bangladesh and Pakistan.

Finally, girls' and women's education in Islamic countries has benefited considerably from the passage of international declarations and conventions. The first was the UN Universal Declaration of Human Rights in 1948, followed by various conventions and declarations regarding education, women's rights, human rights and the rights of the girl child, to mention just a few. Several of these countries have hosted international conferences on women or on education. For instance, at the Cairo Conference on Population and Development (ICPD) in 1994 conferees stressed the importance of girls' education as an end in itself and a means of slowing population growth. Similarly, Amman, Jordan was the site for the Third Global Meeting of the International Consultative Forum on Education for All (EFA) in 1996. The Amman Affirmation stressed the overall importance of educating girls and women, with special emphasis on basic education as a fundamental human right and as a foundation for all forms of development, including economic development, poverty alleviation, and addressing population issues. Governments of Islamic countries and NGO representatives have participated in other conferences on women, including the Fourth World Conference on Women, held in Beijing, China in 1995, and the follow-on conferences. The Beijing Platform for Action obligates all participating countries and donors to take action to implement the strategic objective on girls' and women's education following the strategies and target dates specified in the Platform.

Since the 1970s, international donor agencies have been helping aid-assisted Muslim countries in implementing the international conventions on women's and girls' education. The main contributors to women's education have been the World Bank, United States Agency for International Development (USAID), The Japanese International Development Agency (JICA), the Canadian International Development Agency (CIDA), and the specialized agencies of the United Nations, notably UNESCO, UNICEF and UNDP. These organizations have supported national government and NGO efforts to expand educational opportunities for girls and women in order to achieve the objectives of the international conventions, particularly on Education for All, and the Beijing Declaration and Platform for Action.

Major challenges remain. I have noted the persisting illiteracy and rising numbers of illiterates in several countries, most of which have yet to achieve sustained economic development. The skyrocketing numbers of girls and women graduating from schools and universities have not led to a similar increase in the numbers of employed women. There is a missing link between education and employment, and the numbers of unemployed educated women and men continues to rise. Girls' and women's education has had many tangible and non-tangible benefits for women, their families and communities. Yet the challenges are daunting. Populations continue to rise while resources shrink. Furthermore, structural adjustment measures undertaken in several countries have created new challenges, especially for the poor. There is evidence that poverty levels are rising and there may be some setbacks for girls' education as governments cut social service programmes. The demand for girls' and women's education far exceeds most countries' ability to respond. Gender role stereotypes and divisions are difficult to break, especially under strained economic circumstances. Nobody can tell when education for all will be a reality in all these countries. The poor and disenfranchised, especially girls and women, will continue to be marginalised, unless they get the education and skills they need to become productive members of society. Concerted and collaborative efforts are needed on many fronts if all women and men are to reap the benefits of technological changes in the twenty-first century.

NOTES

1. Computer technology has enabled some Islamic scholars to calculate the occurrence of the word 'knowledge' and its derivatives in the Quran, 860 times.

2. Ahmed Shalabi, *History of Muslim Education*, 2nd edition, Karachi, Pakistan: Indus Publications, 1979.

3. *Madrasah* is the Arabic word for school. Its meaning has been corrupted lately; it has come to refer to the type of *madrasahs* that teach extremist Islam as in Pakistan and Afghanistan.

4. Mehdi Nakosteen, *History of Islamic Origins of Western Education*, Boulder, Colorado: University of Colorado Press, 1964.

5. Joseph, S. Zyliowicks, *Education and Modernization in the Middle East*, Ithaca, NY: Cornell University Press, 1973, p. 142.

6. Justin McCarthy, *The Arab World, Turkey and the Balkans, (1878-1914): A Handbook of Historical Statistics*, Boston: G.K. Hall, 1982, p. 116.

7. Heyworth-Dunn, *An Introduction to the History of Education in Modern Egypt*, London: Frank Cass and Co. Ltd., 1968.

8. Nagat El-Sanabary, 'A Comparative Study of the Disparities of Girls' Education in the Arab Countries,' Unpublished Ph.D. dissertation, University of California, Berkeley, 1973.

9. 'Education of Muslim Women,' in the *International Encyclopedia of Education*, 2nd edition, edited by Torsten Husen and T. Neville Postlethwaite, 1994.

10. El-Sanabary, op. cit.

11. El-Sanabry, op. cit., p. 137.

12. Lawrence H. Summers, *Investing in All the People: educating women in developing countries*, Washington, DC: World Bank, 1994.

13. Nagat El-Sanabary, 'Determinants of Women's Education in the Middle East and North Africa,' World Bank working paper, 1989.

14. Egypt extended the compulsory cycle to include the three-year intermediate cycle in 1989 and Turkey did so in 1990.

15. Nagat El-Sanabary, 'The Saudi Model of Female Education and Reproduction of Gender Divisions', *Gender and Education*, June 1994.

16. El-Sanabary, *Determinants of Women's Education*, 1989, ibid., p. 40.

17. Includes Iran, but does not include the Islamic countries of South and South East Asia.

18. World Bank, *Education in the Middle East and North Africa: A Strategy Towards Learning for Development*, Washington, DC: The World Bank, World Development, 1999, p. 10.

19. According to USAID data and official government sources.

20. World Bank, *Bangladesh: Strategies for Enhancing the Role of Women in Economic Development*, Washington, DC: World Bank Population and Human Resources Dept., 1990, p. 56.

21. Kamel Bahaa El Din Hussein, *Education and the Future*, Cairo, Egypt: Ministry of Education, 1998, p. 30.

22. Andrea Rugh and Heather Bossert, *Involving Communities: Participation in the Delivery of Education Programmes*, Washington, DC: Creative Associates International, Inc. for USAID, 1998.

23. Most countries have three types of secondary schools: the academic college preparatory, vocational education, and teacher training. A few provided nursing education at the secondary level, but this is being phased out in favour of post secondary nurses training. Some countries have phased out secondary teacher training also in order to raise the standard of primary school teachers.

24. El-Sanabary, 1994, op. cit.

25. Statistical Yearbook of Turkey 1983.

26. Ministry of National Education, 'Toward the year 2000: 1991 National Education Report to Parliament', Turkey, December 1990, pp. 46-47.

27. Findings from personal field research in Egypt in 1998-99.

28. World Bank, op. cit., Bangladesh, p. 56.

29. World Bank, *Education and the Future*, Washington, DC: World Bank, 1989, pp. 44-45.

30. Nagat El-Sanabary, 'The Education and Contribution of Women Health Care Professionals in Saudi Arabia. The Case of Nursing', *Social Science and Medicine*, Vol. 37, No. 11, pp. 1331-1343, 1993.

31. Edith A.S. Hanania, *Arab Women and Education*, Beirut, Lebanon: Institute of Women's Study in the Arab World, 1980, p. 25.

32. Ibid., pp. 24-26.

33. Egypt has thirteen public universities, the American University in Cairo and eight new private universities.

34. Kamal Samy Selim, *Children and Women in Egypt, an Information Atlas*, Arab Republic of Egypt: National Council for Childhood and Motherhood, 1996, p. 58.

35. El-Sanabary, 1993, op. cit.

36. Ibid.

37. Jordanian National Committee, Second Report on Implementation of the Convention on Elimiation of All Forms of Discrimination Against Women (CEDAW), Amman, Jodan, 1998, p. 25 (in Arabic).

38. The National Agency for Public Mobilization and Statistics, Illiteracy in Egypt: Future Outlook, 1992, cited in Kamal Samy Selim, *Children and Women in Egypt: An Information Atlas*, National Council for Childhood and Motherhood, 1996, p. 25.

39. El-Sanabary, 1993, op. cit.

5

Remuneration of Nurses in Islamic Countries: An Economic Factor in a Social Context

Hedva Sarfati

INTRODUCTION

This chapter starts with an overview of issues facing the health sector in countries in the Eastern Mediterranean and North Africa (MENA), and where information is available on a number of other Islamic countries. Given the extreme scarcity of statistical data, both currently and in terms of changes over time, the chapter provides the following sequence of considerations:

- It first tries to provide a global picture of the environment in which health operates, noting the relative importance of social or health expenditures, and providing some general health and income indicators.
- It next illustrates the relative shortage of physicians and nurses: indicating, where available, total labour participation rates, with participation rates of women in the labour force, particularly in the health or services sector.
- It then highlights the occupations in which women are concentrated, particularly nursing and teaching, which in turn provide the background for the existing remuneration patterns.

These patterns reflect the low status of women in society, their low status in the health professions and the relatively low pay prevalent for these occupations.

Lastly, an examination of employment data identifies a severe nursing shortage. The chapter concludes by recommending the means to upgrade the status of nursing personnel, putting into focus the provisions of the two unique international standards relative to nursing personnel of the International Labour Organization, which encompass all aspects of health policy planning, training, certification, career paths, working conditions, remuneration, job classification and participation in decision-making.

THE CONTEXT: SOCIAL INVESTMENT AND HEALTH INDICATORS

The general trends in the health sector during the past three decades can be summarized hereafter. A rapid growth rate of the health professions took place in most countries in the world. This rate exceeded the growth rate of the population in many countries while at the same time the resources devoted to health care grew faster than the GNP, especially in the industrialized countries. The medical sector is an important employer the world over, and with the current demographic trends—high birth rates in developing countries and the ageing of the population particularly in industrialized ones, but also in developing countries, notably China and India—demands for health care will remain high, and health care services will continue to expand, creating more employment opportunities in this sector.

At the same time, many governments are struggling with public deficits and debt, and the resulting pressures on health expenditures will force major changes in health care delivery. These changes will also have a substantial impact on the status and working conditions of health care personnel, notably nurses.

In low income countries, the shortage of funds and of trained personnel makes it very difficult to meet the tremendous unmet need for basic health services and infrastructure. Public health expenditure in these countries is low by any standard, amounting on average to 1.4 per cent of GNP in 1990.[1] The UNDP estimated that in 1990-95 an average of 20 per cent of the population in developing countries had no access to health services: the figures were 13 per cent for Middle East States, 22 per cent for South Asia and 42 per cent for South Asia excluding India.[2]

The shortage of trained personnel in the least developed countries is illustrated by the high ratio of population per physician and per nurse estimated by the UNDP for 1988-91 as 19,035, and 13,842 respectively.[3] The situation varies widely among the countries under consideration in this chapter, as will be seen in the tables which give a detailed breakdown by country.

With increasing demands for health care, together with the pressure to limit public deficits, governments face a double challenge of maximizing the impact of existing human resources while at the same time striving to increase these resources by developing training capacity and attracting and retaining qualified personnel, notably women. However, traditional social norms and roles in developing countries, including Islamic countries, may limit the access of women to the health professions, including nursing. Unfortunately, there is very little data available on the employment of women in general and in the health sector in particular for the countries concerned. This chapter will examine some of the available data.

Many governments are reviewing their health policies in the context of their development strategies in the quest for more cost-effective and accessible health care. In this context, the role of preventive, promotive and primary health care—in which nurses can play a vital role—has become evident. Indeed, nurses and midwives constitute about 50 per cent of the world's health care workforce according to the World Health Organization (WHO). The 1996 World Health Assembly of WHO, therefore, passed a resolution aimed at strengthening nursing and midwifery to ensure the best use of nursing staff resources. The resolution calls on Member States to involve nurses and midwives more closely in health care reform, in the development of national health policies, and in formulation and implementation of health plans. They should be involved as well in selecting candidates for fellowships in nursing and health-related fields, in strengthening education and practice in primary health care for these personnel, and in monitoring and evaluating progress towards attainment of national health targets, in particular the effective use of nurses and midwives in the priority areas of equitable access to health services, health protection, promotion and prevention.[4]

A number of governments responding to a 1997 WHO questionnaire[5] indicated their awareness of the important role that nurses and midwives play in the delivery of services, the increasing demands on health services, the shortages of personnel and the frequent inadequate or inappropriate deployment of personnel. A number of countries reported on poor salaries and limited career opportunities which coincided with shortages of nursing and midwifery personnel. While the WHO survey highlights government efforts to remedy this situation by improving salaries and career opportunities as well as increasing the number of budgeted posts for nurses and midwives, several countries stated that due to financial difficulties nurses were sometimes not paid at all for several months.

With the dearth of data and the diversity of situations among and within countries in the Middle East, North Africa and South Asia, it is difficult to draw clear patterns of the health care services. To get a general idea of the major trends affecting the health sector in these countries, selected economic, social and health indicators are reproduced below from UNDP, WHO and World Bank sources.

Table 1 indicates the development of public expenditures as a share of GDP, the relative share of social security and welfare, health and education in central government expenditure, and the ratio of population per doctor and nurse. The figures vary greatly from country to country, depending on income levels, social security coverage and the priority which the health sector retains in government policy. Indeed, while the public expenditure for health as a percentage of GDP has grown significantly between 1960 and 1990 in most of the countries listed, it is still low. It exceeds 3 per cent of GDP only in three countries, namely, Algeria, Tunisia and Saudi Arabia, and varies between 1.0 and 1.8 per cent in seven other countries, as compared with the average of 2.1 per cent for all developing countries and 1.8 per cent for the least developed countries. In contrast, public expenditures for health average 9.7 per cent of GDP for the industrialized OECD countries.

The main challenge to public authorities is, therefore, how to optimize the impact of existing resources—human, material and financial. This involves a re-evaluation of health care systems, assessing the possible role of the private sector, and examining existing inefficiencies in resource allocation, particularly in view of the need to ensure broad access of the population to health care while monitoring costs.

The relevant global indicators affecting health sector policy making in the MENA region and South Asia are clear: demographic trends, income and health indicators, access to health services, trends in public and private health expenditures, distribution of physicians and nurses,

Table 1

Social investment and health profile

Country	Public expenditure on health as % of		Percentage of central government expenditure on						Population per doctor 1988-91	Population per nurse 1988-91
			Social security + welfare		Health		Education			
	GNP 1960	GDP 1990	1980	1992-95	1980	1992-95	1980	1992-95		
Algeria	1.2	5.4	–	–	–	–	–	–	1,064	–
Bahrain	–	–	2.3	4.5	7.6	8.6	9.7	12.0	775	–
Bangladesh	–	1.4	1.7	–	5.7	–	8.8	12.3	12,500	20,000
Egypt	0.6	1.0	12.1	11.0	2.2	2.4	8.6	–	–	–
India	0.5	1.3	–	–	2.0	1.8	1.9	1.9	2,439	3,333
Iran, Islamic Rep. of	0.8	1.5	9.0	10.3	5.4	8.9	15.9	15.9	–	–
Iraq	1.0	–	–	–	–	–	–	–	1,667	1,370
Jordan	0.6	1.8	13.7	15.3	3.8	7.1	7.6	16.3	649	641
Kuwait	–	–	–	16.6	4.9	5.7	9.0	10.9	–	–
Morocco	1.0	0.9	4.6	5.9	3.0	3.0	16.6	17.9	–	–
Pakistan	0.3	1.8	3.4	–	1.6	–	3.1	–	2,000	3,448
Saudi Arabia	0.6	3.1	–	–	–	–	–	–	704	310
Syrian Arab Rep.	0.4	0.4	8.2	2.3	1.1	2.3	7.1	9.8	1,220	1,031
Tunisia	1.6	3.3	8.3	14.3	7.7	6.6	15.3	17.5	1,852	407
United Arab Emirates	–	–	2.5	3.4	6.2	7.3	7.6	17.1	1,042	568
Yemen	–	1.5	–	0.0	3.6	4.7	14.8	20.7	4,348	1,818

Source: UNDP: *Human Development Report 1997*, excerpts from Table 13 'Health profile', pp. 176-177 and Table 18 'Social investment', pp. 186-187.

and gender gaps in education. The tables established by the World Bank, which focus on MENA, confirm the great diversity already noted among the countries in the two regions.

The World Bank data in Tables 2 and 3 provide some insight into the actual per capita health expenditure in dollars and its share in GDP. The breakdown between public and private expenditure provides a useful supplement to the UNDP figures in Table 1.

Tables 4 and 5 illustrate the uneven economic development in the MENA region and the substantially different rates of progress made in the past twenty-five years in reducing infant mortality and improving life expectancy at birth. Almost all the MENA countries have managed to significantly reduce infant mortality during this period, averaging 54 deaths per 1,000 live births, as compared with a rate of 40 per 1000 in East Asia and the Pacific region (Tables 4 and 5). The lower mortality rates, as could be expected, are positively correlated with growth of income per capita, with the six high-income oil exporting Gulf States achieving low infant mortality rates of between 14 and 21 per 1,000 live births.

While most governments of WHO member States have endorsed the organization's objective of Health for All by the year 2000, there is still a significant imbalance in access to health services. This has already been indicated in the UNDP statistics on population per physician and nurse, in Table 1 and by the World Bank 1997 estimates of health expenditures in Tables 2 and 3.

THE HUMAN RESOURCES DIMENSION: LABOUR FORCE PARTICIPATION AND EMPLOYMENT IN THE HEALTH SECTOR

While acknowledging the lack of data regarding the quality of personnel, particularly nurses and paramedical service providers, the World Bank states there is sufficient evidence to suggest that many countries face severe shortages of qualified nurses. Indeed, there is an average of 2.4 nurses and paramedics per 1000 population in the MENA region, as compared to 3.7 in middle income countries and 6.7 in high income countries.[6]

The World Bank 1993 Health Report indicates that public health and minimum essential clinical interventions require about 0.1 physician per 1000 population and between two and four graduate nurses per physician. It notes that given the resource constraints, the

Table 2

Global trends in health expenditure: Regional comparisons, 1994

Region/Income Group	Per capita health expenditure (1994 dollars)	Health expenditure as % of GDP			Public share of health expenditure (% Total)
		Total	Public	Private	
Low & Middle Income Countries	55	5.5	2.8	2.9	49
South Asia	16	5.0	1.2	3.8	24
Sub-Saharan Africa	42	5.6	2.8	3.6	44
East Asia & Pacific	21	3.5	1.5	2.0	43
Middle East & North Africa	54	4.8	2.6	2.2	54
E. Europe & Central Asia	120	5.5	4.5	1.0	81
Latin America & Caribbean	234	7.2	3.0	4.2	41
Low Income Countries	16	4.1	1.5	2.7	37
Middle Income Countries	138	5.9	3.2	3.0	51
High Income Countries	2,329	9.9	6.1	3.9	61

Source: World Bank estimates, 1997.

Table 3

Middle East and North Africa – Health expenditure patterns, 1990-95/[a]

Country	Per capita health expenditure (in exchange rate dollars)	Health expenditure as % of GDP			Public share of health expenditure (% Total)
		Total	Public	Private	
Yemen, Republic	6	2.6	1.1	1.5	42
Egypt, Arab Republic/[b]	38	3.7	1.6	2.1	43
Morocco	40	3.4	1.6	1.7	47
Iran, Islamic Republic	56	4.8	2.8	2.0	58
Jordan	118	7.9	3.7	4.2	47
Algeria	73	4.6	3.3	1.3	73
Tunisia	105	5.9	3.0	2.9	51
Lebanon	124	5.3	2.1	3.3	40
Oman	–	–	2.5	–	–
Saudi Arabia	–	–	3.1	–	–
Bahrain	497	5.7	–	–	–
Qatar	319	2.8	–	–	–
Kuwait	–	–	3.6	–	–
United Arab Emirates	338	2.2	1.9	0.3	86

Source: World Bank estimates, 1997.

Notes: a. Figures in this table are taken from the latest available data between 1990-1995. b. Data for Decision Making Project, 'Egypt National Health Accounts 1994/95', Ministry of Health and Population, Arab Republic of Egypt, 1997.

Table 4

Global income and health indicators[a]

	Per Capita GNP, 1995	Growth in Real GDP Per Capita[b] 1996-2005 (forecast)	Infant Mortality Rate, 1995 per 1000 live births	Life Expectancy at Birth, 1995 Male	Life Expectancy at Birth, 1995 Female
Low & Middle Income Countries	1,100	3.7%	60	63	66
South Asia	350	3.7%	75	61	62
Sub-Saharan Africa	510	0.9%	92	50	53
East Asia & Pacific	800	6.8%	40	66	70
Middle East & North Africa	1,740	0.4%	54	65	68
Eastern Europe & Central Asia	2,130	3.7%	26	64	73
Latin America & Caribbean	3,310	2.2%	37	66	72
Low Income Countries[c]	440	–	69	62	64
Middle Income Countries[c]	2,450		39	65	71
High Income Countries[c]	24,790	2.4%	7	74	81

Notes: a. All regional averages and income group averages cited in this paper are weighted averages. b. World Bank, *Global Economic Prospects and the Developing Countries*, Washington, D.C., 1996. c. Income groups used in this paper are based on 1995 GNP per capita: low income, $756 or less; middle income, $766 to $9,385; and high income, $9,386 or more.

Table 5

Middle East and North Africa: Income and Health Indicators

Country/Region	Per Capita GNP 1995	Infant Mortality Rate[a] 1970	Infant Mortality Rate[a] 1995	Life Expectancy Birth 1995 Male	Life Expectancy Birth 1995 Female
Yemen, Republic	260	188	101	53	54
Egypt, Arab Republic	970	160	57	64	66
Morocco	1,110	130	56	64	67
Syrian Arab Republic	1,120	98	33	66	70
Iran, Islamic Republic	1,446	134	46	68	69
Jordan	1,510	–	31	68	72
Algeria	1,600	141	34	68	71
Palestinian Administration	1,710[b]	–	–	–	–
Gaza Strip	–	–	31	–	–
West Bank	–	–	27	–	–
Tunisia	1,820	124	40	68	70
Lebanon	2,660	50	32	67	71
Oman	4,820	129	18	68	73
Saudi Arabia	6,810	123	21	69	71
Bahrain	7,840	67	19	70	75
Qatar	11,600	71	19	69	75
Kuwait	17,390	54	14	74	79
United Arab Emirates	17,400	87	16	73	76
Iraq	n/a	104	111	59	62
Libya	n/a	124	62	63	66
MENA Regional Average:	1,740	137	54	52	65

Source: World Bank staff estimates, 1997 in 'Health, Nutrition and Population in Middle East and North Africa Region', Nov. 1997.

Notes: a. Rate per 1,000 live births. b. World Bank estimate for 1996.

relatively high ratio of nurses to physicians, for instance in Sub-Saharan Africa, is a positive sign. It acknowledges that 'there is no optimal level of physician per capita or optimal nurse-to-physician ratio, but a rule of thumb is that nurses should exceed physicians by at least two to one.' It further notes that 'the ratio is five to one in Africa, but well under two to one in China, India, Latin America, and the Middle Eastern crescent.'[7]

Table 6 provides a different perspective of the acute staff shortages, indicating the number of physicians, nurses and midwives per 10,000 population based on country statistical profiles published by the WHO Regional Office for the Eastern Mediterranean (EMRO). This usefully complements Table 1. Table 6 confirms the great variation among countries in ratios of nurses per physician. The ratios range from

Table 6

Physicians, nursing and midwifery personnel per 10,000 population

	Physicians		Nurses/ midwifery personnel	
	Rate	Year	Rate	Year
Afghanistan	0.3	96	0.7	96
Bahrain	10.8	95	25.6	95
Egypt	20.2	96	23.3	96
Iran, Islamic Republic	8.2	96	25.9	96
Iraq	5.0	95	23.6	95
Jordan	15.9	95	28.5	95
Kuwait	18.7	95	50.0	95
Lebanon	28.0	96	6.5	96
Libyan Arab Jamahiriya	13.7	93	36.6	93
Morocco	3.8	95	9.5	95
Oman	12.8	96	31.3	96
Pakistan	5.3	96	3.4	96
Qatar	11.2	95	28.6	95
Saudi Arabia	17.0	95	34.0	95
Syrian Arab Republic	10.8	95	20.6	95
Tunisia	7.0	96	29.9	96
United Arab Emirates	16.8	94	32.0	94
Yemen, Rep. of	2.0	95	5.1	95

Source: EMRO: Annual Report of the Regional Director, 1996, Country Profiles, Table 4 'Human and Material Resources Indicators', p. 141.

about 2 to 2.6 nurses per physician in Afghanistan, Bahrain, Kuwait, Libya, Morocco, Oman, Qatar, Saudi Arabia and Yemen to a significantly higher ratio in Iran (3.15), Iraq (4.72) and Tunisia (4.27). There are fewer than two nurses per physician in Egypt (1.5), Jordan (1.79), Syria and United Arab Emirates (both with 1.9). A somewhat unusual situation exists in Lebanon and Pakistan with fewer than one nurse per physician (0.23 and 0.64 respectively).

The World Bank also points out that non-physician primary care providers, for example nurses, nurse practitioners and midwives, provide many advantages to a country. They cost less to train and therefore receive lower salaries, they are more easily attracted to rural areas, and they usually communicate more effectively with their patients. Moreover, in some countries tasks traditionally performed by physicians have been successfully transferred to lower-level primary care providers in order to improve efficiency of health services. Many countries have experimented over the past twenty years with the use of community health workers to provide primary health care as a form of low cost health services. These services include education on sanitation, nutrition, family planning, child health and immunizations, as well as basic health interventions and referrals between communities, health centres and hospitals. Community health workers are central to the successful Aga Khan Health Services in Pakistan, which provides primary health care programmes to remote mountain areas. Mobile teams of physicians and nurses back up these health workers. They collect epidemiological data, provide sanitary education and simple treatment and referrals.[8]

Health care providers in many countries tend to be concentrated in urban areas, and it is difficult to attract primary care providers to rural areas because of professional isolation, lack of additional work opportunities, substandard housing and lack of other amenities. The World Bank points out that culture and tradition prevent Muslim women from participating more actively in health care provision, creating an obstacle to the utilization of health services. It cites the case of Egypt where most physicians are male, and cultural factors constrain women from being seen by men who are not family members. Even when female primary care providers are trained, it is difficult to attract them to under-served areas because of security concerns and the importance to them of staying with their families. In several countries, such as Pakistan, this problem has been addressed by training women to work in their own communities as lady health visitors and lady health workers.[9]

Regarding the actual number of persons employed as nurses or midwives, the existing information is piecemeal, and comparisons are rendered difficult by different definitions, or lack thereof, of categories of nursing personnel (professional nurse, registered nurse, qualified nurse, midwife, assistant nurse, auxiliary nurse, nursing attendant, etc.) and the different educational and practice requirements to qualify for these categories.

The International Labour Office, in its 1992 survey on equality of opportunity in health services,[10] notes that, globally, almost all countries in all regions have experienced growth in the nursing labour force. This overall trend needs to be qualified. First, in a number of developing countries, emigration of health personnel has generated acute shortages, particularly among nursing personnel and physicians. Egypt, India, Pakistan, the Philippines and Sri Lanka thus suffer from a serious drain of manpower to high-income oil-exporting countries, to Europe and to the United States. In Pakistan, only 50 per cent of all trained nurses are registered as practicing in the country, while in the Philippines 62 per cent work abroad. This situation is aggravated by the limited ability of some of the countries to absorb trained health workers in their national health systems. On the other hand, in many countries budgeted positions and posts for nurses and midwives cannot be filled because of financial constraints.

The employment of women in the health sector must be seen within the framework of an overall increase in female labour force participation during the past three decades. All through history women have been largely concentrated in the health sector, in which they constitute the majority of the workforce in most countries. Women's share in the health sector is usually higher than their share in the workforce as a whole. For example, in the Netherlands, Norway, Poland and Sweden, women account for over 80 per cent of the health workforce, while in the Philippines, Turkey and the United Kingdom they constitute between 70 and 79 per cent of the health workforce.

Table 7 provides some comparative data on labour force participation, including the development of women's share in the labour force between 1970 and 1990, and the growth of the total labour force employed in the services sector between 1960 and 1990. In many of the countries, labour force as a percentage of the total population, considering rates in 1990, are rather low. They range

Table 7
Employment indicators in the Middle Eastern crescent and selected South Asian countries

Labour force participation rate, women's share in the labour force and the share of services

	Labour force as a % of total population	Women's share of labour force (age 15 & above) %	Women's share of labour force (age 15 & above) %	% of labour force in services	% of labour force in services
	1990	1970	1990	1960	1990
Bahrain	44	5	17	42	68
United Arab Emirates	51	4	12	42	65
Kuwait	42	8	23	64	74
Qatar	57	4	11	59	65
Malaysia	39	31	36	25	50
Libyan Arab Jamahiriya	29	16	18	26	66
Lebanon	31	19	27	39	62
Iran, Islamic Rep.	29	19	21	21	43
Saudi Arabia	34	5	10	19	61
Turkey	44	38	33	11	19
Syrian Arab Rep.	28	23	25	23	43
Tunisia	35	24	29	23	39
Algeria	28	20	21	19	43
Jordan	27	13	18	26	61
Oman	26	6	12	20	32
Philippines	40	33	37	22	39
Indonesia	44	30	39	18	31
Egypt	35	–	–	–	–
Morocco	38	31	35	17	31
Yemen	30	27	30	11	22
Bangladesh	49	40	42	7	18
Pakistan	35	22	24	19	30
India	43	34	31	14	20
Iraq	26	16	16	25	66
All Developing countries	47	37	39	14	23
Industrial countries	49	40	44	38	57

Source: UNDP, op. cit., Table 16 'Employment', pp. 182-183, collated from ILO data 1996.

between 26 and 31 per cent in nine countries (Iran, Iraq, Jordan, Algeria, Libya, Lebanon, Syria, Oman and Yemen), somewhat higher in thirteen other countries, ranging between 34 and 44 per cent (in increasing order: Saudi Arabia, Egypt, Tunisia, Pakistan, Morocco, Malaysia, Philippines, India, Indonesia, Kuwait, Bahrain, Bangladesh and Turkey). In two countries, rates are higher than the average in industrial countries, with 51 and 57 per cent for the United Arab Emirates ar.d Qatar respectively. Women's share of the total labour market in most of these countries is low, except in four countries where it is close to or surpasses the average of developing countries ranging between 36 and 42 per cent (Malaysia, Philippines, Indonesia and Bangladesh). In most of the countries there has been an increase, sometimes substantial, in women's share in the labour force over the three decades, with two exceptions, where their share declined (from 34 to 31 per cent in India and from 38 to 33 per cent in Turkey).

Richard Anker, who conducted an ILO study in 1998 on gender and jobs, found that the female share of non-agricultural employment is small in the MENA region, averaging 14.8 per cent. It ranges from about 20 per cent in Tunisia and Kuwait, 16.9 per cent in Bahrain, 13.6 per cent in Egypt, and 10.5 per cent in Iran, to 8.1 per cent in Jordan. Generally, women in this region have not entered the labour market in large numbers, although their share of employment has increased over the past few decades. In Bahrain, women accounted for 9.9 per cent of non agricultural labour in 1971 and their share rose to 16.9 per cent in 1991. In Egypt, their share rose only slightly from 9.7 per cent in 1976 to 13.6 per cent in 1986. In India, female share of non-agricultural employment was 12 per cent in 1980, as compared to 28.2 per cent in Malaysia in 1981.

Anker attributes the gender occupational segregation and the low female labour force participation to the societal norms and perceptions associated with Islam and tradition, which limit occupational choices of women and their socially acceptable role in most countries in the region. He points out, however, that the status of women varies greatly across the Islamic countries, and that in some of the countries women are more integrated in professional and educational life. As integration in the labour market also depends on educational attainment, Anker indicates that educational levels are generally lower for women than for men in this region and in a number of South Asian countries. For example, in India, the average schooling is 3.5 years for men and 1.2

years for women. But in Malaysia, there is very little difference between the length of schooling for men and women.[11]

Data provided by Anker on occupational structure and percentage of women by occupational group shows that in various MENA and Asian countries, women outnumber men in service occupations, namely in Bahrain (29.4 vs. 26.7 per cent for men), Jordan (13.4 vs. 7.5 per cent), Kuwait (38 vs. 29.1 per cent), Tunisia (21.45 vs. 11.1 per cent), India (17.9 vs. 10 per cent), and Malaysia (32.1 vs. 14.8 per cent). In Iran, by contrast, the percentage is slightly lower (7.0 vs. 7.2 per cent) and much lower in Egypt (6.0 vs. 11.9 per cent).[12]

The information in Table 8 on the percentage of female workers in four occupations—nurses, teachers (at all levels), stenographers/typists, and bookkeepers/cashiers and related workers—has been extracted from the data presented by Anker on seventeen occupations representing those reputed in Western industrialized countries as being typically 'male' or 'female' occupations. Anker notes that women tend to be over-represented in the professional and technical occupational group when compared with their overall share in the non-agricultural labour force, particularly in the MENA countries.

The nursing profession appears to be a genuinely 'female' occupation world-wide, as about 82 per cent of nurses are women in all twenty-one countries for which data was available. This is consistent with the universal perception of women as better care providers than men. However, male nurses are quite common in non-Asian developing countries. They constitute approximately half of the nursing profession in Senegal and Tunisia and about a third in Bahrain and Mauritius. In 1997, Egypt reported 5.4 per cent of nursing personnel as male, with a decline in female nurses of 6.5 per cent from 1986.[13] On the other hand, Anker underlines the fact that the career choice of women as nurses and men as physicians explains much of the earning gap among medical workers. The higher prestige of physicians also reflects male/female power relationships in society at large.

While teaching has a fairly equal mix of male and female teachers in the twenty-one countries studied, teaching in MENA is a female occupation in all six countries of the sample. He attributes this partly to the existence of separate schools for boys and girls, a common pattern. While stenographers and typists are female-concentrated occupations in virtually all countries surveyed, in six of the countries where this is not the case, (Bahrain, Egypt, Jordan, Kuwait, Tunisia and India), the overall female non-agricultural labour force

Table 8

Percentage of women in comparable occupational groups

	Bahrain 1991	Egypt 1986	Iran Isl. Rep. 1986	Jordan 1979	Kuwait 1985	Tunisia 1989	India 1981	Malaysia 1980
Nurses	64.1	68	n.a.	n.a.	97.9	43.7*	93.1	n.a.
Teachers (all levels)	45.4	39.9	44.7	50.1	56.6	30.4	28.2	45.7
Stenographers/ Typists	74.5**	65.5	n.a.	76.0	58.0	54.5	27.9	90.9
Bookkeepers/ cashiers	25.0***	35.7	n.a.	9.9	13.1	20.6	6.8	49.4

n.a. not available

* includes midwives; ** Stenographers not included; *** cashiers only.

Source: Richard Anker: *Gender and Jobs - Sex segregation of occupations in the world*, Geneva, ILO, 1998, Table 11.1, pp. 254-257.

participation rates are low. Finally, while bookkeepers and cashiers are female-concentrated occupations in the majority of OECD and Asian countries surveyed, this is the case in only three of the twelve MENA and developing countries. This is probably linked to the fact that these jobs are not socially acceptable for women because the work involves public contact with men.[14]

Information in this section clearly illustrates the relative importance of the health sector as an opportunity for women in Islamic countries to enter the labour market. It is now necessary to look at the constraints on such entry which are linked to the low status of women, the low status of the profession, and the relatively low income earned in the nursing profession.

STATUS, ROLE AND REMUNERATION

The growing demands on health care services noted the world over necessitate an increase in health expenditure in which services provided, as well as pay of health care personnel, cannot be separated from macroeconomic budget considerations. Also, the ambitious targets of governments in developing countries to provide broad access to health services require careful examination of the types of services delivered and by whom. In this context, a major emphasis has been made by many governments, in their quest to rationalize public expenditures and to optimize health care delivery, on the provision of community-based primary health care, which emphasizes preventive and promotive along with curative care. The reform process in health care, which implies a shift from hospital-centred curative care to community-based care, is slow and encounters many difficulties— organizational, institutional, and operational. Nurses can play a major role in this reform if properly trained and motivated. This has been acknowledged and promoted by both WHO and the World Bank.

Changing the role of nurses raises a number of issues, such as availability of adequate nursing resources, quality of their training, and the system by which work is distributed between nurses and physicians. These factors vary tremendously among countries. Other issues to consider are entry into the nursing profession as well as retention and turnover, and consequently the status of the profession in society, rewards in terms of career development, job satisfaction, satisfactory working conditions, recognition at work, degree of autonomy and pay.

Remuneration of Nurses

The level of remuneration, especially in relation to earnings in other sectors, is a good indication of the value that society places on its health services, and an important factor in its ability to attract and retain competent staff. As pointed out in the ILO 1992 report on health services,[15] remuneration and salary structure has been a major issue in many industrialized countries, particularly within the public service.

Some significant changes have been introduced to retain staff and allow for greater flexibility, via merit increments, special bonuses or general overtime supplements, and cash and non-cash allowances. Cash allowances include social security provisions such as maternity benefits and a pension. Such allowances are often tied to the cost of living, to family situations, to hardship related to living in remote areas, or to working in difficult or dangerous conditions. Non-cash benefits may include housing, the use of a car and recreational facilities. Bonuses and allowances can constitute a major part of take-home pay. Non-cash benefits also represent a hidden cost which governments do not always take into account. If allowances constitute a high proportion of income, however, the employee can be affected upon retirement since social security benefits are usually linked to basic salary. As noted in an ILO 1995 report on the impact of structural adjustment and public service reform, a pay system in which allowances weigh too heavily can lose its consistency, and can be counter-productive by negatively affecting staff motivation and efficiency.[16]

Special allowances and non-pecuniary incentives were introduced in many countries to improve earnings and make the nursing profession more attractive. In some cases, local bargaining—at regional or hospital level—has replaced central collective bargaining to take account of local conditions and circumstances. While the basic principles governing wage determination are much the same in health services as in other sectors, health services may suffer more from current efforts to contain public expenditures. Where containment is required, it is often achieved by staff reduction, replacement of highly qualified by less qualified staff or an increase of the occupation rate of hospital beds. This has an obvious impact on levels of remuneration, workload, staff de-motivation and the quality of services.

On the whole, however, pay structures in the public health services are based on such criteria as qualifications, degree of responsibility, supervisory functions and seniority. To achieve equity within the public service, different occupations and professions are compared and clustered in the respective salary grades. Significant differences exist in the remuneration of various health occupations and within such occupations, as evidenced by the wage differentials between physicians and professional nurses, and between professional nurses and auxiliary nurses.

In Australia, for example, a medical intern earns more than twice as much as a nurse who, at the top echelon (director of nursing in a large hospital or regional school of nursing), would earn about one-third of a senior doctor's pay in a public hospital. In France, doctors earn about one-third more than nurses at entry level and up to 50 per cent more at a senior level, and the gap widens significantly when allowances are included. In Sweden, a doctor earns on average double the salary of a nurse.[17] Similar comparisons for several Islamic countries are given below.

Pay differentials related to qualifications and the importance of allowances in nurses' pay are complicated and can be illustrated by information provided by the Kuwait Nursing Association. Entry level salaries and allowances are determined by Category and Grade based on the type and level of educational programmes completed. Nurses at each grade receive a basic salary and can also receive a social allowance, an incentive allowance and a professional allowance. The Civil Service Commission has fixed special pay scales for nationals which are different from non-nationals. The highest entry pay level for a BSc nursing graduate of a university programme is three and one-half times that of a graduate of a three-year programme for students who have completed seventh grade.[18]

In Iran, a general pay scale is set for the public sector at Rls 300,000 per month (1US$ = 3,000 Rials).[19] The Act of Harmonizing Method of Payment provides that the basic elements determining pay levels of the three major health care occupations—physicians, midwives, and paramedics—depend on level of education, length of employment, type of job and duties. Under this act, nurses with a bachelor's degree are placed initially in grade 8. During the following six years they are promoted one grade at three-year intervals. Thereafter, promotion takes place at four-year intervals. The final accrued grade is 14 after 22 years of employment.

Beyond their basic salary, nurses in Iran receive: (i) an extra payment as a percentage of the salary; (ii) periodic bonuses for productivity, number of cases treated, specialization, research etc.; and (iii) payments in kind. A nurse recruited in 1998 at Grade 8 will have a basic salary of Rls. 145,000, a job allowance of Rls. 239,112, a housing allowance (if married) of Rls. 12,000 (Rls. 8,000 if single), a family allowance (only men are eligible) of Rls. 50,400, and children allowance (only payable to male nurses) of Rls. 10,080 for the first child and double or treble for two or three children. Therefore, the total pay is more than three times the basic salary. An annual increment of 22 per cent of the base salary is allocated upon approval of the Council of Ministers and the State Administrative and Employment Affairs. Nurses who have worked twenty years in the health centres and contributed for that period may benefit from early retirement. They receive a credit of five extra years of contribution and get full retirement pension, based on twenty-five years' contribution.

In a number of countries, current reforms of pay structures have brought into question some of the basic parameters underlying traditional public sector pay structures, which are increasingly viewed as being too rigid. Efforts have been undertaken to simplify pay and grading and to introduce more flexibility. Salaries for the same job or occupation are no longer necessarily standardized across departments or regions. Job content, professional experience or performance are increasingly being taken into account rather than grade and seniority.[20]

The 1994 ILO study edited by David Marsden on the remuneration of nurses points out that qualified nurses tend to be concentrated in hospitals, whereas nursing auxiliaries and other paramedics are more commonly found in nursing homes and in community or field health work, particularly in developing countries where nurses are scarce. Nurses still represent a big expenditure for the limited resources of these countries.[21]

In most countries where there is a dominant national employer in the health sector, the main source of supply for nursing personnel is new entrants, mainly young women school-leavers. To illustrate the magnitude of the effort needed nationally to attract enough persons to the profession, Marsden states that ensuring a ratio of one nurse or auxiliary per 100 inhabitants (the average in the five industrialized countries covered in the study) would require 5 per cent of the female work force of the country. Given the high turnover in the profession, he assumes that about 10 per cent of the new female entrants to the labour market per year would have to train as nurses or auxiliaries. This would involve a major training effort (usually three years for a qualified nurse and somewhat less for an auxiliary) and further training to meet the growing technical demands on nursing staff.[22] Obviously, the burden is different with a much higher ratio of population per nurse which, as indicated in Table 1, varies significantly among MENA and South Asian countries (310 in Saudi Arabia, 407 in Tunisia, 641 in Jordan, and between 1000 and 3000 in others, reaching 20,000 in Bangladesh).

Although there are few detailed studies on the sensitivity of relative pay to attract persons re-entering the nursing labour market, UK data suggests, according to Marsden, that National Health Service (NHS) employers have to compete with employers in other activities to attract re-entering nurses. Also, a number of nurses are leaving the NHS each year for other jobs. While pay is not the only motivator, data collected on school teachers suggest that starting salaries and mid-career salaries play a role in attracting and retaining staff. Besides recognition and autonomy, the possibility of combining professional and family responsibilities is also important. This element has contributed to the development of part-time work in the nursing profession in various countries.

Marsden emphasizes that international comparisons of pay levels for nursing personnel are extremely difficult since there is a great variation among, and even within, countries of the parameters that determine pay. The levels of qualifications required for nursing practice, the number of grades within the nursing profession, the distinction between qualified nurses and managerial/supervisory posts, the difference between a qualified nurse and an auxiliary nurse, and the borderline between nurses and other health occupations, are often blurred. Marsden, therefore, tried to give an appoximation of the relative pay of nurses as compared to physicians and other occupations. In Canada, the United States and the United Kingdom, qualified nurses' pay was higher than the average of female workers, and in the US it was above that of all full-time workers (male and female). In contrast, nursing aides (male and female) earned much less than the average of all workers (male and female). In the UK, qualified female nurses earned more than full-time adult white-collar women and much more than blue-collar women (+55%), but less than blue-collar men, and much less (-36%) than white-collar men. Marsden noted that, despite the strong demand for nurses and the prevailing shortages in many countries, nurses' pay remains generally low in several countries with the exception of the US.

These findings are confirmed by more recent data from the ILO's 1997 October Inquiry, which provides statistics on occupational wages and hours of work in selected countries and in occupations, including the health sector.[23] For the sake of comparison, data was included on pay and hours of work for book-keepers/accountants and stenographers/typists in banking; stenographers/typists in public administration; teachers (third level and second levels as well as kindergarten); auto mechanics; and health occupations, including physicians, dentists, professional nurses, auxiliary nurses and where available other health occupations and ambulance drivers. For countries of the MENA and South Asian region, comparative data was available for Bahrain, Bangladesh, Tunisia and Yemen.

In Bahrain, the pay of professional nurses—for which only male nurses data is given—is 38 per cent that of physicians and about 51 per cent that of dentists, but about 57 per cent of the pay of a bank accountant, and about 64 per cent that of teachers at all levels, including kindergarten. Male professional nurses earn more than both male stenographer/typists in the banking sector and male ambulance drivers (+37%), but only slightly more than female ambulance drivers (+13%) who earn more than their male colleagues.

In Bangladesh, both male and female professional nurses earn an average of 75 per cent of the pay of physicians and dentists, and 84 per cent of 3rd level teachers of mathematics and languages. They earn the same amount as accountants and 2nd level language and literature teachers as well as technical education teachers, but more than kindergarten teachers (+60%), stenographers/typists in the banking sector (+52.3%), X-ray technicians and auto mechanics (+31%).

In Tunisia, a professional nurses' pay represents 35.2 per cent of a physician's pay, 42.7 per cent of a dentist's, 78 per cent of a medical X-ray technician's, 52 per cent of a 3rd level teacher's and 61 per cent of a 2nd level teacher's. It is higher than the pay of public administration stenographers/typists (+29%), ambulance drivers and auto mechanics (+37%). But it is lower than the pay of kindergarten teachers (-6.5%).

In Yemen, the pay of professional nurses is 84.2 per cent that of physicians and dentists. The gap here is rather low but represents merely 40 per cent of a banking accountant's pay, 76 per cent of a second level technical education teacher's, and 80 per cent of banking stenographer/typist'. It surpasses the pay of kindergarten teachers and X-ray technicians (+14.3%) and ambulance drivers (+23%).

The survey also gives an indication of normal weekly working hours, which in Bahrain total thirty-six in all sectors. In Bangladesh, weekly hours are forty-five in banks and thirty-nine in insurance, public administration, education and health services. In Tunisia there is a great variation among sectors in normal working hours, with thirty-nine hours in public administration and eighteen for education services at all levels except kindergartens where it stands at twenty-five hours. In the health services it varies between thirty-six hours for physicians and dentists, thirty-nine for nursing personnel and laboratory technicians, and forty-eight for ambulance drivers. In Yemen, normal working hours in banks stand at forty-eight per week with forty-two hours in public administration and thirty-six in education services, but forty-eight hours in health services.

Clearly, therefore, something needs to be done in the area of pay policy. However, too low pay may not always be revealed by recruitment difficulties if the workers concerned are constrained in their choice of occupation or are crowded into a narrow segment of the labour market and thus have little alternative.

Pay Differentials and Occupational Segregation

In the countries under consideration the public sector is a major employer of the health care workforce. Despite national and regional variations, public services in most countries share common features related to remuneration: i.e. pay structure is usually centrally determined as are across-the-board pay increases. Pay scales are based on grade rather than on job content, occupational category or individual merit. Progress on the scale is usually related to seniority rather than individual performance. Salary scales generally cover health and medical personnel, which apply the principle of equal pay.

In practice, however, for a variety of reasons, differences of remuneration are important, with women workers earning less than their male colleagues in the same occupations. The reasons for these differences are numerous. One reason is that the pay packet or basic pay is only a part of public service remuneration. A broad range of benefits and allowances constitute a significant part of take-home pay. ILO studies of civil service pay found allowances make up 6.2 to 106 per cent of total salary in Africa,[24] and a generally higher ratio in South Asia, often exceeding 100 per cent.[25] Cash allowances and other benefits introduce a degree of flexibility in a generally rigid pay structure, and provide some leeway in negotiating pay, but they reduce the transparency that is expected in public service pay.

Other reasons for pay differentials among men and women in the health sector, indicated in the 1992 ILO health care report,[26] include the lower qualifications and less vocational training that women have as compared with men, and more limited opportunities for upgrading their skills or attending further training courses. In addition, men generally work longer hours and are more likely to work overtime with higher pay rates. Formal seniority systems reward employees who remain on the job for an uninterrupted full-time career, whereas women often interrupt their careers for child-rearing. They acquire less seniority at similar stages of their career, and hence have lower pay and less advancement opportunities. Career breaks also mean that women may lose certain skills associated with uninterrupted professional experience and may become out of touch with new working practices and technologies. Working part-time is also associated with similar negative impacts on a woman's career path.

These differences in skill upgrading and uninterrupted presence at work on a full-time basis also result in women being under-represented in higher managerial and supervisory positions. For example, male nurses in the United Kingdom earn on average 21 per cent more than female nurses, while among auxiliaries women earn only 54.94 per cent of male auxiliary earning. In Brazil, in 1980, 70 per cent of health professionals who earned less than three times the minimum salary were women. Only among qualified nurses did a small proportion of women earn higher salaries than men. Among the intermediate and lower qualified nursing personnel, men were better represented in the intermediate income groups, while the great majority of women (84.9%) in this category had incomes below three times the minimum salary. Among the exceptions, besides the case of the United States mentioned earlier, women paramedics and assistant nurses in Sweden who are employed by the county councils have higher average earnings than males.

Another important source of pay inequality in many countries and regions of the world is the persistent under-valuation of professions that are female-dominated. The caring functions are usually associated with nursing and often considered of secondary importance as compared to the diagnostic functions of physicians. Culturally, the nursing profession has its origin in charitable and voluntary service. These services are looked at as an extension of family and household care functions and hence associated with low status and low pay. This under-valuation has been maintained in spite of the increasing level of qualifications, skills and experience required for practising the profession and the increasing responsibilities that nurses can and do assume in many countries.

The increasing decentralization of management and authority in the health services has an important impact on pay determination and the introduction of different pay rates based on local recruitment and retention needs. This fragmentation makes pay comparability more difficult and hence also hinders the means to adhere to the principle of equal pay for work of equal value.

Nursing Personnel: Shortages and Status

The limited choice of alternative occupations for women seems to characterize the situation prevailing in South Asia, the Middle East and North Africa where female participation rates in the labour force are low. The nursing profession, as we have seen, is one of the areas, together with teaching, which is socially acceptable for women. So the competition with other activities may not be relevant. Other factors may, however, militate against attracting and retaining women in the profession, particularly the low social status of the profession, and the fact that social and cultural values discourage re-entry to the labour market after marriage and child-rearing. These attitudes may now be changing in some countries, with the rising awareness of the need to address nursing shortages. Several examples of countries can be provided.

In Egypt, the ILO 1994 study on remuneration of nurses notes that because of the tremendous shortage of nursing staff, a great number of nurses are actually working in more than one institution, even sometimes on a full-time basis. This is seen to cause a heavy personal strain on these nurses and is said to explain the high rate of attrition and turnover. The authors of the study note that among the problems that negatively affect the nursing profession in Egypt are:

(i)   the dependency of nurses on physicians for decision-making;
(ii)   a burden of work incommensurate with preparation;
(iii) low financial and moral remuneration (sic) as compared with the attributed responsibilities;
(iv)   unsatisfactory working conditions;
(v)   uncertain career structure and promotion opportunities; and
(vi)   poor community acceptance of nursing as a profession as compared with other professions.

The study includes a report presented to the Egyptian People's Assembly in 1989 regarding factors causing attrition among highly qualified nurses, particularly in government institutions. These include:

(i)   salary deductions for rent when nurses live in hospital premises;
(ii)   cuts in the budget preventing nurses from having a hot meal while working, especially during night and afternoon shifts;
(iii) very low bonuses for special work and overtime;
(iv)   no/or low budget allocation for uniforms;
(v)   absence of facilities for nurseries preventing nurses with young children from working;
(vi)   non-availability of continuous education and higher education among employees;
(vii) lack of opportunities for transfer of nurses to their home governorate;
(viii) overload of non-nursing jobs to be performed by qualified nurses because of absence of auxiliary assistance:
(ix)   shortage of facilities, which is reflected in the performance of nurses; and
(x)   shortage of nurses in certain governorates giving rise to a deterioration in the quality of care provision.

These constraining factors result in a high number of nurses leaving the profession, high absenteeism and turnover, errors, frustration and absence of responsibility. The situation also results in emigration: some 8000 Egyptian nurses work in other Arab countries and another 1000 leave the profession every year.[27]

The nursing shortage in Jordan led to the creation in 1983, by the Supreme Jordanian Health Council, of the National Nursing Committee to study the situation. They found that not enough applicants were attracted to nursing because of perceived lack of recognition and little autonomy of the profession. A later study by Zuraikat and McCloskey recommended that hospital administrators should improve benefit packages and make salaries more attractive, provide more opportunities for part-time work, more choices of hours and shift work, provide child care facilities and ensure transportation for weekend work. Maternity leave and weekly days off should be increased. To address the psychological factors of dissatisfaction, a career ladder should be introduced as a high priority, based on annual evaluations to reward creativity and dedication to work. Opportunities for continuing education should be given with both refresher courses and in-service training, as well as time to carry out research, to write and to publish.[28]

REGIONAL PERSPECTIVE

A WHO publication on nursing practice, which includes a global international overview and regional chapters, notes that there are differences in nursing practices among countries, but that often the reasons for these differences lie outside the direct control of nursing. In contrast, it highlights the common influences on nursing practice world-wide which are related to cultural factors:

> Chief among these [factors] is that most nurses are women, and so the position of nurses in society and the power they hold, the respect in which they are held and the value which is given to their work, is usually closely aligned to the position of women. Inevitably, if nursing work is not respected and valued, nurses will be denied positions of influence in health care planning and implementation. Education for nursing will not be seen as important and deserving of resources if nurses' work is seen as women's work, when women's contribution to the development, culture and maintenance of a society is not perceived as significant. In common with all female-dominated professions, nursing attracts low salaries, and often poor working conditions.[29]

Another factor contributing to the low status of the profession results from the traditional subordination of the nursing profession to the medical profession, which is usually dominated by men. In this context, nurses have accepted tasks transferred to them from physicians, while continuing to assume the caring and 'housekeeping' functions traditionally associated with women. This subordination prevents nurses from developing their autonomy, acquiring further specialization and thus contributing more fully to the quality of health care. At the same time, achieving this type of 'emancipation' requires access to appropriate basic and further training both in specialized disciplines and in management and leadership. While many recognize the need for such changes, much remains to be done.

Thus, for example, the WHO regional office for South-East Asia notes in the same study that the role of nurses as health promoters has been developed in six countries: Bangladesh, India, Myanmar, Nepal, Sri Lanka and Thailand, where Public Health Nurses have a role in health promotion in the community. However, the expansion of health promotion and direct service to villages and communities is only in its early stages. A major constraining factor in such deployment is the lack of adequate housing and security, particularly for unmarried young female nurses. While some of these countries tried to overcome this problem by training some male nurses for work in rural and other difficult areas, it proved difficult to attract and retain them to work there because of poor career prospects and lack of schooling and other facilities for families.[30]

The WHO regional office in the Eastern Mediterranean (EMRO)[31] also acknowledged that in the region the low status of women compounds the low status of nurses who have no control over the health service rendered. 'The lack of power and prestige and the lack of a role in decision-making have contributed to low self-esteem of nurses and poor image of the profession.'[32] EMRO states that nursing education, therefore, needs to be upgraded since the current nine years of preparatory education do not provide students with the basic scientific knowledge nor with the general education required for nursing practice. Moreover, as nursing graduates are rather young (15-17 years old), they do not have the maturity to cope with caring responsibilities or with health problems of families, and hence they often leave the profession.

In hospitals, the organization of nursing services follows a fragmented distribution of tasks. As a result, the 'caring' component of nursing services, which requires a holistic approach to the patient's and the family's needs, is often missing. In addition, nurses are not represented on decision-making bodies relating to resource allocation, nursing personnel and other key organizational issues. Nor are they empowered by the decision-making process to plan, implement and evaluate nursing actions. This is perceived as detrimental to the development of clinical and public health nursing practice in the region.

On the whole, public health nursing services and community nursing care are not well established, and approximately 90 per cent of the nursing workforce in the region is employed in hospitals. This leaves preventive and health promotion activities understaffed, aggravating the shortage of nursing staff in the community. This means that the poor and rural population, who have the greatest need for comprehensive care and nursing services, are under-served, and generally receive care from lesser qualified personnel, if at all. This situation causes concern about the risk of an influx of unqualified personnel, low quality of services and increased demand for supervisory posts to monitor unskilled staff. A related concern is the general lack of strong cohesive leadership to formulate policies and focus strategies to enhance the professional status of nurses and contribute to the development and quality of nursing services. A concurrent need is the introduction of adequate legislation to support nursing practice by establishing a uniform accreditation system and validation of standards of practice, which reflect modern nursing practice and correspond to the demands of health systems.[33]

The EMRO survey also points out that: 'the shortage of nurses in most countries of the region is a fundamental cause of low standards of nursing care. As the demand for nursing care outpaces the ability of countries to produce or provide additional personnel, the work load for existing personnel increases, quality of care suffers, and morale among nurses declines, leading to high attrition in the workforce.' The situation is exacerbated by the fact that 'nurses spend a sizeable percentage of their time in non-nursing activities. For example, in Bahrain, 22 per cent of nursing activities observed were personal, clerical, indirect or training activities. A similar study in a university hospital in Egypt found that nurses spent more than two-thirds of their time in indirect care activities. In a study in Kuwait, only 60 per cent of the activities of nursing personnel were patient-centred. Nurses are often assigned to non-nursing jobs in laboratories, the X-ray department, pharmacy and administration, depleting the nursing workforce and affecting the quality of services.'[34]

Last, but not least, the current centralized decision-making processes in the health services inhibit the ability of managers to innovate and improve the quality of practice. It is, therefore, necessary to give nurses not only managerial responsibilities but empower them to take and implement decisions. The current practice of assigning nurses to managerial positions on the basis of seniority or degree qualification needs to be improved by providing opportunities for appropriate management training, in areas such as problem-solving, research-based learning, total quality management and quality assurance.[35]

EMRO concludes that governments are trying to address the issues and are taking steps to assess their needs for nursing and midwifery services and to develop a structure to meet these needs. Lebanon has undertaken a study to assess nursing workforce and training institutions. Pakistan set up a task force of nursing leaders to analyze problems that hinder nursing education and services. Syria organized a national conference for policy makers, health officials and nursing leaders to formulate a plan for upgrading the nursing profession. Bahrain, Egypt, Jordan, Kuwait, Sudan and the United Arab Emirates have developed national strategic plans for nursing and midwifery services. A regional strategic plan for nursing development was adopted in 1993 by the six Gulf countries. Several EMRO countries have established a comprehensive registration system with standards of practice to guarantee that only properly qualified staff can practise nursing. And a number of countries in the region have targeted activities for the forthcoming five years to strengthen nursing and midwifery, particularly through improvement of education, further training and curriculum development, including development of nursing management and quality assurance.[36]

MIGRATION OF NURSES

International migration of health workers, of physicians and nurses in particular, has been a traditional practice of health care occupations. Globalization and the liberalization of the movement of people across borders facilitate this trend, particularly in the process of regional integration in Europe (EU), the Americas (NAFTA) and the Gulf States. To assess the magnitude of such migration, the 1993 World Bank World Development Report recalls that the main flow of physicians and nurses has been from developing to industrialized countries, with the former donating as much as 56 per cent of all migrating physicians. More than 90 per cent of nurses who migrate go to North America, Europe and the high-income countries in the western Pacific. Only about 7 per cent emigrate to developing countries. Migration of health workers, mostly from the developing countries of Philippines, Egypt, Bangladesh and India, also plays an important role in the Gulf States.[37]

Migration is often motivated by the desire to find employment or get better paying jobs. A Filipino nurse, for example, would be paid

US$ 146 per month in a state-run Philippine General Hospital as compared to US$ 2500 in the United States.[38] The ILO 1994 study on nursing personnel in its chapter on the Philippines indicates that wages of nurses in private hospitals are comparable to those of motor vehicle mechanics and drivers, while those of book-keepers and accounting clerks, elementary and secondary school teachers, plumbers and pipe-fitters are relatively higher. The author, E. Ortin, concludes that 'in both public and private sectors the basic salary of P 3,000 annually is clearly inadequate. Many private hospitals pay nurses, attendants and midwives even lower salaries. This amount can be considered low even when compared with the cost-of-living allowance which averages P 4,515.28 to P 5,992.5 (1988) and the poverty line of P 4,320 during the same year[...] Many hospitals do not offer shift differential pay, hazard pay, difficulty pay and other incentives[...] Many nursing personnel in private institutions have no security of tenure and are more at risk of redundancies[...] A high turnover rate due to poor conditions can prove costly in a developing country and can lead to social problems.'[39]

This description, and the earlier one on the situation in Egypt, epitomize the supply-side set of causes for nurses' preference for migration in general, and more particularly in developing countries. But the picture would not be complete without mentioning the demand-side, particularly the motivation by governments to respond to severe shortages of nursing personnel by facilitating immigration. But while such policy helps to cope with shortages, there is a risk of failing to adapt the national training and education facilities and their 'outputs' to the needs of the health sector labour market. Immigration is also not without its own problems of adaptation of immigrant nurses to cultural and social values of 'host' countries, as well as their limited understanding of the language and customs to adequately communicate with patients and their families. Quality nursing care cannot be assured because of the differing standards of practice and levels of training of immigrant personnel. And for the nurses concerned, there is the need to ensure acceptable working conditions and career development opportunities.

For the 'exporting' governments, the expected income from nurses' remittances can be very advantageous. The Philippines, for example, received an estimated US$ 680 million from expatriate workers in 1986, the majority of whom were nurses. Some 2000 to 3000 nurses emigrate each year from the Philippines. Although detailed figures are not available, Egypt is also known to be an important source for emigrating nurses who relocate to the Gulf States.

The drain on trained human resources in a developing economy implies a distortion in the uses of the limited health care budgets, and a threat to the quality of health care.

A 1993 WHO survey on nursing personnel resources states that among twenty-five countries reporting emigration, the negative consequences were that 'the clinical expertise of experienced nurses was lost, positions could not be filled, more training of new nurses was required and some services had to be curtailed.' In Pakistan, for example, as a result of emigration there was sometimes only one nurse per sixty patients in large hospitals. In Lebanon, emigration of nurses between 1989 and 1990 approached 60 per cent, leaving major health care services in a dire state. For the Philippines, nurses make up 93 per cent of the Filipinos working overseas, 80 per cent of whom migrate to the oil-rich Gulf States, particularly to Saudi Arabia. In 1987, some 23,000 Filipino nurses migrated to the Gulf and some 3000 to the United States. About 2000 Bangladeshi nurses were working abroad, largely in the Middle East. There were 1160 nurses in Bahrain, but only 27 per cent of whom were Bahraini; 65 per cent were Indian and 6 per cent were Filipino. Egypt reported that relocation of nurses from public to private hospitals and emigration to the Gulf States and the United States affected the quality and workload of those who remained (as pointed out in the ILO 1994 study). In Oman, 85 per cent of the nurses were non-Omanis and efforts were being undertaken to develop a national workforce.[40]

ICN Views on Migration

The International Council of Nurses (ICN), located in Geneva, Switzerland, is an organization whose affiliates consist of 118 national nursing professional organizations, including many from Islamic countries of the Middle East, South Asia and North Africa.

Given the constraining factors that push nurses to emigrate, and the frequent imbalance of the nursing workforce almost everywhere—shortages or over-supply—the ICN believes that quality health care is directly dependent on an adequate supply of qualified nursing personnel. It notes that the majority of WHO member States report a shortage, maldistribution and misutilization of nurses, and that many countries experience difficulties in recruiting and retaining sufficient numbers of registered nurses. At the same time, financial constraints force some governments to close health facilities despite the need for services, while career structure, conditions of employment and pay exacerbate the nursing shortages experienced by health institutions.

The ICN acknowledges that nurse migration is a reality of life and an international phenomenon. While recognizing that individual nurses have the right to migrate, it also acknowledges the potential negative impact of international migration on the quality of health care. Massive recruitment campaigns by some member states for foreign nurses delay effective local measures that would improve recruitment, retention and long term human resource planning. Governments and health authorities must address the shortcomings that cause nurses to leave the profession and which discourage them from returning. It, therefore, considers that, in line with the provisions of the ILO Nursing Personnel Convention No. 149 and Recommendation No. 157, national nurses associations have an important role to play in ensuring quality health care and satisfactory conditions of work for nurses.[41]

UPGRADING THE STATUS OF NURSING PERSONNEL: WHO RECOMMENDATIONS AND ILO STANDARDS

Persistent low status, poor conditions of work and low remuneration are the main reasons for growing shortages of nursing personnel. A broad range of measures is needed to address these problems, as pointed out in the aforementioned 1997 WHO study, and more particularly in the section relating to the Eastern Mediterranean Region. These measures include: policy priority for strengthening the nursing profession and improving its role in health care delivery in hospitals and communities; formulating national health plans; improving access to education and further training; diversifying and enriching the education curriculum; improving leadership and management training; improving conditions of work; and adopting measures to raise levels of remuneration to those in comparable professions requiring similar or equivalent qualifications and responsibilities. Last but not least, nurses must be involved in health policy formulation and decision-making at the different levels that concern health services delivery, whether care in hospitals, or preventive and health promotion activities in the community.

These policy recommendations which relate to all aspects of the nursing career and its development, are spelled out in the two international labour standards adopted in 1977 by the International Labour Organization, formulated in close co-operation with the World Health Organization, namely the Nursing Personnel Convention No. 149 and its accompanying recommendation No. 157, the main provision of which are summarized below.

The ILO Nursing Personnel Convention

Convention No. 149, adopted in 1977, applies to all categories of persons providing nursing care and nursing services wherever they work. It calls upon ILO member States who ratify it to formulate and apply a national policy concerning nursing personnel and nursing services designed to provide the quantity and quality of nursing care necessary for attaining the highest possible level of health for the population. This policy shall be formulated in consultation with the employers' and workers' organizations concerned, where such organizations exist. It should be included within a general health programme (where such exists), and within the resources available for health care as a whole. Furthermore, it is to be co-ordinated with policies relating to other aspects of health care and to other workers in the health sector.

More concretely, it states that governments must adopt the necessary measures to:

- provide nurses with education and training appropriate to the exercise of the profession. The basic requirements for such education and training and their supervision is to be laid down by national laws or regulations or by the competent authority or professional bodies, empowered to do so by such laws or regulations. Nursing education and training is to be co-ordinated with that of other health workers;
- nursing personnel should enjoy employment and working conditions, including career prospects and remuneration that are likely to attract persons to the nursing profession and to retain them in it. Their conditions of work at least be equivalent to those of other workers as regards hours of work, compensation of overtime,

inconvenient hours and shift work, weekly rest, paid annual leave, educational leave, maternity leave, sick leave, and social security;

- laws and regulations on occupational safety and health should be improved by adapting them to the special nature of nursing work and of the environment in which it is carried out;
- national laws or regulations should specify the requirements for the practice of nursing, limiting it to the persons who meet these requirements; and
- nursing personnel should participate in the planning of nursing services and should be consulted on decisions which concern them, in a manner appropriate to national conditions.

The Convention states that terms and conditions of employment should preferably be negotiated between employers and the workers' organizations concerned. Where disputes arise in connection with the determination of these terms and conditions, settlement shall be sought through negotiations between the parties, or in a manner that ensures the confidence of the parties involved, through independent and impartial machinery such as mediations, conciliation and voluntary arbitration.

The Convention is an international treaty that is applicable to ILO member States which have ratified it. So far thirty-six ILO member States have ratified Convention 149, including major nursing 'exporting' countries like Egypt, Jamaica and the Philippines. Other ratifying countries among those covered in this chapter are Bangladesh and Iraq. Azerbaijan, Kyrgystan and Tajikistan have also ratified it.

The ILO Nursing Personnel Recommendation

Recommendation No. 157, adopted at the same time, provides more details on the different topics covered by the Convention. Thus, for instance, it states that the policy concerning nursing should include measures to facilitate the effective utilization of nursing personnel in the country as a whole in various establishments and sectors, and promote the fullest use of their qualifications. For this purpose, legislation and regulations related to education, training and practice should be introduced and adapted to developments in the qualifications and responsibilities required of nursing personnel to meet the demand for their services.

To ensure greater uniformity of employment structure in the various establishments, areas and sectors employing nursing personnel, a rational nursing personnel structure should be established, based on an occupational classification containing a limited number of categories determined by reference to a broad range of factors including: education and training; the level of functions and authorization to practice; the level of judgement required; the authority to take decisions; the complexity of the relationship with other functions; the level of technical skill required; and the level of responsibility for the nursing services provided. As an example of such occupational classification, the Recommendation suggests that it may include three categories of staff—professional nurses, auxiliary nurses and nursing aides. For each of these it provides details on the level of training and responsibilities.

It stipulates that nursing personnel of a given category should not be used as substitutes for nursing personnel of a higher category; except in case of special emergency, on a provisional basis, and on condition that they have adequate training or experience and are given appropriate compensation.

A substantive section of the Recommendation deals with education and training, which specifies, *inter alia*, that measures should be taken to provide the necessary information and guidance on the nursing profession to persons wishing to take up nursing as a career. It gives details on legal prescriptions that should exist on basic educational requirements. It specifies that such education should be organized by reference to recognized community needs, taking account of resources available in the country. It should, moreover, be co-ordinated with education and training of other health care professionals and include both theory and practice. Such training should be given in approved preventive, curative and rehabilitation services, under the supervision of qualified nurses. Continuing education and training both at the workplace and outside should be an integral part of this education and training, and it should be available to all in order to ensure updating and upgrading of knowledge and skills, in order to enable nursing personnel to acquire and apply new ideas and techniques. The duration of basic education and training should be related to the minimum educational requirements for entry to training and to the purpose of training.

There should be two levels of approved basic education and training:

(a) an advanced level to train professional nurses, having sufficiently wide and thorough skills to enable them to provide the most complex nursing care and to organize and evaluate nursing care, in hospitals and other health-related community services. Students accepted at this level should have the general educational background required for entry to university; and

(b) a less advanced level, to train auxiliary nurses able to provide general nursing care which is less complex, but which requires technical skills and aptitude for personal relations. Students accepted at this level should have attained as advanced a level as possible of secondary education.

In addition, the Recommendation states that there should be programmes of higher nursing education to train nurses for the highest responsibilities in direct and supportive nursing care, in the administration of nursing services, in nursing education and in research and development in the field of nursing.

As regards nursing aides, they should be given theoretical and practical training appropriate to their functions.

Continuing education and training should include programmes which (a) would promote and facilitate the advancement of nursing aides and nursing auxiliaries, and (b) would facilitate re-entry into nursing after a period of interruption.

As the majority of nursing personnel in many countries consists of a female workforce between the age of 35 and 45, the provisions on continuing vocational training and programmes for returning to work, often after child-rearing, assumes a particular relevance.

Like the Convention, the Recommendation underlines the importance of nurses' participation in decisions concerning national health policy in general and their profession in particular, including the principles related to education and training and the practice of the profession.

The Recommendation emphasizes that nursing personnel should not be assigned to work that goes beyond their qualifications and competence. On the other hand, they should be able to claim exemption from performing specific duties, without being penalized, where performance would conflict with their religious, moral or ethical convictions and where they inform their supervisor in good time of their objection.

Representatives of nursing personnel should participate in the determination of any disciplinary rules applicable to these personnel and should guarantee fair judgement and adequate appeal procedure, including the right to be represented by persons of their choice at all levels of the proceedings, in a manner appropriate to national conditions.

In the area of career development, the Recommendation states that measures should be taken to offer nursing personnel reasonable career prospects, by providing for a sufficiently varied and open range of possibilities of professional advancement, leadership positions in direct and supportive nursing care, in the administration of nursing services, or in nursing education or research and development. A grading and a remuneration structure should recognize the acceptance of functions involving increased responsibility and requiring greater technical skill and professional judgement. The importance of functions involving direct relations with patients and the public must also be recognized.

Other measures recommended in this area include:

- advice and guidance on career prospects and on re-entry into nursing after a period of interruption;
- taking into account of past nursing experience and the duration of interruption in determining the level at which a re-entering nurse will be recruited;
- provision by employers of staff and facilities for in-service training, preferably at the workplace; and
- provision of facilities to help nurses wishing to participate in education and training programmes and able to do so, including paid or unpaid educational leave, adaptation of hours of work, and payment of study or training costs.

Remuneration of nursing personnel should be fixed at levels commensurate with their socio-economic needs, qualifications, responsibilities, duties and experience. It should take account of the constraints and hazards inherent in the profession, and factors which are likely to attract persons to the profession and retain them in it. Financial compensation should be given to nursing personnel who work in particularly arduous or unpleasant conditions. In determining the remuneration, the principle of comparability with other professions requiring similar qualifications and carrying similar responsibilities is recommended. The periodic adjustment of pay to take account of variations in the cost of living and rises in the national living standard is also recommended. Pay should preferably be determined by collective agreement. Pay should be payable entirely in money and deductions should only be permitted under conditions prescribed by national laws or regulations or fixed by collective agreement or arbitration award. As regards work clothing, medical kits, transport facilities and other supplies required for the performance of the work, the employer should provide and maintain free of charge.

The Recommendation and its annex contain numerous provisions on the arrangement of working time, including part-time and temporary employment, occupational health protection, social security, basic rights and freedoms for nursing students.

A special section deals with international co-operation and staff exchange programmes. The Recommendation points out that where organized exchange programmes exist, these are the best way of extending the possibility of education and training abroad. However, in the light of the important migration flows that characterize the profession, an intended and negative result for the country of origin has been that some trainees from developing countries used the exchange training programmes as a way of finding permanent employment abroad. This has exacerbated the needs of community nursing shortages.

CONCLUSIONS

This overview of the health sector in Islamic countries and the role nurses can play in improvement of the quality of services and access to such by the population at large, focuses on an important policy issue for countries involved in a development effort. General education, particularly basic schooling for girls, is an essential precondition in this process of improving health care and living standards, and more generally, in combating poverty. Access of girls to technical and higher education in the health professions is also important in this context. Once qualified, they need satisfactory working conditions and income, and opportunities for career development and social recognition. While most governments recognize these needs, budget constraints often limit their capacity to take the appropriate measures to reach these objectives.

As a result, those who qualify for entry into the nursing profession are often likely to leave it, with no incentives to re-enter. There is, therefore, an urgent need to improve the work environment, terms and conditions of employment and career perspective.

Remuneration is an important factor since the decline in the real value of public sector wages in general has been almost universal, leading to poor morale and performance, moonlighting, and difficulties in recruiting and retaining qualified staff. Competitive pay rates, therefore, need to be established for public sector health services. Pay levels, and particularly bonuses and allowances, should be made comparable to those of jobs with similar qualifications, skills and responsibilities as well as hardships, and should reflect the prevailing labour market situation. They should also reflect productivity gains to ensure more efficient and cost effective service delivery.

Since remuneration is related to levels of education, training and experience, nurses would benefit from continuing education, training and skill-upgrading opportunities in order to diversify their skills and acquire specialization in nursing practice, as well as in health management or in primary health care. Career planning and counseling also needs to be undertaken in close consultation with nursing personnel and their professional organizations. Due account must be given in this context to facilitating the re-entry of nurses to the profession after marriage and child-rearing and helping them reconcile employment with family responsibilities.

Professional associations and trade unions can facilitate a greater involvement of nurses in policy formulation, in strengthening the status of the profession and improving conditions under which it is practised. They can provide useful inputs to curriculum development. They can motivate nurses to improve their qualifications and guide them in their professional orientation. And, of course, they can negotiate better outcomes in terms of working conditions and career advancement.

But career development and job satisfaction also depend on the degree of autonomy given to nurses to make decisions at the workplace and beyond, in areas that relate to health policy and health environment. Assurances of social recognition, autonomy and increased responsibilities are essential to ensure adequate entry of staff into the profession.

The World Bank points out that nearly all countries face the fundamental problem of inadequate numbers of primary care providers and too many specialists, and that most health care workers are concentrated in urban areas. Policy makers should therefore recognize the value of programmes in which nurses receive education and in-service training to work in primary health care, public health, health policy and management. Indeed, many tasks performed by physicians can be successfully delegated to nurses, midwives and community health workers at substantial reduction in costs.[42]

As pointed out in this chapter, there is a dramatic absence of basic data on the health sector in the countries covered, and more particularly, on nursing personnel. Any policy improvement in this area would therefore urgently require the establishment of a reliable database with up-to-date statistics on employment, pay and conditions of work in health services, in general, and for nursing personnel in particular. Data should be included on career paths of the major categories of nursing personnel, doctors and paramedical staff, as well as movement in and out of the profession, migration patterns, and working hours and remuneration.

More transparency is needed in existing pay scales, particularly as regards fringe benefits and allowances, and more options for career advancement and promotion are necessary to motivate and retain staff in the profession. Such information is essential for human resources planning in the health sector, for policy formulation which aims at strengthening the status of nurses, and for dealing with severe staff shortages.

A number of efforts are now being made in the Gulf States to start database collection of information on some of these aspects. This will be invaluable for both policy-makers at national levels, and hospital management and personnel responsible for primary health care services at the community level.

In the absence of such data it is difficult to accurately assess supply and demand and to determine the need for remedial action in areas of training and education, in deployment of scarce resources to provide optimum health service to the population, in developing and implementing an appropriate human resources policy, and in adapting conditions of work and remuneration to aspirations of existing and new staff.

As a final statement, it can be said that the widespread acknowledgement of the problems confronting the nursing profession, the readiness of governments to revise policies, and the growing leadership within are setting the stage for improvements throughout the world, including in Islamic countries.

NOTES

1. UNDP, *Human Development Report 1997*, New York, Oxford: Oxford University Press, 1997. 176-177.
2. Ibid., p. 56.
3. Ibid., pp. 176-177.
4. WHO, *Strengthening Nursing and Midwifery*, Resolution adopted by the 49th World Health Assembly, 23 May 1996.
5. WHO, *Strengthening Nursing and Midwifery—A Global Study*, Geneva, 1997.
6. World Bank, *Health, Nutrition and Population in the Middle East and North Africa Region*, November 1997, p. 10.
7. World Bank, *World Development Report 1993. Investing in Health*, New York: Oxford University Press, 1993, p. 139.
8. Ibid., p. 139.
9. Ibid., pp. 141-143.
10. ILO, *Equality of opportunity and treatment between men and women in health and medical services*, Report II, Standing Technical Committee for Health and Medical Services, First Session, Geneva: ILO, 1992, pp. 2-6.
11. Richard Anker, *Gender and Jobs—Sex segregation of occupations in the world*, Geneva: ILO, 1998, pp. 145-147.
12. Ibid., pp. 170-173.
13. Information provided to the ILO Office in Cairo by the Egyptian Ministry of Health, Nursing Sector, in March 1998 and June 1998.
14. Anker, op. cit., pp. 264-269.
15. ILO, *General Report*, Report I, Standing Technical Committee for Health and Medical Services, First Session, Geneva: ILO, 1992, pp. 44-46.
16. ILO, *Impact of structural adjustment in the public services (efficiency, quality improvement and working conditions)*, Joint Meeting on the Impact of Structural Adjustment in the Public Services, Geneva: ILO 1995, pp. 43-44.
17. ILO, *General Report*, 1992, op. cit., pp. 44-46.
18. Reply to the author's questionnaire from the Kuwait Nursing Association, March 1998.
19. Personal communication from the International and Public Affairs Department of the Social Security Organization, Tehran, Iran, 25 August 1998.
20. ILO, *Impact of Structural Adjustment*, 1995, op. cit., p. 44.
21. David Marsden (ed.), *The Remuneration of nursing personnel: An international perspective*, Geneva: ILO, 1994.
22. Ibid., pp. 5-6.
23. ILO, Bureau of Labour Statistics: *Statistics on occupational wages and hours of work and on food prices, October Inquiry results 1997*, Special supplement to the Bulletin of Labour Statistics, Geneva: ILO, 1998.
24. Derek Robinson, *Civil service pay in Africa*, Geneva: ILO, 1990.
25. David Chew, *Civil service pay in South Asia*, Geneva: ILO, 1992.
26. ILO, *Equality of opportunity and treatment between men and women in the health and medical services*, Report II, 1992, op. cit., pp. 22-27.
27. Cheherzade M.K. Ghazi, Nassar Shafika, Ismail Mahassen, Nihad E. Fifry and Selim Mogha A.A., 'The remuneration of Egyptian nurses,' in D. Marsden (ed.), *The remuneration of nursing personnel*, op. cit., p. 144.

28. Nashat Zuraikat, and J. McClosky, 'Job satisfaction among Jordanian registered nurses', *International Nursing Review*, vol. 33, no. 5, 1986, pp. 143-145.

29. WHO, *Nursing practice around the world*, Geneva: WHO, 1997.

30. Ibid., pp. 15 and 21.

31. Ibid., pp. 12-18.

32. Ibid., p. 62.

33. Ibid., pp. 14, 20-25 and 53-56.

34. Ibid., p. 57.

35. Ibid., p. 27.

36. Ibid., pp. 64-65.

37. World Bank, *World Development Report*, 1993, op. cit., p. 141.

38. ILO, *Terms of Employment and Working Conditions in Health Sector Reforms*, Report to a Joint Meeting of the ILO, Geneva, 21-25 September 1998, Geneva: ILO, 1998, p. 37.

39. E. Ortin, 'The remuneration of nursing personnel in the Philippines,' in *The remuneration of nursing personnel*, D. Marsden (ed.), op. cit., p. 217.

40. Miriam Hirschfeld, Beverly Henry and Hurdis Griffith, *Nursing personnel resources—Results of a survey of perceptions in ministries of health on nursing shortage, nursing education and quality of care*, Geneva: WHO, September 1993, (ref. WHO/HRH/NUR/93.4), pp. 30-31.

41. ICN, *Position Statement: Nurse Retention, Transfer and Migration*, adopted in 1977 and 1989, last reviewed in 1992, Geneva: ICN, 1992.

42. World Bank, *Investing in Health, World Development Report 1993*, op. cit., p. 139.

ACKNOWLEDGEMENTS

The author wishes to express appreciation and thank the following persons and organizations for their contributions to this chapter: Ms Fadwa Affara, the International Council of Nurses (ICN) (Geneva); the International Labour Office (Geneva), in particular, Mr Ashagri, director of the Bureau of Labour Statistics, Ms Gabriele Ullrich, public service and Health sector specialist at the Salaried Employees and Professional Workers' Branch, Ms Naziha Gaham-Boumechal, human resources expert at the Labour Administration Branch and Ms Loretta de Luca, senior employment specialist, ILO Multidisciplinary Team, (Cairo, Egypt); Mr Dalmer Hoskins, Secretary General, International Social Security Association (ISSA) (Geneva); Mr Mike Waghorn, Assistant General Secretary, Public Service International (Ferney-Voltaire, France); Dr Atskuo Aoyama, health specialist at the World Bank (Washington, DC); and the World Health Organization, in particular Dr Miriam Hirschfeld, Director, Division of Human Resource Development and Capacity Building, Dr E. Abou Youssef, Regional Adviser, Nursing and Paramedical Development, WHO/EMRO (Alexandria, Egypt).

My thanks also goes to the national institutions who provided information, namely: Ms A. Khaksar-Fard, Assistant Director General at the International & Public Affairs, Social Security Organization, Tehran, Iran; The Tunisian National Social Security Fund (CNSS), Ministry of Social Affairs, Ms Lateefa Al-Mansour, Secretary General, Kuwait Nursing Association, Safat, Kuwait; and Ms Afaya Bzeouich Belgacem, Secretary General of the Health Federation of the General Union of Tunisian Workers (UGTT), Tunis, Tunisia.

6

Violence Against Nurses: Violation of Human Rights

Mireille Kingma

Violence—being destructive towards another person—is increasing. According to the World Health Report of 1997, violence in all its forms has increased dramatically worldwide in recent decades. Apart from civil conflict and war, violence can be interpersonal, self-directed, physical, sexual as well as mental, including acts of exclusion. This chapter will look at the manifestations of violence towards women and female nurses in particular. Contributing factors involved in the generation of workplace violence in the health sector and nurses' coping mechanisms will be identified. Strategies developed to reduce violence in the health sector will be summarised in order to stimulate local and national action:

1. Domestic violence is a pattern of behaviours that may start with palpable tension and intimidation in the relationship and progresses to physical assault with injury to the woman (or man) and sometimes the children. It is a pattern of meaningful, purposeful, coercive behaviour directed at achieving control over the victim.
2. Sexual harassment: Any unwanted, unreciprocated and unwelcome behaviour of a sexual nature that is offensive to the person involved, and causes that person to be threatened, humiliated or embarrassed.
3. Bullying is offensive behaviour through vindictive, cruel, malicious or humiliating attempts to undermine an individual or groups of employees.

VIOLENCE

Violence is a generic term that incorporates all types of abuse—behaviour that humiliates, degrades or otherwise indicates a lack of respect for the dignity and worth of an individual. Violence crosses all boundaries, including age, race, socio-economic status, education, religion, sexual orientation and workplace.

In many countries, violence is endemic and the leading cause of death among males aged 15 to 34. It is acknowledged, however, that the burden of violence is disproportionately borne by young people and women. More often than men, women are targets of violence. They are subjected to domestic violence[1] and workplace violence that can be manifested through physical and verbal abuse, sexual harassment[2], and bullying.[3]

Gender violence is considered a universal plague even though it continues to be grossly under-reported. Despite its high costs, almost every society in the world has social institutions that legitimise, obscure or deny abuse. Many cultures have beliefs, norms, and infrastructures that authorize and therefore perpetuate violence against women (Heise et al., 1999). Societal tolerance of such abuses has been a contributing factor to the widespread existence of such behaviours.

WHAT ARE SOME OF THE STATISTICS?

- Around the world, at least one woman in every three has been beaten, coerced into sex, or otherwise abused in her lifetime (Heise et al., 1999).
- Worldwide, it is estimated that more than 16 per cent of women will be raped in their lifetime (UNICEF).
- In the USA, 2-4 million women are victims of domestic violence every year. Nearly four in ten female emergency room patients have been victims of physical or emotional domestic abuse sometime in their lives, and 14 per cent have been physically or sexually abused in the past year.
- In the developing countries, one-third to over one-half of women report being beaten by their partner.
- In a suburb of a Middle-East capital, 30 per cent of the women respondents reported having been beaten every day and 34 per cent

once a week during the period under review (World Organization Against Torture).

- One Caribbean island survey revealed that one in three women have been sexually abused as a child.
- Eighty per cent of the women in a central African village reported having suffered violence from their husbands (World Organization Against Torture).
- The Human Rights Commission of a country in South-East Asia affirms that rural women are denied their rights to inherit property, get education, decide about their future and get employment (Klasra, 1997).
- Worldwide, the great majority of sexual harassment victims are women.

A recent report undertaken by the International Labour Organization concludes that workplace violence has also gone global, crossing borders, work settings and occupational groups. The 1992 British Crime Survey found that the workplace was the fastest growing of all locations for violent crime. Incidents of work-related violence recorded by successive surveys doubled between 1991 and 1995 (NHS *et al.*, 1998). In the United States, violence in the workplace ranks as the leading cause of occupational death for women (Neurath, 1996).

The Declaration of Alma Ata (WHO/UNICEF, 1978) recognizes the right to health. Violence is destructive by nature and has profoundly negative health implications on observers as well as the victims. Violence can, therefore, be considered a violation of the basic right to health. While the dramatic statistics above paint an alarming picture, the exact magnitude of the physical and psychological harm inflicted is unknown. It is estimated that less than half the female victims of violence report the abuse. Violence has become a public health *and* labour concern of epidemic proportion with extensive health care implications.

WHY IS THIS RELEVANT TO NURSES?

Known to be a serious problem in many countries in the industrialised world, new research indicates that violence in the health care workplace is actually a global phenomenon. Crossing borders, cultures, work settings and occupational groups, violence in the health care workplace is an epidemic in all societies, including the developing world.

What happens in the workplace is often a reflection of cultural norms. A World Bank report concludes that violence against women is rooted in the social relationships of patriarchy that are based on a system of male domination and female subordination (Samath, 1997). There is a range of norms and beliefs that are particularly powerful in perpetuating violence against women. These include 'a belief that men are inherently superior to women and that men have a right to 'correct' female behaviour' (Heise *et al.*, 1999).

While the workplace is outside the realm of personal relationships, individuals are conditioned to treat women in a certain way (Ahmad-Aziz, 1998). These attitudes are manifested when dealing with female nurses who suffer from the societal tolerance of violence against women. It should not be surprising that 'health care providers typically share the same cultural values and societal attitudes toward abuse that are dominant in the society at large' (Heise *et al.*, 1999). While patients and their relatives perpetrate the majority of cases of reported physical violence against nurses, there is a significant amount of abuse generated by colleagues.

The International Labour Organization as a normative body addressing workplace conditions and protocols has created a network of interrelated occupational health conventions that guarantees workers the right to a safe work environment. In some countries, even when laws defending the rights of men to use violence against women are repealed, the culture that created them continues to exert a tremendous influence over behaviour—even in the workplace.

When nurses have initiated legal proceedings against abusers, the courts have on several occasions refused to grant compensation to nurse victims. This was justified on the principle that to practise nursing was to accept the risk of personal violence. Nurses are often made to feel that they are 'legitimate targets' and that violence is 'part of the job'.

VIOLENCE AGAINST NURSES

Although it is true that male nurses have been victims of abuse and violence in the workplace, this is less frequent and not within the scope of the present chapter. In fact, 95 per cent of nurses around the world are women. Attitudes towards women are often reflected in interactions with the profession. What are some of the relevant statistics?

- Health care staff is at greater risk from work-related violence than the general population (NHS *et al.*, 1998).
- Health care workers are more likely to be attacked at work than prison guards or parole officers (Mahoney, 1990).
- The Health and Safety Executive has identified nursing as the most hazardous occupation in the United Kingdom. Nurses are more likely to be on the receiving end of violence than policemen (HSC, 1997). Nursing staff were more than twice as likely to be involved in a violent incident compared with all other staff (NHS, 1999).
- In the US, it is estimated that between 1 and 2 million workplace assaults occur annually. Almost half of these assaults occur in health care institutions. Nurses are more likely to suffer nonfatal injuries while at work than are members of any other profession. According to the Bureau of Labor Statistics data bank, 27,800 nurses received injuries severe enough to take time off work in 1995. Forty-five per cent of those injuries were the result of assaults or aggressive acts committed by patients and directed toward the nurse. By 1997, the percentage of injuries incurred by patient assault of staff had grown to 55 per cent. The majority of these caregivers were female nurses and nursing assistants (Erickson *et al.*, 2000).
- In the US, 82 per cent of emergency nurses surveyed had been assaulted during their careers. In the year preceding the study, 56 per cent of nurses had been assaulted; 29 per cent of these assaults were unreported. Only two nurses (3.6%) felt safe from the possibility of patient assault at work 'all of the time' (Erickson *et al.*, 2000).
- Ninety-seven per cent of nurse respondents to a UK survey knew a nurse who had been physically assaulted during the preceding year. 47 per cent of nurses polled had been physically attacked in the preceding year and 85 per cent had been verbally abused. Up to 95 per cent of nurses reported having been bullied at work. Approximately 75 per cent of nurses reported having been subjected to sexual harassment at work (*Nursing Times*, 1998).
- More than six out of ten violent incidents that took place in the National Health Service (UK) over 1999 were aimed at nurses. On average, there were eleven violent incidents per 1,000 nursing staff

each month. Almost 50 per cent of nurses had been physically attacked in the preceding year (*Nursing Times*, 1999).

- More than three in four mental health nurses in Scotland (UK) have experienced a violent event at work in the year preceding the study. One in ten of the 760 nurses questioned said the event had been so serious that medical assistance had been necessary, while almost half had required first aid (*Nursing Standard*, 1999).
- In Nova Scotia (Canada), 80 per cent of nurse respondents reported experiencing some form of violence in their nursing careers; 63 per cent reported having experienced harsh or insulting language; 25 per cent had been verbally threatened with physical harm; 35 per cent had attempts of physical harm made against them; 24 per cent were sexually harassed in the workplace; and 21 per cent were victims of a physical attack (RNANS, 1997).
- Fifty-six per cent of staff working in the emergency care unit of a major hospital in Barcelona (Spain) reported being exposed to verbal aggression by patients or their relatives (Chappell *et al.*, 1998).
- In Sweden, 75 per cent of the health staff reported having been exposed to threats, 93 per cent to minor physical violence and 53 per cent to severe physical violence during the previous twelve months (Chappell *et al.*, 1998).
- A survey in Adelaide (Australia) found that 91 per cent of all staff and 96 per cent of all personal care attendants in nursing homes or hostels stated that they had experienced aggressive behaviour from a resident (Chappell *et al.*, 1998).
- Eighty-five per cent of Australian nurses reported being victims of verbal and/or physical abuse with 43 per cent of these nurses experiencing abuse on 1-4 occasions in the previous twelve months, and 15.8 per cent experiencing abuse more than twenty-five times in the same period (Fisher, 1998).
- A study in Australia found violence against remote area nurses was extreme and nearly all remote area nurses had experienced severe episodes of violence within twelve months prior to the study. Verbal threats and abuse were experienced by 82.1 per cent, 46.7 per cent had experienced property damage, 45.1 per cent had experienced physical assault, 31.8 per cent had experienced sexual harassment, 17 per cent had telephone threats, 10.8 per cent had experienced sexual abuse, and 8.3 per cent had been stalked (Fischer, 1998).

- Over 46 per cent of the nurses surveyed by the Irish Nurses Organization reported having been assaulted at some stage during their careers and that those who were assaulted in the past year were assaulted an average of three times. Eighty per cent of the nurses reported witnessing nurse to nurse bullying and more than half reported having been personally bullied.

Few studies in the area of violence, including sexual harassment, have been conducted in developing countries. The documentation available, however, suggests that violence against nurses exists and is often sanctioned by societal norms.

- In Turkey, 75 per cent of the nurse respondents reported having been sexually harassed during their nursing practice. These incidents were perpetrated by physicians (44%), patients (34%), patients' relatives (14%) and others (9%). The study concluded that sexual harassment was a significant problem in this country (Kisa *et al.*, 1996).
- Male physicians were identified as the major perpetrators of sexual harassment in a study undertaken in Pakistan. As the instigators of sexual harassment against nurses, patients and patients' relatives were reported less frequently but in a significant number of cases (Shaikh, 2000).
- Recent cases of abuse against nurses (1990) are not isolated incidents, but form a long history of violence that has been associated with the nursing profession in Pakistan. 'The recent uprising of nurses was reported to be the direct result of an armed attack by a gang of four doctors on two nurses who had earlier complained about the doctors' alleged misbehaviour.... While most nurses suffer such degradation silently, the ones who protest by taking the issue to the police are said to be subjected to terrible punishment—ranging from torture to even murder at the hands of implicated influentials' (Bokhari, 1990).
- According to recent research, more than half of the health care workers surveyed had experienced at least one incident of physical or psychological violence in the twelve months previous to the survey: 61 per cent in South Africa, 56 per cent in Portugal; 54 per cent in Thailand. In Lebanon, the study showed that the prevalence of verbal abuse was the highest (41% of the respondents), followed by bullying/mobbing (22.4%), physical violence (6%), racial

harassment (5%), and sexual harassment (2.4%) (ILO/ICN/WHO/PSI, 2002)

- Many nurses in Pakistan feel that they are being exploited just because they are women working in a world of men (Shamin, 1998).

- There is a clause on misconduct of workers in the West Pakistan Industrial and Commercial Standing Orders Ordinance 1968. No provision, however, is made for addressing the misconduct of employers and management. This leaves women feeling vulnerable in an already hostile environment. Even women from the upper class working in corporate organizations do not have a law which can protect them from sexual harassment at work (Ishfaq, 1998).

- 'The nature of the work of nurses requires them to have contact with non-family males such as doctors and other health care workers, patients and their relatives. Such contact is contrary to the socio-cultural norms in many sectors of Pakistani society which govern the behaviour of women. Studies have shown that this aspect of nursing contributes to its low social status.... Women living or working outside the protection of their family are vulnerable targets for sexual harassment' (Amarsi, 1999).

- In Lebanon, research showed that the patient or a relative was the main perpetrator of physical violence while colleagues or managers were the main perpetrators of bullying, verbal abuse, sexual and racial harassment (ILO/ICN/WHO/PSI, 2002)

- A government ban on the 'export' of female nurses and housemaids from Bangladesh was under fire from human rights and women's organizations and labelled a violation of human rights. According to an official at the Ministry of Manpower, the ban was prompted by numerous reports of sexual harassment of female domestic workers (Islam, 1998).

- 'The most important strategy to recruit and retain sufficient numbers of nurses in Pakistan is to check the sexual exploitation of nurses. Society must start viewing nurses as professionals, and not as objects of desire who can be harassed through brute force' (Bokhari, 1990).

'The nurses are essentially an abandoned breed, a friendless community. Hospitals exploit them to the hilt and pay them meagre salaries, doctors often treat them badly, paramedics hate them, society feels they are 'untouchables', and for all pleasure seekers, they are objects of carnal desire. And then, on the other extreme, the patients demand that they behave like angels.... In addition to the doctors, nurses' matrons also constantly humiliate their wards by imposing various restrictions on them.... The imposition of curbs were felt to be necessary in order to avoid the involvement of nurses in 'unsavoury' incidents.... The attitude of the matrons is indicative of the hospital establishment's peculiar strategy for dealing with incidents of brutality against nurses. The implicit assumption is that the nurses themselves are mainly responsible for inviting trouble'. (Bokhari, 1990)

In summary, violence against nurses is world-wide and appears to be increasing although the degree of under-reporting continues to be very high. Of great concern is the widespread practice of colleagues, co-workers and administrators of blaming the victim of violence for provoking the incident (Fisher, 1998). Societal values, the treatment of women and the status of nursing as a profession determine the framework or context within which nursing is practised. In addition, they influence the level of work-related violence experienced by nurses.

Twenty-three-year-old F.S. was a staff nurse working on the night shift at a Karachi hospital when she was raped at gunpoint by two male visitors to a private patient. 'I reported the attack to the hospital matron and was told to keep my mouth shut. The patient was a prominent one,' F.S. told me. 'I received the same response when I went to the hospital's medical superintendent. I was too afraid to go to the police in case they raped me again.'

Ten days later, F.S. was arrested, charged with *zina*, and she spent two months in Karachi's Central Jail. At her court hearing, where she was able to identify her attackers, she was found guilty, sentenced to five years' imprisonment, five lashes, and a 10,000 rupees fine. Her attackers were never charged. On appeal in a higher court, F.S. was acquitted of all charges. But by then she had lost her job because her reputation was now 'tarnished', and her fiancé had broken off their engagement because he didn't want to marry 'a woman who was no longer pure'. Says her mother, 'I was so proud of my daughter when she became a nurse. It is good to work for suffering people. But men in Pakistan think that because a nurse has to go out of the house at night to work, she must be a bad woman. These men who have ruined my daughter's life should be hanged. Instead, they went totally unpunished. Why is there one justice for men and another justice for women? (from Jan Goodwin, *Price of Honour*, Little Brown and Company. NZ, 1994).

RISK FACTORS IN THE HEALTH SECTOR

While cultural values and societal norms may have a significant impact on the existence of violence in the health sector, there are also risk factors associated specifically with the health and nursing services. These would include:

- Staff working in isolation.
- Staff working outside normal hours, especially at night.
- Staff handling valuables (e.g. drugs, cash).
- Staff exercising authority, (e.g. providing/withdrawing a service, enforcing legislation).
- Inadequate staff coverage.
- Lack of staff training (e.g. nature of violence, coping mechanisms).
- Inter-relationships within the work environment (e.g. managers' disinterest, horizontal violence—aggressive behaviours directed horizontally within an oppressed group).
- Patients/clients with high and sometimes unrealistic expectations.
- Lack of adequate communication between staff and patient/client.
- Dealing with people who have been drinking or taking drugs.
- Dealing with people under stress, frustrated, emotionally/mentally unstable, violent or grief-struck.
- Environments that are not client-friendly (e.g. crowded, busy, uncomfortable).

Each of these health sector risk factors needs to be examined and its potential impact in a given work environment assessed. Effective prevention strategies depend on recognising the dangers, their possible impact and the measures likely to eliminate (or at least reduce) the hazards.

THE CONSEQUENCES OF NURSE ABUSE

The impact of physical violence, verbal abuse and sexual harassment is of great concern in view of its prevalence. The consequences of such acts may manifest themselves on the individuals involved but also on the health care services provided.

Personal impact:

- Shock, disbelief, guilt, anger, depression, overwhelming fear;
- Physical injury;
- Increased stress levels;
- Physical disorders (e.g. migraine, vomiting);
- Loss of self esteem and belief in their professional competence;
- Paralysing self-blame;
- Feelings of powerlessness and of being exploited;
- Sexual disturbances;
- Negative effect on interpersonal relationships;
- Loss of job satisfaction;
- Absenteeism leading to job insecurity;
- Anxiety of loved ones.

Impact on health services:

- Deterioration of the quality of care provided (e.g. increased medical errors);
- Breakdown of communication channels;
- Absenteeism;
- Deterioration of the work environment (e.g. loss of staff morale);
- Abandonment of the profession, reducing health services available to the general population;
- Negative effect on recruitment to the profession;
- Perpetuation of unacceptable societal behaviours;
- Increasing health costs;
- Increasing administration costs (e.g. litigation expenses);
- Anxiety of patients and staff.

The impact of verbal abuse must not be minimised. The consequences are similar to the effects of physical assault and have serious repercussions on provision of care. At least 18 per cent of the nursing turnover rate is related to verbal abuse, with many nurses choosing to leave the career as a result (Worthington, 1993). The loss of qualified nurses inevitably intensifies the stress placed on an often short-staffed health unit. It has been demonstrated that co-workers who had not witnessed the violent incident also displayed post-traumatic stress response symptoms, once informed.

These incidents leave memorable traces over the long as well as short-term. A study showed that 18 per cent of nurse victims of physical assaults by patients continued to experience moderate to severe traumatic responses six weeks following the assault. Long-term follow-up highlighted that 16 per cent of those responding after one year were still suffering (Poster, 1993). Violence harms nurses both personally and professionally, altering their lives and the quality of their contributions to health services.

NURSES' RESPONSE TO VIOLENCE

The immediate reaction of nurses, as individuals, will be dictated by:

- Personality type;
- Learned coping and problem-solving mechanisms (conscious and unconscious);
- Physical environment; and
- Societal expectations (cultural and professional).

Immediate responses may range from highly passive to highly active (see Figure 1). Nurses too often passively accept abuse and violence as 'part of the job'. To avoid violence, many nurses ignore abuse, as was the case for some 30 per cent of the nurse respondents to a survey in Canada. Of these nurses, 25-35 per cent found this measure helpful (MARN, 1989). However, such action is likely to interfere with the nurse/patient relationship or may inhibit patient-related communication between co-workers and the consequences must be seriously considered.

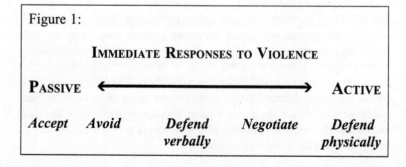

Figure 1:

IMMEDIATE RESPONSES TO VIOLENCE

PASSIVE ⟷ ACTIVE

Accept   Avoid   Defend   Negotiate   Defend
                    verbally   physically

In the same survey, verbal defence was used by most respondents and found to be generally helpful in preventing further violence (except for extended/personal care institutions). Interestingly, this study showed that benefit from any of the wide range of mechanisms used depended to a great extent on the category or type of health care setting and patient involved.

Negotiation or conflict resolution was used by the majority of nurses in all health care settings and was found to be most helpful in psychiatry, ambulatory care and community care.

Physical defence was used the least. However, 80 per cent of the nurses having resorted to this response mechanism reported the action as being helpful. The use of physical intervention is controversial, as it touches on ethical and legal concerns. While the main defence to assault available to staff is said to be self-defence, many nurses are reluctant to use this mechanism and much ambiguity is reported. For example, 70 per cent of surveyed nurses in the Ontario study felt that it was inappropriate for nurses to deal physically with violent behaviour even if they had received self-defence training. Yet over half of these same nurses (76%) supported self-defence training as a strategy for reducing violence in the workplace (RNAO, 1991).

RESPONSE CONTINUUM

Once the violent incident is terminated, treatment of injuries, if required, takes precedence. Whether or not in need of treatment, during the follow-up period nursing personnel tend to choose among the responses below:

- *Avoidance* – This may involve avoidance of the problem or avoidance of the perpetrator of violence. Interference with the performance of duties becomes apparent and no resolution to the problem is possible.
- *Denial* – Frequently, traumatic events are suppressed. No resolution of the problem is possible and maladaptive behaviours may appear.
- *Discussion* – The incident is informally discussed with team members, family and/or friends. One study showed that discussion with team members was used most often and found to be helpful in preventing future occurrences of violence. Discussion with family

and/or friends was not found to be helpful in prevention (MARN, 1989).

- *Reporting* – Only one-fifth of cases are estimated to be officially reported. Most nurses who denounce such incidents feel they are not taken seriously and consider the effort not worthwhile. In one study where direct observation was used, it was noted that of 686 witnessed episodes of violence, only seven incident reports were filed (Erikson *et al.*, 2000). These researchers also found that the more prior assaults nurses had been subjected to, the less likely they were to report patient assaults. The phenomenon labelled 'habituation' may represent a formidable barrier to reporting violent incidents. At the same time, employers exert great pressure to withdraw such reports to avoid giving the institution a poor image for future patients, rather than facilitating reporting of all violent incidents and refraining from using hidden disincentives, threats or reprisals.

- *Counselling and debriefing* – Only 14.9 per cent of the respondents to a UK study reported having received counselling/follow-up support after an incident of violence (RCN, 1994). The positive impact of counselling services has been confirmed for both the victims of violence and persons indirectly involved in the incident. Debriefing techniques have been developed to 'enable the victim to re-experience the traumatic incident in a controlled and safe environment.... By giving the perception of control over their life back to the victim, debriefing can prevent the development of adverse reactions to the trauma' (RCN, 2000). Combining emotive and psycho-education techniques appears to facilitate emotional stability. Emotional care must 'aim to convey acceptance, respect and understanding; communicate empathy, reassurance and support; encourage ventilation of feelings; preserve dignity; empower the victim; provide anticipatory guidance and ensure adequate follow-up' (MacFarlane *et al.*, 1993). Legal counselling is often also advisable to assure that the rights of all those concerned in the case are interpreted correctly should legal action be pursued.

- *Prosecution* – Although nurses are not legally required to tolerate abusive behaviour, prosecuting offenders is rare. When a patient initiates violence, prosecution is often considered to be unprofessional and unethical. Nurses often blame themselves for being unable to cope with aggressive behaviour and feel ill prepared to defend their competence and legal rights in court. However, prosecution may be considered part of the nurse's healing process as well as a means to file compensation claims. Yet, prosecution is not viable in all cases; for example, psychotic patients are not considered responsible for their actions.

Effective responses to violence need to be developed. Prevention, however, is the best strategy. There needs to be a concerted effort to eliminate violence and its negative consequences. A zero-tolerance campaign must be widely introduced and reinforced.

SECURITY IN THE WORKPLACE

Where do we go from here? How do we ensure security in the workplace? Employers must provide—and employees have the right to expect—a safe work environment. This depends on the following six factors (see Figure 2). Each of these must be thoroughly investigated and appropriate measures taken to attain the highest level of safety against violence. Strategies adopted by the International Council of Nurses, a federation of over 120 national nurses' associations worldwide, include:

Social structure

As mentioned above, traditionally many cultures have covertly accepted physical violence, sexual harassment or verbal abuse against women. Complaints lodged by female nurses have frequently been minimised, ridiculed or considered useless in the light of 'human nature'. Violence directed toward male nurses appears to be less frequent but is in no way more tolerable. The pressures on female and male victims to remain silent are great and under-reporting has hampered the development of effective strategies to eliminate or at least reduce violence in the workplace. Respect of an individual's right to personal dignity and privacy must be integrated in the social norms and behaviour codes.

Legal context

Legislation must be introduced that will support all individuals' right to a safe work environment, including health care workers. Specific

Figure 2:

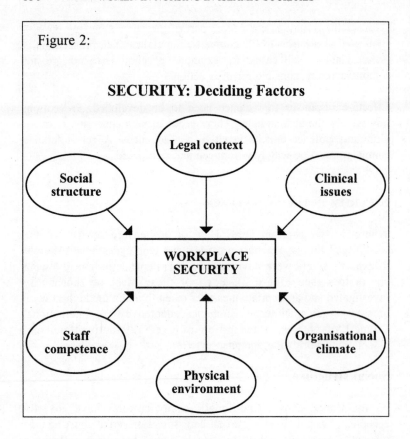

SECURITY: Deciding Factors

legislation dealing with security questions would mean that measures could be imposed on employers, mechanisms put in place to monitor their implementation and disciplinary steps taken in cases of non-compliance. Legislation can, for example, demand that hospitals perform a safety or risk assessment, analyse the incidents of violence observed or reported, develop a plan to correct the problems identified, impose specific educational requirements for certain high-risk employees or supervisors and discipline persons interfering with the reporting of any act of assault or violence. Legislation can also increase the penalties for assaults (verbal or physical) against health care workers.

Clinical issues

Research has not yet provided a reliable tool to predict the potential for violence although progress has been made (e.g. Brennan's Two-Minute Risk Assessment). Studies, however, support the theory that health care workers are at greatest risk of future assaults with the small percentage of patients who have a history of violent behaviour and who are, in fact, responsible for the majority of assaults.

Of particular significance is a history of violent behaviour within the past several hours. This has proved to be a strong predictor of assaults in the emergency department. By flagging charts of patients with a history of assaultive or disruptive behaviour, assaults against staff were reduced by 91 per cent in one study, highlighting the importance of taking a complete patient history.

The most useful criteria in indicating a potential for immediate violence have been changes in the patient's autonomic nervous system. Sweating, flushed face, changes in the size of the pupils of the eye, muscle tension are some of the subtle cues that can be identified by nurses. Other warning signals include a changed tone of voice (e.g. louder or sudden lowering in volume), a clenched fist, a tightened jaw, threatening language, pointing or jabbing with a finger, staring or avoidance of eye contact, invasion of personal space and increased activity (e.g. pacing in the hallway) (RCN, 2000). Nurses must learn to assess from a distance and to trust their instincts.

The majority of injuries from surveyed violent incidents have been sustained while containing patient violence, underlining the need for more appropriate containment techniques and/or staffing levels. Furthermore, the workplace should develop protocols and procedures with regard to chemical and medical restraint as well as seclusion, taking into account the therapeutic justification as well as the rights of the health care worker and the patient.

Organizational climate

An organization's formal policies and management attitudes greatly influence the climate in the workplace. The degree to which an individual's safety and dignity are considered important will greatly influence security within the work environment.

Management's traditional 'paternalistic' attitude towards nursing personnel has made many nurses feel dependent and helpless and thus guilt-ridden when unable to cope with violent incidents—encouraging the process of punishing the victim. Contrarily, management must send a strong, consistent message of zero-tolerance of abuse, sexual harassment and violence in the workplace. Supported by clear written policies and procedures—including confidential grievance machinery —this attitude must be integrated in the behaviour code of all employees and management.

A positive organizational climate includes the following aspects:

- Management ensures that staff are aware of their rights, legal requirements and responsibilities;
- Acknowledgement is made that violence will not be tolerated.
- Development of security policies are multi-disciplinary in their approach (administrative, nursing, medical, security, ancillary and maintenance staff).
- Decisions regarding violent patient admission and discharge are made jointly by the physician and the nurse.
- Security factors are regularly investigated to identify hazards and develop strategies to reduce them.
- Continuing education programmes are developed on containing occupational hazards, including violence, and sufficient work time is allocated for attendance (see also *Staff Competence* below).
- Staffing levels are determined to assure security of employees, as short-term and temporary staffing have been associated with increased incidents of violence in health units.
- The quality of care and competence of staff are maintained at optimal levels.
- Responsibility for unskilled workers is rationally allocated to professional staff.
- The health team skill mix meets patients' needs.
- Staff is allowed to introduce safe work protocols and organize their work accordingly.
- Professional staff is given some flexibility so that rules and policies are not interpreted by patients as intolerable constraints.
- Funds are allocated for the implementation and maintenance of security measures (i.e. security personnel, adequate lighting, alarms, telephone, guarded parking).
- Support structures (e.g. medical services, confidential grievance machinery, counselling services with debriefing teams

comprising mental health professionals) are easily accessible to workers.

- The responsibility and accountability for management of pre- and post-aggressive incident strategies are clearly outlined.
- Transportation policies take into account security risks for personnel.
- The movement and management of patients through various health units/services are rationalised and clear to those involved. For example, long waits in emergency rooms and the inability to obtain needed services or explanations have been cited as contributing to violence.
- High-risk activities and locations are identified and dealt with specifically (e.g. on-site storage of narcotics, cash-handling functions).
- Policies specific to field workers have been developed to deal with particular risks, e.g. regular reporting to base, visits in pairs to high-risk areas, police support for certain assignments, written protocols on when to stay or leave a high-risk situation.

Physical environment

All measures must be taken to reduce the physical environment aspects that accentuate stress and trigger violence. While these approaches have previously focused on hospitals and health centres, they can be applied to other health care settings as well. Examples of such measures include:

- Provide safe access to and from the workplace.
- Minimise access or entry points used by the public to health care facilities, including staff living quarters.
- Facilitate visitors' transit route from one main visitors' entrance.
- Place security services at main entrance, near visitors' transit route and emergency departments.
- Place staff parking areas within close range of workplace.
- Provide adequate and effective lighting.
- Facilitate appropriate routing of patients.
- Provide spacious and quiet reception areas, with sufficient space for personnel.
- Provide public toilets.
- Choose colours that do not encourage aggression.

- Allow observation of reception areas by staff.
- Reduce boredom by providing activities (e.g. reading materials, television).
- Choose furniture, fixtures and fittings that cannot be used as weapons. Pens, stethoscopes, cords and chairs can become dangerous in incidents of violence.
- Climate control.
- Install duress alarm systems at appropriate locations.
- Separate treatment rooms from public areas.
- Provide appropriate communication equipment for staff (e.g. mobile phones).
- Screen incomers through metal detectors.

Staff competence in dealing with violence

Inadequate training has been identified as a contributing factor to the prevalence of assaults and, in fact, research has shown that training in the management of assaultive behaviour can reduce injury from assault.

Attitudes are important in dealing with violence. The nurses' tendency to automatically blame themselves for such incidents must be eliminated. Nurses must openly recognise that violence and harassment are intolerable in the workplace and no longer accept such incidents. An attitude of zero-tolerance is essential if sound policies are to be developed and conscientiously implemented. A comprehensive educational programme would, therefore, include:

- Level of risk based upon historical data.
- Legal and ethical rights and responsibilities of workers and management.
- Employer's policy and procedures related to aggressive patients (i.e. prevention, management and follow-up).
- Medical/psychiatric/social causes of aggressive behaviour.
- Triggers that provoke violence in the health care setting.
- The assault cycle.
- Recognition of impending violence.
- Techniques to interrupt escalating violent behaviour.
- Techniques of negotiation and conflict resolution.
- Communication skills, including assertiveness training and debriefing skills.

- Techniques of medical and physical restraint.
- Post-incident management and analysis.

CONCLUSIONS

Supported by the research previously mentioned, various points can be highlighted:

- Violence in society is an increasing problem.
- Violence is highly destructive and has long-term, as well as, short-term effects on its victims.
- Health personnel in general and nursing personnel in particular are victims of abuse and violence in the workplace.
- Society and health sector stakeholders have responded in various ways to incidents of violence and with varying degrees of success.

Violence in society is a challenge of already epidemic proportions. Women are often considered legitimate targets of violence and this attitude must change. Health care workers, especially nursing personnel, are recognised as being at higher personal risk. Nurses, predominantly women, are victims of the rise in domestic as well as workplace violence. Particular attention needs to be placed on the elimination of abuse and violence against nursing personnel, as they represent a category of workers considered most vulnerable. It must be stressed that such acts perpetrated against any category of health personnel, employed person or private citizen, must be strongly condemned.

Once violence in the workplace is identified as a concern, as a professional issue and as a labour priority, the stakeholders need to develop appropriate strategies to eliminate, or at least reduce the number of such incidents. The mechanisms listed above when adapted to a given work setting may assist this process and advance the zero-tolerance campaign against violence. Attention needs to be focused on social structure, legal context, clinical issues, organizational climate, physical environment and staff competence.

Violence in the health sector is highly destructive and has a negative impact not only on the professional and personal lives of health care providers but also on the quality and coverage of services delivered. All stakeholders, including patients, must be concerned and take action now.

156 WOMEN IN NURSING IN ISLAMIC SOCIETIES

BIBLIOGRAPHY

Chappell, D. and Di Martino, V. (1998). *Violence at Work*. Geneva: ILO.
Health & Safety Commission. (1997). *Violence and Aggression to Staff in Health Services: Guidance on assessment and management*. London: HSE.
ICN. (1997). *Guidelines on Coping with Violence at the Workplace*. Geneva: ICN.
Occupational Safety and Health Administration. (1993). *Guidelines for Security and Safety of Health Care and Community Service Workers*. Washington: US Department of Labor.
————. (1996). *Guidelines for Preventing Workplace Violence for Health Care and Social Service Workers*. Washington: US Department of Labor.
RCN. (1998). *Dealing with Violence Against Nursing Staff: An RCN guide for nurses and managers*. London: Royal College of Nursing.
RCN/NHS Executive. (1998). *Safer Working in the Community: A guide for NHS managers and staff on reducing the risks from violence and aggression*. London: Royal College of Nursing.
Registered Nurses' Association of Nova Scotia. (1997). *Violence in the Workplace: A resource guide*. Ottawa: RNANS.
Reinhart, A. (1999). *Sexual Harassment: Addressing sexual harassment in the workplace—a management information booklet*. Geneva: ILO.

REFERENCES

Affi, L. Arraweelo. (1995). 'A Role Model For Somali Women.' Presentation: Somali Peace Conference.
Amarsi, Y. (1999). 'Key Stakeholders' Perceptions of NHRD in Pakistan.' Unpublished doctoral dissertation. McMaster University.
Bokhari, A. (1990). 'Nursing Grievances.' *The Herald*. February: 60-63.
Carroll, V., Morin, K. (1998). 'Workplace violence affects one-third of nurses.' *Nursing World*. September-October.
Crossette, B. (2000). 'Unicef Opens a Global Drive On Violence Against Women.' *New York Times*. 9 March.
Erickson, L., Williams-Evans, A. (2000). 'Attitudes of emergency nurses regarding patient assaults.' *Journal of Emergency Nursing*. June: 210-215.
Goodman, E. (2000). 'Honour Killers of Woman Get Away With Murder.' *Herald Tribune*. 28 March.
Goodwin, J. (1994). *Price of Honour: Muslim women lift the veil of silence on the Islamic world*. NY: Little Brown & Co.
Graydon, J., Kasta, W., Khan, P. (1994). 'Verbal and physical abuse of nurses.' *Canadian Journal of Nursing Administration*. 7(4):70-89.
Heise, L., Ellsberg, M. and Gottemoeller, M. (1999). 'Ending Violence Against Women.' Population Reports. Baltimore: Johns Hopkins University School of Public Health.
Hirschfeld, M., Henry, B., Griffith, H. (1993). 'Nursing Personnel Resources.' Results of a survey of perceptions in ministries of health on nursing shortage, nursing education and quality of care. Geneva: WHO.
HSC. (1997). 'Violence and Aggression to staff in health services. Guidance on Assessment and Management.' Norwich: HSC.

ICN. (1994). 'Guidelines on Coping with Violence in the Workplace.' Geneva: ICN.

ILO. (1998). 'Violence at Work.' Geneva: D. Chappell and V. Di Martino.

_____. (1999). 'Sexual Harassment. Addressing sexual harassment in the workplace.' A management information booklet. An ILO survey of company practice. Geneva: A. Reinhart.

ILO/ICN/WHO/PSI. (2002). 'Joint Programme on Workplace Violence in the Health Sector.' Geneva: ILO.

Islam, T. (1998). 'Population-Bangladesh: Ban on Export of Nurses Criticised.' *World News.* 17 August.

Jan, R. (1996). 'A Cultural Dilemma. Pakistani Nursing.' *Reflections.* 4th Quarter: 19.

Jawaid, A. (1998). 'International Women's Day. The march forward.' *The Review.* 5-11 March: 4-11.

Khan, N. (2000). Islam and Feminism. Video. 3 April.

Kisa, A., Dziegielewswki, S.F. (1996). 'Sexual Harassment of female nurses in a hospital in Turkey.' *Health Services Management Research.* 9(4):243-53.

Klasra, M. (1997). 'Women's Rights in a Man's Society.' *Dawn.* 20 June.

MacFarlane, E., Hawley P. (1993). 'Sexual assault: Coping with crisis.' *The Canadian Nurse.* June: 21-24.

Mahoney, B.S. (1990). Doctoral dissertation.

Manderino, M.A., Berkey, N. (1997). 'Verbal abuse of staff nurses by physicians.' *Journal of Professional Nursing.* 13(1):48-55.

Manitoba Association of Registered Nurses. (1989). 'Nurse Abuse Report.' Winnipeg: MARN.

Neurath, P. (1996). 'Violence stalks the health-care field.' *Puget Sound Business Journal,* 16 September.

NHS. (1999). 'Managers' Guide—Stopping Violence Against Staff Working in the NHS.' London: NHS.

Nurse Assault Project Team. (1991). 'Executive Summary.' Registered Nurses Association of Ontario.

Poster, E.C. and Ryan, J. (1993). 'Nursing staff responses to patient physical assaults.' Presentation at Conference. *Violence: Nursing Debates the Issues.* American Academy of Nursing.

RCN. (1998). 'Safer Working in the Community: A guide for NHS managers and staff on reducing the risks from violence and aggression.' Nottingham: Phil Leather, Tom Cox, Diane Beale and Bridgette Fletcher.

_____. (2000). *Nursing Standard.* 14(28): workbook.

_____. (1998). 'Dealing with Violence Against Nursing Staff. An RCN Guide for nurses and managers.' London: RCN.

_____, Australia. (1998). 'Violence and Nursing.' Australia: Jan Horsfall.

Registered Nurses' Association of Nova Scotia. (1996). *Violence in The Workplace: A Resource Guide.* Nova Scotia: RNANS.

Reuters. 'Beating Women Isn't a Crime in Many Places, Report Finds.'

Royal College of Nursing. (1994). 'Violence and Community Nursing Staff.' London: RCN.

Samath, F. (1997). 'Neglect will stop economic takeoff: WB'. *Dawn Journal.* 23 October.

Shaikh, M.A. (2000). 'Sexual harassment in medical profession—perspective from Pakistan.' *Journal of the Pakistan Medical Association.* 50(4):130-1.

Shamim, A. (1998). 'Changing images of unsung nightingales.' *The News on Sunday.* 5 April.

Taylor, D. (1999). 'Student preparation in managing violence and aggression.' *Nursing Standard.* 14(30): 39-41.

The Frontier Post. (2000). 'Minister eulogises nurses' services.' 10 February.

US Department of Labor. (1996). 'Guidelines for Preventing Workplace Violence for Health Care and Social Service Workers.' Washington: US Dept. of Labor.

UNISON. 'Violence at Work. A Guide to risk prevention for UNISON branches, stewards and safety representatives.' London: UNISON.

APHA. (2000). 'Violence against world's women is widespread.' *The Nation's Health.* Washington, DC: APHA. March.

Whitehorn, D., Nowlan, M. (1997). 'Towards an aggression-free health care environment.' *Canadian Nurse.* 93(3):24-6.

Worthington, K. (1993). 'Taking action against violence in the workplace.' *The American Nurse.* June: 12.

7

Women of Pakistan:
Trapped but Struggling

Kausar S. Khan

INTRODUCTION

The women of Pakistan present a tragic picture, and the evidence is everywhere. It is to be found in the local newspapers, in reports of human rights groups, both local and international, and in the scanty research undertaken in the country.

Pick up any local newspaper any day, and there will be reports of grossly unfair treatment of women placidly tucked away in the inside pages, and not too infrequently there will be the sensational case that is splashed on the front page. Newspaper coverage suggests that the literate class (about 20 per cent of the population) are well aware of the injustices meted out to women in Pakistan, while the vast majority, the semi-literate and illiterate masses, seem to silently accept the status quo. The bulk of the literate population does not react, and at best there is a quiet stirring of discomfort voiced in cocooned privacy. This is not to say that nobody reacts, for there is a persistent reaction, even if from a tiny minority of concerned persons and groups. And this is where the paradox of Pakistan is to be found: gruesome reality that is known, reported and talked about; an overall tacit acceptance by society at large which reads and ignores the issues; and the persistent protest and activism of non-government organizations, individual activists, writers and poets committed to women's rights and human rights.

The newspapers of Pakistan bring, every day, news that shares a common theme—i.e., women must not make choices, even for their own lives. The newspapers report: a woman killed because she was seeking divorce; two women of the same family shot dead by a male

---

Excerpt from Amnesty International Report, 1999

According to the non-governmental Human Rights Commission of Pakistan (HRCP), 888 women were reported deliberately killed in 1998 in Punjab alone. Of these, 595 killings were carried out by relatives; of these, 286 were reportedly killed for reasons of honour. The Sindh Graduates Association said that in the first three months of 1999 alone, 132 honour killings had been reported in Sindh. Everyone contacted by Amnesty International about the incidence of honour killings in Pakistan held that the real number of such killings is vastly greater than the number reported.

In a total of 196 cases reported in Sindh, 255 persons were killed, including 158 women and 97 men. The data does not in all cases include information about the perpetrators, but of 154 persons killed for reasons of honour where the relation of the perpetrator to the victim is given:

- *In forty-six instances exactly one-half of the killings were carried out by the husband and the other half by male relatives of the murdered women.*
- *Of the eighty-one women killed alone, forty were killed by their husbands, thirty-six by male relatives, including brothers, fathers, uncles or sons, and five by others including their fathers-in-law or brothers-in-law.*
- *Of the twenty-seven men killed, three were killed by the husbands of the alleged kari (sic woman killed), and twenty-one by other male relatives of the women, with three killed by others, including the husband's relatives.*[2]

---

family member after being brought back by those who abducted them; a woman shot to death by her brothers; a woman hacked to death by her father; a woman strangulated by her husband; a woman shot dead by her son, and so on and so forth. As Hina Jilani, a woman and a human rights lawyer says, '*The right to life of women in Pakistan is conditional on their obeying social norms and traditions.*'

Thus, although the harshness of women's existence in Pakistan is very visible, silence prevails over its more murky depths and the scale of protest and demands for change are abominably inadequate.

In order to fully understand the struggle to change the socio-cultural and legal environment that affects women negatively one needs to understand the following:

a) What constitutes the realities of the women of Pakistan.
b) The issues of safe motherhood.

A Mosaic of Some Hard Facts

'The status of women is considerably worse in South Asia than in most of the world. And within South Asia, Pakistan has one of the worst records in female health and education. Pakistan's fertility rate of 5.4 is considerably higher than that of any other large Asian country, and as many as 1 in every 38 women die from pregnancy-related causes—compared, for example with 1 in 230 women in Sri Lanka.'[3]

'We all know that women have a very unequal status in Pakistan—30% of our population lives below the poverty line and women bear the brunt of this because their access to resources is less than that of men..... Only 23% of adult women are literate compared to 49% of men; 49% of girls are enroled in primary schools compared to 80% of boys. Some 28% of women participate in the labour force compared to 72% of men and as far as their income is concerned, women's income is 19% compared to men's income of 81%. Only 3% of administrative and management positions are occupied by women, compared to 97% by men and women's representation in Parliament is only 2% compared to 98% for men.[4]

'An important aspect to be examined is the contradiction between their (sic women) legal status on the books and their legal status in actual practice. Even where the constitution or the laws accord women a high or equal status, social norms and customs make their constitutional and statutory rights seem like a mockery. Forced marriages, restrictions on their right to work or educate themselves, denial of inheritance of property and lack of control over their earnings are some of the most common examples of socially accepted practices within the country. In actual fact, the majority of women in Pakistan are not even aware of their legal rights and they live in accordance with the cultural norms and traditional laws which regulate their lives, even overriding religious injunctions.'[5]

'Pakistan's political history, like many of its neighbours, is one of frequent crisis and incomplete resolution. These crises are woven into the texture of its history, its concepts of itself and its sense of political possibility. The country has fought foreign wars...and domestic wars...the disruptions and discontents of civil society have often skirted the edges of state violence, and have given continued cause for citizens to re-examine their relationships to the state in which they live. Its history and future alike are intricately linked to its overlapping ideological moorings, its economic and social conditions, and the instrumental goals of the state. For almost five decades, conflicts over the role of religion in society, democracy in the polity and the transformative capacities of state institutions in the economy have been the underpinnings for a politics of unique opportunity and often, profound division and dismay.'[6]

'In the fifty-five years since its independence, Pakistan has struggled with constitutions, governments and the structure of the state. It has swung between the poles of dictatorship and democracy, and between civilian and military rule. Although it was established with a parliamentary system of government, the military has seized power four times since 1947, ruling directly and indirectly for more than half the life of the country. Intervening periods of elected, civilian government have responded to popular fears of renewed military rule by accommodating the army to prevent its re-emergence in politics. Each permutation of power has therefore embodied deep popular concerns and ambivalence about government, its patrons and its beneficiaries.'[7]

'Among the most lethal forces which impact (on) women's dignity and security are customary practices which aim at preserving female subjugation. Often defended and sanctified as cultural tradition, they are usually fiercely defended by those who practice them, shrugged off by society and condoned by law-enforcing agencies and the courts. As a result, most of these inhuman practices continue unabated.'[8]

The above quotes are self-explanatory in the sense of laying down the larger context within which the women of Pakistan live out their lives. The outcome of this context is perhaps best represented by the idea of 'the missing women'. Compared to Sub-Saharan Africa, where the female-male ratio (FMR) is 1.022, the ratio in Pakistan is 0.905 (it is 0.933 in India and 0.940 in Bangladesh and 0.941 in China). According to the calculations given by Amartya Sen,[9] there are 5.2 million women missing in Pakistan, a proportion of 12.9 per cent (the proportion is the 'ratio of missing women to the actual number of women in a particular country'). This figure is the highest in the world; the proportion of missing women in China is 8.6 per cent. In India it is 9.5 per cent and in Bangladesh it is 8.7 per cent. In lay terms it means that though economically Pakistan may be better off than Sub-Saharan Africa, there are more women dying in Pakistan than anywhere in the world. If death is to be the ultimate metaphor for social injustice towards women in any society, then it is Pakistan which tops the list. This is the hardest fact to grapple with if the well-being of women is to be brought to the centre-stage of Pakistani society.

WHAT HAS CHANGED—UNDERSTANDING THE ISSUES THROUGH THE GENDER LENS

In view of the rudimentary sketch of the social picture presented above, one now needs to understand the bluntness of the efforts for improving women's health.

We must understand the complexity of the issues that surround a woman's existence, and make visible the gaps in the efforts for safe motherhood. This understanding should not only be an intellectual grasp of a tragic situation (for the intellect is often at a loss to understand the existential nuances of life), but going beyond the intellect one would need to pause, and allow a woman's life to speak to us. As we listen—and not only to the words, but also between the words, we wonder how safe *really* is her motherhood. If we can begin to sense the apparently hidden dimensions of motherhood on which are predicated the risks to her very existence, we may begin to understand why the interventions in her name are not as effective as justice would demand.

In the last fifty years, the number of health facilities has increased, both in the urban and rural areas. Today, there are far more health care providers than there were fifty years ago. One can safely state that every decade has made available something new, something useful for women. Yet the question remains, how have changes in society touched women like Fatima, who are a majority today, just as Fatima's mother and grandmother were a majority during the prime of their lives?

ADVANCES IN HEALTH CARE AND LIMITED BENEFITS

Even if there is not much significant difference in the day to day lives of the Fatimas of today and of yesteryears, there is definitely a substantive difference in the context of their lives. Around them, there

---

Fatima

It is Fatima's tenth pregnancy, and she has been married for barely 12 years. Fatima is 27 years old, but looks to be much older. She is always tired though her emaciated body continues to work for 18 hours a day.

Fatima is neither despondent nor disgusted with life; she is neither a skeptic nor a cynic; she is simply a woman who is driven to care for her children, her husband, and her family which includes her in-laws, but excludes her parents and brothers and sisters. She herself is not the centre of her life, but she definitely is the central figure in the lives of those she supports through her responsibilities towards them. Whether her role is valued is a different matter. That she is taken for granted and never appreciated is a reality she seldom considers.

Fatima has studied till class three, and laments without any bitterness at being removed from the school by her father. She had accepted her fate, and was not like the few in her village who had protested and pestered their families for the continuation of their schooling. Fatima felt obliged to acquiesce by helping her mother, who was always busy. In so doing she had been moulded and prepared for her role as a woman in Pakistan.

Fatima's mother had over ten pregnancies. She does not remember the exact number. She likes to focus on the number of boys she has.

Fatima's grandmother was also married very young, and too had a large brood of children.

Fatima's daughter was ten years old, and was studying in class four at the school near her village. The middle school was 20 kilometres away...chances of Fatima's daughter studying beyond primary school seemed bleak. It was immaterial whether she continued her studies; it would not make much difference to her life, Fatima would tell her daughter.

---

are more options (for schools and health facilities) in terms of sheer numbers. There are more trained health staff, and even the *dais* (the traditional birth attendants) today are trained, and more advanced technologies are now available. There are also more people talking of safe-motherhood than there were in the 1970s and 1980s. The media, too, especially the electronic media, has expanded in leaps and bounds; there are more surveys and more research being conducted now than twenty years ago. Yet, what have been the gains of the Fatimas of our society?

How safe is the motherhood of Fatima? Most healthcare providers are likely to focus on services available, and many would be concerned with the quality and effectiveness of the services. Some could go beyond the technical issues, and look for the issues of access to available services: why a woman does not come for ante-natal check-ups, why does she delay accessing the services, why does she not take food according to her need, why does she not use contraceptive services, etc. These providers may even consider the attitude of the health care providers as a factor that discourages a woman from accessing services; and they may also look at the timings and duration of the services made available. In so doing they may be taking a hard and thoughtful look at the behaviour of women who, according to them, should access the available services for their own good. Some of them may even launch an 'information, education campaign' so that women's behaviour may change for the better. There is probably adequate evidence that such campaigns have brought about change in women's behaviour, and have enhanced the safety of their motherhood. Whether such behaviour becomes an integral part of women's lives is not very clear (researchers could perhaps have the answer). However, it is debatable whether behavioural change is rooted in drumming a message (like selling a product), or if it is more likely to be sustainable when it becomes part of a belief-system—a system where a woman's perception of her rights and responsibilities is not blindly lived, but understood, negotiated, interpreted and consciously chosen.

If the concern for safe motherhood is to go beyond the issues of health services, and to go beyond the mere description of the enigma of women not accessing available services, it could mean a new venture. It would then require working with concepts that could help understand the barriers to women's access to available services, irrespective of the issues of quality and effectiveness, and affordability and cultural sensitivity of the services. It would amount to venturing into the gender related determinants of women's health behaviour and health-seeking behaviour. This would require a clear understanding of *how* what she does has something to do with her *position and status in society,* and what safe-motherhood interventions try to address are her *practical needs,* and not her *strategic interests* (which are linked to her *status* in society). This conceptual dyad of *practical needs* and *strategic interests* is but one analytical tool that helps one to comprehend the critical shift from the narrow focus on women, to gender and social relations. This is but one of the fruits of the advances in the thinking on women and gender.

There have been considerable advances in the thinking on gender and development, and many efforts are being made to apply the understanding of gender to health. (This is still not so in the mainstream of the health sector, even though the word 'gender' has entered the discourse of health but is often limited to just the desegregation of the data). It would thus perhaps be useful to conduct a gender analysis of safe motherhood by relating some of the central concepts in gender-thinking to women's health.

GENDER ANALYSIS OF THE CONTEXT OF SAFE MOTHERHOOD

Three sets of concepts can be evoked to examine the context of safe-motherhood—the context being the larger social milieu. This social context constitutes the web of relations which govern women's lives and within which each woman plays out her life—most of the time according to the script prepared for her by society. Fortunately, all women do not live according to the script society has prepared for them. Many women, from different classes, have rewritten the pre-given scripts by accessing their own strength and vision. Whenever a woman does this, or is supported/facilitated to do so, her *strategic interests* can be said to have been met.

Practical needs and *strategic interests:* this is one set of gender-concepts that has already been mentioned. While considerable material exists on these concepts, suffice it to say that in the health context, addressing women's *practical needs* is to consider their immediate needs of: addressing gynaecological morbidity; safe delivery; nutritional needs, especially during pregnancy and lactation period; use of contraception; immunisation against tetanus; etc. Women's *strategic interests*, on the other hand, would be for a woman to be able to decide how many children she wants; to be able to say 'no' to her husband, if she does not want to have sex; to be able to take action when inflicted with violence; *to have a say* in their children's education, especially their daughter's, etc. In short, women's strategic interests entail acquiring a status or position in society that is equal to a man's in terms of rights and dignity. Thus, whereas women's practical needs relate to the concrete conditions (multiple pregnancies, anaemia, illiteracy, battering, etc.) all these factors contribute to what can be called 'at risk motherhood'. For motherhood to be safe and sustainable, women's status in society would have to change.

Women's status in society will improve when their strategic interests are addressed and met, and when this happens their health conditions too will improve. Right now, most interventions for promoting safe-motherhood focus on women's practical needs, and it seems a tacit assumption that this would lead to changes in women's status. One seldom, if ever, comes across interventions that deliberately work for women's strategic interests, and then consider the impact on women's practical needs.

Access and control are the two other categories of thought that are significant in the analysis of gender and development. The issues of access and control are to be seen in the context of resources—whatever they may be. At the household level, the resources could be food, money, time, and the assets related to a household: land, furniture, jewellery, physical space in the house, etc. The question thus is, what is the status of a woman within her household? Does she have equal access to the resources in the household? Furthermore, does she have equal control over the resources?

The same questions can also be raised for the larger society within which the woman lives. Here, in the larger context, the resources would include services like health, education, credit, information, training, transport, etc. How much access do women have to the resources available, and do they exercise any control over the resources?

There is likely to be a great variety in the extent of access and control that women may have. Detailed analysis can be done for specific groups of women or for larger communities and/or population groups—an exercise that is not within the scope of this chapter. Here it will suffice to say that women, by and large, experience considerable internal and external barriers to accessing resources, and have minimal, if any, control over the resources. With respect to the health of women, it would be useful to consider how many women have control over their own bodies—irrespective of their class, ethnicity, religion, profession, etc. When women do not have control over something as intimate as their own bodies, and also encounter major hurdles to accessing resources, what difference does even the best of health services make to their lives? This is not to say that health services should not be improved, or that quality and effectiveness and affordability are not significant issues for promoting women's health.

The concern here is whether such realisation could help us begin to question the distribution of two most critical resources, the time and money of the policy makers and implementers. What portion of time and money is allocated to addressing service-issues, as compared to the issues of gender relations, and the related socio-economic issues?

Another set of concepts in gender analysis revolve round women's roles. Two roles are taken into consideration, namely: *productive* roles and *reproductive* roles. (Sometimes 'community management' is also listed as a role, but in the present context the other two roles will suffice.)

Even a very simple tabulation of activities in which women and men are involved, reveals that women invariably are more involved in reproductive roles, which seems to be their prime responsibility. (Reproductive roles are all those activities which reproduce and sustain life and relations. In short, all that would go under 'caring' for the family members). Men, on the other hand, are primarily involved in productive activities (except when they are unemployed), and reproductive activities are more often than not optional for them. Furthermore, besides this division of male-female labour into types of activities, it is also important to note that there are economic returns in productive activities, while reproductive work is primarily unpaid work (except when it is sold as a service by either men or women, for example, cooking, washing clothes, etc. When a traditionally reproductive activity is sold as a service, it then falls in the category of productive work.) Societies world-wide place greater value on activities that are productive, and there is little or no value attributed to reproductive work. (The verbal appreciation that is often bestowed on reproductive work needs to be re-assessed by relating it to the extent of access and control a woman has to resources.)

Women's reproductive health is often interpreted only in the context of 'producing babies,' and the biological hurdles or difficulties she may encounter. The challenge that the gender-perspective provides lies in seeing how women's gynaecological morbidity and safe delivery of babies can be related to the issue of the larger reproductive roles and activities and the lack of value of these roles and activities. It would also be useful if health care planners were to analyse why and how the division of labour takes place, whereby less valuable work (that which does not have economic returns) is assigned to women and more valuable work to men, and how do these factors affect women's health? Once this is understood, perhaps health planners and implementers will start looking for ways that could bring changes in the division of labour.

The reproductive health package that the Government of Pakistan has developed for the women of Pakistan focuses entirely on women's practical needs. It does not indicate any awareness of the importance of the issue of division of labour, whereby women's roles are socially confined to reproductive roles while the society values productive roles.

The pursuit of safe-motherhood should not lead one only to health services (even though considerable work is still pending in this area). If women are themselves to be involved in their own safety, then the gender issues also need to be addressed. Health providers often do not see the need for creating an 'enabling environment' for women. Without this environment, women's access to resources will be minimal, and control over resources would be even less. If health providers concern themselves only with service-delivery, they may succeed in meeting some of the practical needs of women, but women's strategic interests would still be neglected and would continue to engender hurdles to their health. Unless efforts are also made for larger changes in the value-systems in society (i.e. where the productive and reproductive roles are equally valued, so that hierarchies are not created between men and women) women will continue to be trapped in their reproductive roles, and these roles will continue to be less valued. Different values are associated with differences in rights; and with differences in rights comes imbalances in relationships whereby one is subordinated (i.e. women) and the other dominates (i.e. primarily men, but often assisted by those women allies who also see the world from their existing social-lens and not through the gender-lens.)

Can there *really* be safe motherhood without tackling larger and long-term issues of division of labour, in which men and women are blindly trapped because their society has so constructed their roles? Is it fair that all efforts be made for addressing *only* the practical needs of women? Would Fatima's health be ensured without raising the gender issues?

TRAPPED BUT STRUGGLING

Women of Pakistan have shown an admirable resilience to struggle for better opportunities in their lives. As individuals, small groups and coalitions of groups, they have lobbied with the government of the day; protested and demonstrated on the streets; questioned discriminatory laws and petitioned against them; internationalized issues as and when needed; kept a vigil on attacks by misogynists; and lobbied with progressive elements of society, whether they be trade unionists, cultural groups or other interest groups. The strategy all along has been to be vocal and to be peaceful. Women have persevered but the struggle has not been easy. They have had to struggle against the State, as well as the parliamentarians (for example, in 1999, women's groups and human rights groups lobbied the Senate of Pakistan to condemn the killing of women in the name of honour, but the Senate failed to do so). The judiciary too has not always been forthcoming, and perhaps the greatest adversary has been the politicised religious groups seeking political power and striving to espouse their ideals through control of women. Moreover, even the apparently 'progressive' individuals and groups have not been as supportive as was hoped. To illustrate one has only to recall what a senator said in defence of the Senate's failure to allow a debate on the issue of killing of women in the name of honour: he opined that the government could not permit the debate because of the 'political reality on the ground.'[10]

This section will try to capture the quagmire in which the women of Pakistan are trapped, and also present some examples of the resilience and strength of these women.

In 1989, a rape case in one of the leading teaching hospitals in Karachi lead to a flurry of activities by women activists of the city. A student nurse and a resident nurse had been raped by a fourth year medical student and his friends in a private room of the hospital. There was instant reaction by women's group and human rights groups. Activism had started, even though nurses in the concerned hospital were apprehensive about taking direct action for fear of reprisal. Support was provided to the two nurses and leading lawyers were consulted. There was a protest march and a street play was performed on the hospital premises to highlight the injustice and motivate people to join the protest. The case was followed in the courts, and monitored in the press.

The case became centre stage of the women's movement in Karachi. Its impact in generating activism within the nursing profession was witnessed a few months later when in another government hospital in Karachi nurses protested against sexual harassment by some physicians. Women's groups closed ranks in support of the nurses and a private school of nursing joined the protest in full force.

The report of the National Commission for Women, 1997, stated:

Among the most lethal forces which impact [on] women's dignity and security are customary practices which aim at preserving female subjugation. Often defended and sanctified as cultural traditions, they are usually fiercely defended by those who practice them, shrugged off by society and condoned by law-enforcing agencies and the courts. As a result, most of these inhuman practices continue unabated.[11]

Such reports reflect the concern of the State that something needs to be done to ameliorate the status of women in Pakistan. Unfortunately, the inability of the State to bring significant improvement to the lives of women is indicative of a deep-rooted incompetence and lack of will. Pakistan's brief history presents distinct periods of sensitivity to the quagmire of unfairness in which women were trapped and other periods, dark and nauseating, when the State itself became belligerent and tried to clobber women into narrow peripheries of human existence.

The three main periods identified by a women's resource group Shirkat Gah were: 1947–1970: The Initial Years; 1971–1977: Impetus for Women; and 1977–1988: A Period of Reversals.

Life in Pakistan has not been a smooth unfolding of events ensuring a progressively better life for women (and other vulnerable groups, i.e., the poor in general). Socio-economic progress has not been impressive, and political instability has been the chief identifying feature of Pakistani society. The outcome has been a rapid rise in the incidence of violence and insecurity. Pakistan's priorities have continued to ignore the poor and disadvantaged, with the defence 'needs' of the country and its nuclear programme siphoning its meagre resources.

Women of Pakistan have used whatever avenue was available to them to forge new pathways for the betterment of women. They have also created new space for advancing their cause. A review of research on women reveals a steady progress in the development of critical

Critical Periods in the History of Women in Pakistan

1947–1970: The Initial Years

With independence, women were granted the right to educational, political and economic participation; but the demand for 'equal rights' was opposed by conservative factions who had enough (or were perceived by other political forces to have enough) leverage to prevent a consensus on women's greater participation in the development process. The fact that only a small number of women were lobbying for women's rights facilitated the side-tracking or overshadowing of women's issues by what were seen as greater policy matters. For example, in 1948 women members of the National Assembly proposed a bill to secure women's economic rights. The bill was dropped from the agenda until thousands of women marched on the Assembly of Chambers in protest. The ability of women legislators to publicly mobilise women resulted in the passage of the West Punjab Muslim Personal Law (Shariat Application Act 1948 IX of 1948) which recognised women's right to inherit property, including agricultural holdings.

1971–1977: Impetus for Women

The 1971–1977 Z.A. Bhutto era was a period of progress for women. Widespread politicalisation of women was undertaken by Bhutto's Pakistan People's party. Begum Nasim Jahan, a PPP founder member, mobilised educated women to impart the party message in Lahore *mohallas* (neighbourhoods). The political sensitisation of women was extended when the PPP set up a Women's Wing with provincial links. In 1972 all government posts and services were opened to women and for the first time women were appointed as Provincial Governor, University Vice Chancellor and Deputy Speaker of the National Assembly.

1977–1988: A Period of Reversals

In July 1977 the coup d'etat that brought in martial law under General Zia-ul-Haq heralded in a period of reversal for women. Retrogressive laws such as the Hudood Ordinances (1979) and the Law of Evidence (1984) were brought on the statute book, others were proposed and directives curtailing women's participation in public life introduced. Paradoxically, by sharply focusing attention on gender issues and discrimination, the reversals of women's right galvanised a wide spectrum of women and women's groups to form a women's rights lobby.... In the following decade WAF (Women's Action Federation) remained the most active women's rights lobby and pressure group.[12]

thinking and analysis of issues revolving around women.[13] The '50s and '60s represent what the reviewer called the Budding Thoughts, wherein it was foreign researchers who undertook anthropological studies on women. The '70s saw a beginning in the development of local concerns. Women's and development issues were raised and discussed in this period. The '80s saw the rise of critical thinking among women activists. 'There is also a growth of feminism, of multi-disciplinary approaches that reflect and resemble changes the world over. Possibly too, the generation of young women politicised during the seventies started to write seriously and to publish in the eighties.'[14] The '90s, despite the socio-political uncertainties, saw more steady work on women and by women. Issues of violence against women, reproductive health and rights, women and law, etc, started to be pursued in a more systematic manner.

Swimming against the current of religious intolerance and political uncertainties, the women of Pakistan continue to work for increasing choices, for their rightful place as equal members of society, and for social justice and peace.

NOTES

1. Amnesty International's Report, 'Pakistan: Violence against women in the name of honour', *Slogan*, Vol. 10, No. 12, September 1999, p. 10.
2. Amnesty International's Report, 'Pakistan: Violence against women in the name of honour', *Slogan*, Vol. 10, No. 12, September 1999, p. 15.
3. A.G. Tinker, 'Improving Women's Health in Pakistan', *Human Development Network*, Health, Nutrition, and Population Series, Washington, D.C.: The World Bank, 1998, p. 5.
4. M. Hussain, Review of Services Available to Women, 'New Directions in Research for Women', Proceedings: National Conference on New Directions in Research for Women, May 1997, p. 9.
5. S. Zia, 'The Legal Status of women in Pakistan', in F. Zafar (ed.), *Finding Our Way—Readings on women in Pakistan*, Lahore, Pakistan: ASR Publications, 1991, pp. 29-30.
6. P.R. Newberg, *Judging the State–courts and constitutional politics in Pakistan*, New Delhi: Cambridge University Press, 1995, pp. 2-3.
7. Ibid., p. 9.
8. Report of the Commission of Inquiry for Women, August 1997.
9. Amartya Sen and Jean Drèze, *Hunger and Public action*, Oxford: Clarendon Press, 1989, p. 52.
10. Quoted in *Slogan*, Vol. 11, Issue 1, Oct. 1999, p. 8.
11. Report of the Commission of Inquiry for Women, August 1997, set up on the basis of a resolution of the Pakistan Senate.

12. F. Shaheed et al., *Women in Politics*, Lahore: Shirkat Gah Publication, May 1994, pp. 5-7.
13. Proceedings from The Aga Khan University Conference, Farida Shaheed, 'New Directions in Research on Women', 1997.
14. Ibid., p. 14.

8

Nursing Education in the Eastern Mediterranean Region: A World Health Organization Initiative

Fariba Al-Darazi

The nursing profession in the Eastern Mediterranean Region (EMR) has developed in a varied manner in the twenty-two countries that comprise the region.[1] Factors determining the characteristics of nursing and nursing education are numerous and diverse, including influences of: nursing heritage from the colonial era; missionary health workers and educators from an assortment of mission societies of western Europe and North America; cultural and traditional views about education of girls and women; national and local customs about women's roles in the home vs. a career; and slowness of impact of efforts within each country to achieve significant change.

Among the many factors at work, the following have compromised the quality of nursing and nursing education: a lack of power and control by nurses over nursing education; a lack of quality standards; failure to attract or in some cases even allow males into the profession; upper age limits excluding adult learners; variation in entrance requirements from six years of general education to twelve years; variation in curriculum length from twelve months to five years; curriculum content that is oriented toward the medical model with little involvement in activities related to health promotion and prevention of disease; inadequate emphasis on community orientation; inadequate teacher preparation; and isolation of nursing education from practice.

To better serve the nursing profession, the WHO office in the EMR formed an Advisory Panel on Nursing which was composed of a nursing leader from each of the twenty-two countries, the WHO

Nursing Adviser, and consultants. The need to examine the status of nursing education in the EMR became a priority for the Advisory Panel on Nursing in 1995. A meeting of the panel was held in Tunis, Tunisia in September of 1995 to address the following objectives: (1) recommend relevant standards for basic and post-basic nursing education in the EMR, and (2) develop guidelines for countries to establish speciality programmes in priority areas of nursing practice.[2]

Dr Hussein A. Gezairy, Regional Director, EMR, noted the achievements that had occurred in nursing and midwifery development at country and regional levels since the panel last met in 1993. He made reference to Regional Resolution EM/RC41/R.10 on the need for national planning for nursing and midwifery in EMR, which stressed the importance of having sufficient numbers of well qualified nursing and midwifery personnel to implement strategies for achieving health for all, as well as the need to locate nursing schools within smaller communities beyond the major cities, and to enact legislation on nursing and midwifery.

The panel first addressed the needs of basic and post-basic nursing education and then the issue of regional standards for basic education. The following presents several examples of country and regional situations in regard to basic and post-basic nursing education.

BASIC NURSING EDUCATION

In recent years all member states in the EMR have established nursing schools, launched mass media campaigns to attract young males and females to the professions of nursing and midwifery, introduced incentive schemes to reduce attrition among nursing employees, and provided training opportunities for nurse educators and managers. However, many member states still suffer from a shortage of qualified nursing personnel despite a multiplicity of nursing categories.

Country reports indicate that, at present, the types of basic nursing and midwifery education programmes vary among member states, and sometimes several types of basic nursing courses exist in the same country. For example, Kuwait has a three-year nursing programme for students who have passed nine years of basic general education; a two and a half year associate degree programme in nursing following completion of secondary school; and a four-year Bachelor of Science in Nursing curriculum at Kuwait University. Similarly, in Egypt there are three types of educational programmes to prepare future nurses: the secondary technical schools offer a three-year course after nine years of general education; the technical health institutes offer a two-year basic course after completion of secondary education; and university programmes are four years in length followed by a one-year internship. In Sudan, three-year programmes in the ministries of health of the twenty-six states are open to students who have completed twelve years of general education; in addition, the nursing branch of the technical secondary school for girls is now offering a three-year programme after nine years of general education: and three universities offer four-year B.Sc.N. programmes after twelve years of general education.

Lebanon, Saudi Arabia and Iraq all have three programmes of basic nursing education. In Somalia, nursing students were initially admitted after eight years of general education to a three-year programme, but this was reduced to two years in the 1970s, leading to a continuing deterioration in the quality of nursing care. In 1988, the Ministry of Health raised admission requirements to twelve years and re-instituted a three-year programme, but the civil war began before the first group graduated.

In Jordan there are two categories of registered nurses, one prepared at the university level with a four-year baccalaureate degree, and one prepared with a three-year diploma. In addition, there are associate nurses prepared in a two-year programme, and two categories of practical nurses, one prepared after ten years of general education and one after twelve years. Basic nursing education in Yemen has developed at two levels: the diploma nurse and the B.Sc. nurse, though entrance requirements for the diploma programme vary between north and south, and programmes in the south are in English while in the north they are in Arabic.

Iran has a four-year university-level baccalaureate programme following twelve years of general education, and a shorter practical nursing programme. And Cyprus now has only a three-year diploma programme, with plans to upgrade the school of nursing to a four-year university-level degree.

In addition to the problems of multiple categories of personnel resulting from these diverse basic programmes, in several countries the largest number of nursing students are attending programmes that require only nine years of schooling for admission. It is generally agreed that nine years of preparatory education do not provide sufficient knowledge of basic sciences or general education to study modern nursing. Furthermore, when students graduate, they are only 17 years old, emotionally too young to cope with the responsibilities of caring for the sick in hospitals or for families in the community. This leads to a high attrition rate, adding to the chronic nursing shortage.

In most countries of the region, nursing curricula were founded on the Western medical model, stressing individual and curative hospital care. Thus, graduates of many nursing programmes are not prepared to participate in the strategy of Health For All through primary health care (PHC). In recent years a number of countries have adopted more relevant community-oriented programmes with emphasis on PHC. For example, the new community-oriented B.Sc.N. programme in Iran is designed to prepare graduates who are sensitive to the health needs of the country, who have the knowledge and skills to preserve and restore health and prevent illness, and who have developed problem-solving attitudes.

In Cyprus, the basic nursing programme now includes experience in caring for people of all age groups and emphasizes the concept of primary health care in all areas of practice. However, in many countries efforts to implement more community focused curricula have encountered problems arising from the affiliation of nursing schools with hospitals and the needs of hospitals for the services of students to make up for the shortage of nursing personnel. Also, teaching staff are not fully prepared to undertake training in the community, and in some programmes physicians remain a dominant force. Educational resources vary widely. Few institutions have adequately qualified teachers. Clinical training is a particular problem in some countries due to the shortage of clinical trainers to supervise students, the absence of role models and clear standards of nursing care, and the unavailability of equipment and resources. Field practice in community settings is often lacking.

The majority of nursing schools also have inadequate teaching-learning materials that are in national languages and culturally relevant. Some countries also report a shortage of journals related to nursing in the college libraries. This lack of resources compromises the quality of the training.

The quality of basic nursing education in almost all twenty-two countries is also compromised by the lack of a systematic approach to the accreditation of nursing education programmes. While periodic curriculum reviews are carried out in some programmes, there is no system for monitoring the implementation of nursing education against identified standards. Clearly, basic nursing education in the region needs a set of standards to ensure the graduation of competent nurses who will deliver comprehensive care and contribute effectively to the health services of countries in the EMR.

POST-BASIC EDUCATION

Because of the complexity of health services at all levels, qualified nurses with advanced knowledge and specialized skills are also required. Intensive care nursing, management of cancer patients, accident and emergency care, infection control, diabetes education, occupational and mental health nursing—to name a few—are specialty nursing fields needed in most countries of the region. Global forces driving the creation of speciality areas in nursing include the increasing complexity of health care, structural changes in health care delivery, new technologies and new consumer demands as well as changing health needs. For many countries interest in nursing specialization is high, but there is immense diversity in regard to what constitutes a specialist, how long specialty training takes and at what level it is appropriate.

Generally it is agreed that a nurse specialist needs to possess advanced up-to-date knowledge that enables her (usually a female) to analyze complex problems, take critical decisions and move on to appropriate actions. In her practice she is innovative, flexible and responsive to rapid changes in the conditions of patients, clients or groups of individuals. In working with her colleagues, she exhibits leadership qualities to develop nursing practice. She is accountable and responsible for her interventions. And finally, she is self motivated for personal growth. The specialist nurse is above all a skilled practitioner. In addition, the specialist manages the nursing care of groups of clients working with nurses with lesser qualifications; acts as a consultant to other staff on practice problems; is a researcher, educator, and manager of a specialized unit; and facilitates practice development through innovative approaches to care delivery.

Educational programmes leading to nursing specialization extend from three months special training programmes to post-basic certificate or diploma programmes or to a graduate masters level programme.

With such diversity one also finds variations in entrance requirements, curricula content and competencies developed. The challenge to the Eastern Mediterranean Region now is to systematically place, develop, implement, and monitor nursing specialization programmes in a way that responds to the demands of the region and at the same time assures professional development.

Some countries in the EMR are now developing training in specialized areas. However, as with basic programmes, the programmes vary greatly in length and scope as well as entrance requirements. For example, in Pakistan, one-year post-basic courses are taught in the specialized fields of ward administration and teaching, obstetrics, cardiology, ophthalmology, community health, anesthesia and urology, among others. All nursing colleges in the country plan to add more specialization to their existing programmes.

In Kuwait, until the mid-1980s, one-year programmes were offered in midwifery, surgical nursing and community health nursing to those who had completed a three-year basic nursing programme. In their place, the country now offers four-week certificate courses in medical/surgical nursing and continuing education in mid-level management, ward management and clinical teaching. Jordan offers programmes ranging from nine to twelve months in length for specialization in a variety of areas, including a diploma in midwifery for registered nurses. There are also shorter programmes in narrow areas such as kidney dialysis, burns, etc.

Bahrain offers a one-year post-basic programme in midwifery, psychiatric nursing, cardiac care and community nursing to associate degree nursing graduates. Sudan offers a one-year post-basic programme in nurse midwifery, a two-year programme for health visitors, and a two-year programme for nurses to become medical assistants. In Tunisia, specialization occurs in three different ways: a) diploma nurses with five years of experience can receive specialized training lasting from one to two years; b) nurses can be prepared as specialists in paediatric nursing, psychiatric nursing, intensive care nursing, operating room nursing or general care nursing in a three-year basic programme; c) or students who have completed the baccalaureate may be trained in three-year programmes as high technicians of public health specializing in obstetrics, anaesthesia, radiology, therapy or biology.

DIRECTIONS FOR CHANGE

In some countries, weak undergraduate programmes have been upgraded into specialty programmes as a short-term solution to fill acute needs for health services. In other cases nurses have been used as the pool for developing para-medics. Both of these developments raise questions about what constitutes specialist training and what constitutes a specialist nurse.

To avoid the chaotic proliferation of programmes in specialized areas, post-basic programmes, similar to basic nursing education programmes, need to be guided by a comprehensive approach to the development of quality nursing, with integrated and interrelated activities.

At the macro or national level, a strong nursing structure in the ministry of health is needed to be responsible for policy and planning. Clear policies on the contributions of nursing to health care and on the responsibilities of nursing personnel are crucial. On the basis of such policies, a strategic plan of action can be developed to meet each country's needs for nursing care.

Good legislation is needed to govern both nursing education and nursing practice, and there must be a regulatory body to enforce the legislation, provide direction to the profession, and undertake the necessary validation and accreditation of training programmes. The regulatory body should not be a part of the ministry of health, nor should it be headed by a high ministry official.

Sound basic nursing education that is relevant to health services needs, follows trends in nursing and health care and is based on approved standards, is an integral part of this comprehensive approach, as is an up-to-date registration system for all categories of nursing personnel. At the micro level, or the actual working situation, a sound management system is needed to define jobs and roles, indicate how they are to be created, specify working conditions and clarify supervision—in other words, ensure that nurses can practice what they have been taught. A system of quality assurance based on relevant and applicable standards of nursing care is a part of sound management.

In addition, sound programmes for post-basic, graduate and continuing education are needed to prepare specialized nurses. Further, practice-based research is needed to advance nursing knowledge and continually improve nursing practice.

Finally, it is crucial to develop collaborative relationships within the profession, for example, through the development of nursing associations, and to build relationships with other professional groups. The ultimate aim is to develop collaborations for health.

REGIONAL STANDARDS FOR BASIC NURSING EDUCATION

Sound basic nursing education programmes are part of a comprehensive approach to strengthening nursing. However, without standards to guide the development and evaluation of basic education programmes, it is impossible to say what is sound and what is not sound.

Standards provide a means of measuring the degree of excellence of an educational programme and of comparing the degree of excellence of one programme to that of others. Many countries around the world have developed national standards for nursing education, and the current trend is toward setting regional standards for groups or subgroups of countries.

Regional standards for nursing education in the EMR are crucial to:

- Ensure that existing programmes of nursing education and those now being developed follow current trends in nursing education, respond to health needs in the Member States, are in line with technological advances and produce graduates who are competent and accountable for their practice;
- Guide institutions in Member States in improving existing educational programmes and provide a basis for developing new programmes;
- Consolidate the multiple programmes now available in existing Member States;
- Promote a regional level of nursing education and performance and thus advance the uniform development of nursing;
- Allow free mobility of students and graduates among Member States;
- Guide the activities of students and teachers in nursing education programmes;
- Demonstrate the uniqueness of the professional preparation of nurses;
- Attract capable candidates to the profession; and
- Monitor regional progress in developing nursing education.

LEVELS OF PRACTICE

Deciding on the levels of nursing practice is a prerequisite to setting standards for the education of practitioners. There are currently twenty-two levels of nurses and midwives in the Eastern Mediterranean Region. The range is from one to five per country and the mean, three per country. The Regional Advisory Panel agreed that one level of nursing practitioners—the professional nurse—is the goal for the region. The rationale for setting one level is based on the vision statement set forth by the panel in its first strategic plan for nursing development in the region, for the years 1995–2000: 'To have nurses capable of meeting the challenges of the rapidly changing world and meeting the present and future health needs of the people in an efficient and cost-effective manner as members of the health team, with the ultimate goal of contributing to the maintenance and/or improvement of quality of life.'[3]

The specific reasons for having one level of nursing practitioners prepared in a baccalaureate programme include:

- practitioners who can work at all levels of health care—primary, secondary and tertiary,
- need for active involvement in country development,
- promotion of healthy life styles,
- work in a variety of settings,
- the increasing complexity and costs of health care,
- continuing advances in science and technology,
- the rising expectations of health care consumers,
- the need for practitioners who can participate in health services research and nursing research,
- the need for practitioners who can function as teachers and as leaders in nursing,
- the need to improve the image of nursing and attract more qualified students to the profession,
- the need to prepare nurses for continuing self-development,
- the importance of working in health care teams and collaborating with other disciplines,
- the importance of inter-regional and international collaboration,
- the need to prepare nurses who are better client advocates, and
- the need to provide a solid foundation for cost-effective specialization.

Given the resource constraints and consequent difficulties in revising existing educational programmes and developing new programmes to produce this level of practitioner, the panel also agreed to a transitional period of fifteen years during which there may be two levels of nurses—the professional nurses prepared in a four-year baccalaureate programme and the technical nurses prepared in a two and a half year programme with twelve years of schooling.

The transition period will continue until 2010, by which time the technical nurse should be phased out. During this period, countries need to develop or expand bridge programmes that enable technical nurses to move into baccalaureate programmes without overlap and repetition, provide incentives and support nurses as they complete their education as professional nurses, and set penalties for failure to do so.

STANDARD SETTING

Standards for nursing education must be based on the aims and objectives of educational programmes. In the Eastern Mediterranean Region the first aim of basic programmes is to provide quality care in all types of settings—hospitals, primary care clinics, homes, schools, industry, etc.—for all age groups. Further, the aim is to produce nurses who are not only practitioners but are also active as citizens and members of their community, sensitive to political and social development, and able to play a role in policy and politics. The objective of preparing these nurses is to have an impact in improving the health of the people, developing nursing as a profession and promoting sustainable development in countries.

The second aim is to develop the capacity of nursing educational institutions through linkages with institutions of higher education and educational authorities, through integration with hospitals and health services, and through collaboration with health-related institutions, the mass media, religious groups and political leaders. The objective of this capacity-building is to provide broad learning programmes as a basis for meeting the lifelong learning needs of the nursing workforce.

Success in achieving these aims requires a legal framework for nursing education and practice, a regulatory system, standards for educational programmes, accreditation (validation) of programmes and a registration system for graduates. Success also requires high calibre students, adequate resources and a clear educational process that includes educational philosophy, curriculum, extra-curricula activities that are a part of preparing citizens, teaching-learning strategies, clinical/field work and continuing education.

Standards for basic nursing education are of three types: structure, process and outcome. The Regional Advisory Panel further extended these into educational training institutions, teaching staff, administrative support, physical facilities, entrance requirements, curriculum and evaluation.

PRIORITIES FOR NURSING SPECIALIZATION IN THE EASTERN MEDITERRANEAN REGION

The Advisory Panel on nursing considers that specialization should be developed in accordance with national health plans and country needs. The Advisory Panel agreed that the four top priorities for nursing specialization in the region are midwifery, community health nursing, psychiatric/mental health nursing and critical care.

The rationale for making midwifery a priority includes the fact that fertility rates in the region are high and still rising; morbidity and mortality rates for women and children remain high; many women live in poverty and suffer from poor living conditions, pollution and illiteracy; the current quality of maternal child care is often poor because qualified midwives are lacking; and good midwifery care is both cost effective and culturally appropriate. The specialist midwife is viewed as a person who cares for women throughout the life cycle and for children up to the age of five years.

The rationale for giving community health nursing top priority is similar to that for midwifery, since community health nursing overlaps with maternal and child nursing. In addition, changing demographics and health care delivery patterns mean that there are growing numbers of people who need to be cared for in the community—the elderly, AIDS patients, the disabled, those with chronic diseases and those needing home care after hospital discharge. Also, community health nurses are needed to improve immunization rates, well child care and adolescent care, and to develop occupational health nursing services in the growing industrial sector.

Specialization in psychiatric/mental health nursing is a priority for numerous reasons. The population experiences increasing problems from the growing pressures of life in the region, and more specifically, from internal and external political conflicts and the increase in substance abuse and emotional disorders that accompany development. In the past, patients with emotional problems were isolated and often stigmatized and psychiatric nursing was a neglected speciality. Therefore, there are few qualified nurses in this area of specialization. Furthermore, basic nursing education in this field is insufficient for effective care.

Critical care is also a priority area for specialization because of the increasing acuity of hospitalized patients, both adult and paediatric; the rise in the number of trauma victims as vehicular accidents continue to increase, and changes in disease patterns resulting from economic development and the growing elderly population. In addition, continuing advances in technology and the increasing numbers of critical care units make it imperative to prepare nurses to handle these patients.

CONCLUSION

The recommendations from the Advisory Panel meeting were further developed into 'A Strategy for Nursing and Midwifery Development in the Eastern Mediterranean Region,' which was published by WHO as a EMRO Technical Publications Series 25 in 1997.

The strategy for action includes a vision statement for nursing (in box),[4] outlines the need for a strategy and indicates the necessity for a joint effort 'involving governments, educational institutions, health service management and nursing leadership.'[5] In addition, the strategy urges countries to develop regulations for the profession, reinforcing the points put forward by Affara's chapter on Control and Standards.[6] The strategy also emphasizes the need to professionalize nursing and midwifery through improved and established educational standards and by increased development of nurse leaders qualified to participate in the governance and management of health organizations.

Another issue covered by the strategy is the challenge faced by the profession for promoting nursing research in order to incorporate nursing innovations and make use of advances in technology. A significant part of the strategy deals with the improvement and development of a country's nursing structure, a structure that recognizes the capabilities of practitioners, develops strong nursing leadership and promotes 'flexible approaches to the management of nursing.'[7] This structure of nursing, so essential to the improvement of all aspects of nursing in EMR, will require action on the part of government officials in appointing qualified nurse leaders to positions of influence and responsibility.

The Vision

In a changing world, nursing professionals will offer efficient and effective practice of the highest possible standard and safety, founded on up-to-date research and knowledge. They will meet the present and future health care needs of the people as members of the health team in a cost-effective manner in a variety of settings, with the ultimate goal of contributing to the maintenance and /or improvement of quality of life.

NOTES

1. The Eastern Mediterranean Region of the World Health Organization includes twenty-two countries extending from North Africa, across the Middle East and into Pakistan.
2. This chapter is a summary of the 'Preliminary Report of the Third Meeting of the WHO Regional Advisory Panel on Nursing and Midwifery,' Tunis, Tunisia, September 1995.
3. Vision statement, ibid., p. 12.
4. A Strategy for Nursing and Midwifery Development in the Eastern Mediterranean Region, EMRO Technical Publications Series 25, World Health Organization, Regional Office for the Eastern Mediterranean 1997, p. 9.
5. Ibid., p. 10.
6. Fadwa Affara, 'Issues of Control: The Role of Nursing in the Regulation of the Profession', in *Women in Nursing in Islamic Countries*, Nancy Bryant (ed.), Oxford University Press, Karachi, 2003.
7. EMRO Technical Publications Series 25, op. cit., p. 22.

9

Nursing Health Human Resources in Pakistan

Yasmin Amarsi

BACKGROUND

The World Health Organization (WHO) recommends that health human resource development (HHRD) 'takes place within a context of interdependent social, educational, political and cultural influences'.[1] There is no doubting the weight of such factors in relation to HHRD in Pakistan, including its political and administrative systems, socio-economic and educational dimensions of society, demographic patterns and trends, cultural trends and status of women, impact of external donors, and the current health situation.

OVERVIEW OF PAKISTAN

A country with a population of approximately 148 million, Pakistan is located on the Arabian Sea between India and Iran in the south, and is bordered by China and Afghanistan in the north. The country is comprised of four provinces: Balochistan, the North-West Frontier Province (NWFP), Punjab and Sindh; also the Northern Areas, and the disputed territories of Jammu and Kashmir.

While Urdu is the most commonly spoken language, multiple languages and dialects are used throughout the country.[2] English is widely used for instructional purposes in higher education, including professional institutions, as well as commercial, legal, government, and official businesses in the country.

Political and Administrative Systems

After a turbulent political history, Pakistan has until recently been a multi-party, parliamentary democracy. The majority of public policies are formulated at the federal level under the Planning Commission. The federal government provides policy guidance, but implementation of public policies relevant to social development such as education, health, water supply, and sanitation are provincial responsibilities.

Pakistan and India were ruled as one country by the British until 1947 when Pakistan achieved its independence.[3] Pakistan has since faced several periods of instability due to political unrest and natural disasters such as floods and famine and it has also been involved in three wars with India. Difficult relationships between India and Pakistan have resulted in high defence spending, leaving scarce financial resources for the social sector, including health. In addition, the presence of about 3.5 million Afghan refugees (the result of Russia's invasion of Afghanistan and on-going civil disturbances) has placed an additional burden on the country. Associated with this large refugee population has been an increase in drug abuse, free flow of arms and ammunition resulting in increased violence, as well as accidents and stress due to insecurity.[4]

Recent developments in Afghanistan have increased the complexity of relationships with India, and added to the numbers of the Afghan refugees.

Socio-economic Dimensions

Pakistan has achieved a substantial rate of growth in its economic and agricultural sector over the last three decades with its Gross Domestic Product (GDP) growth rate averaging 5.8 per cent from 1985-1990. During the 1980s, Pakistan was the sixth fastest growing economy in the world.[5,6] Despite its per capita income, which compares favourably with some of the developing countries such as India and Bangladesh (See Table 1), Pakistan is still classified as one of the lowest income countries of the world. It has made only marginal improvement in development of its social indicators, particularly in the fields of health, education and women's development, which are among the worst in the world.[7] The quality of life among its people has not corresponded to the economic growth[8] as the country has not translated its economic progress

Table 1

Key Social Indicators for Pakistan and Selected Countries

Country	TFR	PGR (%)	IMR (1,000)	PCGNP (US$)	FLR (%)	MMR (1000,000)	Contraceptive Use (%)
Pakistan	5.9	2.9	95	430	21	600	18
Bangladesh	3.4	2.2	94	220	22	650	45
India	3.4	1.9	81	300	34	420	41
Indonesia	2.9	1.6	71	740	75	400	55
China	2.0	1.1	35	490	68	95	83
Egypt	3.9	2.2	46	660	34	266	47
Kenya	5.4	3.6	61	270	59	500	33
Canada	1.8	1.3	6.2	20,510	96	7	73
USA	2.0	1.0	7.6	22,340	80	13	74
UK	1.9	0.2	–	16,600	79	11	81

TFR = Total Fertility Rate   PCGNP = Per Capita Gross National Product
PGR = Population Growth Rate   FLR = Female Literacy Rate
IMR = Infant Mortality Rate   MMR = Maternal Mortality Rate

Source: Adapted from Rosen, J.E., & Conly, S.R., 1996, *Pakistan's population programme: The challenge ahead* (Country Study Series No. 5, p. 13), Washington, DC: Population Action International.

Table 2

Government Expenditure (% of Total)

Country	Defence	Education	Health	Social Welfare	Economic Services
Pakistan	27.9	1.6	1.0	3.4	11.6
Bangladesh	10.1	11.2	4.8	8.0	43.4
India	17.0	2.5	1.6	6.9	20.8
Indonesia	8.2	9.1	2.4	1.8	27.1
Iran	9.6	20.9	7.9	15.5	16.1
Nepal	5.9	10.9	4.7	6.8	43.0
Philippines	10.9	16.1	4.2	3.7	24.7
Sri Lanka	9.4	8.3	4.8	18.4	24.6
Thailand	17.1	20.2	7.4	5.9	24.3
Canada	2.0	7.4	9.9	–	–
USA	5.1	7.0	13.3	–	–
UK	4.2	5.3	6.6	–	–

Source: Adapted from World Bank, 1993a, *World Development Report 1993*. Washington, DC: The World Bank and Oxford University Press.

into human development. In comparison with other countries in South Asia, budget allocations for the social sector in Pakistan have remained consistently low. As indicated in Table 2, Pakistan's allocations for education (1.6%) and health (1%) are the lowest among the listed developing countries such as Bangladesh and Nepal. Allocation for military spending (27.9%) is the highest among these countries. These budget allocations are indicative of the value placed on the social sector by the policy makers and decision makers.

Social indicators are directly proportionate to the government's budget allocation. Pakistan ranks 134th out of 174 countries on the Human Development Index (HDI), which uses life expectancy, education, and income as its three measures.[9] It also ranks lowest in the South Asian region in most of the gender-related human development indicators.[10] It has been estimated that 30 per cent of the population lives below the poverty line.[11]

Educational Dimensions

Education plays a critical role in promoting the cultural, social, economic, and political development of a country. As Lockheed[12] states:

> Education improves income distribution, increases savings and encourages more rational consumption, enhances the status of women, and promotes adaptability to technological change...a diverse body of literature demonstrates that the adults in developing countries who have a higher level of educational attainment have more paid employment, higher individual earnings, greater agricultural productivity, lower fertility, better health and nutritional status, and more modern attitudes than adults who have lower educational attainment. They are also more likely to send their children to school. These characteristics are dimensions of development (p. 2).

There is a marked difference in basic education between Pakistan and other low-income countries.[13] The current overall literacy rate is officially 37 per cent, with female literacy approximately 21 per cent; among rural females the rate was reported to be as low as 0.8 per cent in rural tribal areas.[5] Official estimates of total enrolment in the primary schools indicate not only low enrolments among girls, but also high dropout rates, particularly in the rural areas.[14]

Demographic Patterns and Trends

Pakistan is the ninth most populated country[6] with an annual population growth rate of 3.1 per cent, one of the highest in the world.[15] Currently, 3.7 million people are being added annually to the existing population; 9.4 babies are born and 2.4 deaths occur every minute.[11]

Approximately 70 per cent of the population lives in rural areas. The urban population has been steadily increasing since the 1960s (about 4.4% a year); this unplanned urban growth has led to pockets of severe urban poverty.[15] Official estimates are that the population of Pakistan in 2000 reached more than 148 million, a nine-fold increase in the century compared to the world population increase of four-fold over the same period.

High population exerts strong pressure on social facilities such as education, health, sanitation and water, and on the environment through excessive congestion in urban areas.[8] Employment opportunities also become limited because of the increase in those eligible for the labour force. The country's population is predominantly young, resulting in a high proportion of a dependent population; 50-60 per cent of the population consists of persons less than 15 years of age and women in the childbearing period of life.[11]

Cultural Trends and Status of Women

Although the constitution of Pakistan guarantees equal protection for women and men, the realities illustrated in the country's law and dictated by social norms present quite a different picture. Shaheed and Mumtaz[16] describe the cultural norms in Pakistan:

> Gender specific roles are very clearly demarcated by culture: women are responsible for the reproduction of the society and servicing this collective within the home; men are responsible for their families' financial and physical needs and carrying out chores outside the household...women's mobility is greatly restricted, early marriage for girls encouraged, and women's employment in remunerated activities negatively valued. To facilitate the maintenance of 'honour' codes, society operates according to the rule of purdah: gender segregation and female seclusion.

These socio-cultural constraints negatively impinge on women's human resource potentials and their economic progress.[17,18] Saeed[19] further explains the phenomenon:

> Attitudes and perceptions, deeply rooted in patriarchal social traditions, shape behaviour patterns toward women, cast their shadows on legislation and colour value judgments involving women. It is mostly the men who interpret religious injunctions as set out in the Quran. Thus male conservative perceptions and whims hold sway, even though many of the practices these give rise to are contrary to the injunctions of Islam.

The injustices perpetuated by social and traditional norms are reinforced by discriminatory laws such as the Hudood Ordinance. Pakistan is one of the few countries in the world where women are prosecuted for adultery and after reporting being raped, condemned to death by stoning if unable to produce four male witnesses. This has resulted in imprisonment of thousands of women on charges of adultery.[20,13]

In addition, motherhood poses a great risk to a woman's life as many of her potential illnesses are pregnancy related. Only 24 of every 100 pregnant women have access to a health professional for childbirth. Their access to health care, especially reproductive care, is further limited because of cultural restrictions which prevent women from seeking care from male providers. For example, women have to be accompanied by a male when accessing health services or gaining access to services.[8,21] Similarly, female health care providers are often not able to practice in rural areas because of cultural restrictions and lack of security.[22] Consequently, until the early 1990s, Pakistan was one of the very few countries in the world where women had a lower life expectancy than men, although the current life expectancy rate is estimated to be 63 years for females and 61 years for males.[21] The average life expectancy of women in most countries is 5-10 per cent longer than that of men.[14]

Women's position in society has not changed in any significant manner in Pakistan since independence in 1947; the majority of women (76%) remain illiterate. Primary school enrolment of females was 49 per cent in 1993, but 55 per cent drop out by the time they reach grade four. Furthermore, female enrolment at the secondary level is only at 13 per cent.[23,24] International evidence shows that the social and economic benefits of female education are very significant.[13,25]

Educating females is potentially a cost-effective method of reducing health problems as women are essential health care providers to the entire family. Women can be educated to detect and prevent diseases of infancy and childhood and to practice better hygiene, sanitation, and nutrition in the household.[26,13] The low education rate for females also impacts on the number and calibre of female health care workers available to a country.

Current Health Situation

As indicated in Table 3, the health indices in Pakistan have shown some improvement, but the pace of improvement has been slow. In comparison with average low income countries, the health status of its people remains poor. The composition of Pakistan's burden of disease indicates that about 50 per cent are communicable diseases and maternal and peri-natal conditions. Nutritional deficiencies account

Table 3
Pakistan's Health Indicators: 1960-1970 and 1990

Health Indicators	1960-1970	1990
Life expectancy (years)	43	62
Fertility rate	7.0	6.1
Crude death rate (per 1000)	23	9
Infant mortality rate (per 1000)	137	95
Maternal mortality rate (per 100,000)	n/a	340
Under 5 mortality rate (per 1000)	221	137
Low birth weight babies	27%	25%
Malnourished babies	72%	40%
Contraceptive prevalence rate	4%	12%
Access to health services	51%	55%
Access to safe water	29%	50%
Access to sanitation	14%	35%
Birth attended by health personnel	–	35%
Population per doctor	3,780	2,000
Population per nurse	10,040	3,448

Source: Adapted from Mahbub ul Haq. (1997). *Human development in South Asia*. Karachi, Pakistan: Oxford University Press.

for a further 6 per cent.[21] The total government expenditure on health as a percentage of GNP is approximately 1.0 per cent which is very low.

Health Human Resources Development (HHRD)

Health human resource development is the key to an efficient and effective health care system in any country and plays a predominant role in the socio-economic and technological development of nations.[27] The ultimate goal of human resource development (HRD) is to improve the quality of life of all its people.[28] Human resource development has three major components: planning, production, and management.[28,29,30] (See Figure 1) Health human resources include all persons engaged in any capacity in the production and delivery of health services. In current times of economic restraint, health human resource strategies are developed or re-examined to ensure more efficient, effective, and equitable provision of health services. Reorganizing and restructuring of health human resources is a complex phenomenon which requires commitment, political will, well-qualified staff, and sufficient resources, as well as being dynamic in nature.[1] Health human resource development historically has evolved from an emphasis on increasing numbers of health personnel to improving their quality.

A rudimentary form of human resource development existed in Pakistan at the time of independence in 1947, but to date Pakistan has not been able to develop effectively its human resources in the field of health. Consequently, HHRD has generally remained inadequate. This is illustrated by imbalances in production as well as in the distribution of health personnel, and by a skewed staff mix. Imbalances are evident in that only 17 per cent of all health professionals are employed in rural areas where 70 per cent of the population resides, a number insufficient to meet needs in the rural areas.[15] Further, the health care system is characterized by a predominance of physicians, an orientation to curative services,[31] poor management of health personnel, and a centralized bureaucratic system.

Since 1973, human resource development policy has been consistently documented by the federal government in its five-year plans (FYPs) and in the national health policy of 1990. The policies have primarily emphasized the numbers and types of health care workers and neglected factors such as quality of education and improvements in the work environment. While HHRD policies have addressed all health personnel, implementation has generally focused on increasing the number of doctors; the supply of nurses and other female cadres has lagged behind.[11]

Within any health care system, registered nursing personnel are important human resources.[32,33,34,35] They usually constitute one of the largest groups of health professionals,[36] and make up approximately 70 per cent of the total health service workforce.[37,34,38] In 1989, an American survey asked 663 hospital chief executive officers to rank order the ten most important factors which they believed contributed to quality of patient care. In 97.3 per cent of the cases, nursing was ranked as the most important factor.[39]

In 1993-1994 a worldwide survey was conducted by the International Council of Nurses (ICN) regarding nursing issues, priorities, and activities. Some 107 national nurses associations of seven regions were surveyed. The response rate was 43 per cent (n=46). The member states were concerned with nursing shortages, nursing legislation, salaries, and working conditions of nursing personnel. Nursing education was ranked as the top priority.[40]

In Pakistan, nursing human resources include Registered Nurses (RNs), Registered Midwives (RMs), and Lady Health Visitors (LHVs). In the fifty years since Pakistan obtained independence, the number of nursing personnel has increased but has not kept pace with increased demand. The increasing demand for nurses is associated with rapid population growth, advances in health technology, shift in the patterns of diseases, rising social expectations, and rapid growth of the health industry.[11] A major challenge to the health sector in the country is inadequate nursing human resources which has persisted for the last five decades.[11,41] Nursing continues to face critical problems, both in the quality and in the number of trained nurses. The Economic Survey of 1995-1996 showed 22,531 registered nurses (RNs) and 69,694 registered physicians for a population of approximately 133 million, i.e. one physician for every 1,837 persons and one RN for every 5,681 persons. In contrast, Brihaye[32] reported a ratio of at least three nurses per 1,000 persons in the developed countries and one nurse per 1,000-5,000 persons in the developing countries.

World Health Organization (WHO)[42] and Asian Development Bank (ADB)[43] consultants emphasized the absence of accurate and reliable data on distribution and utilization of nursing staff, nursing human resource flows, and number of available registered nurses. Zaidi explains the contradictory nature among numerous inconsistencies in government published data: 'Thus the extreme unreliability of data…makes analysis suspect, and can often lead to manipulation of the statistics to suit one's own purposes'.[3, p.171] A situational analysis would provide further understanding of the complexities of health human resource development. Timely and reliable data on nursing personnel numbers, mix, distribution, and characteristics are essential for monitoring trends in the health care delivery system. Abdellah and Levine[44] suggested that to make full utilization of existing technologies and resources in achieving effective patient care, research on nursing human resource development be considered a priority for the twenty-first century.

A Study of Human Resource Development for Nursing

The Coordinated Health Human Resource Development (COHHRD)[1] model is one of the few models recommended for development of comprehensive HHRD plans at the macro or country level (Figure 1). It addresses all three components of HHRD and emphasizes the importance of coordination between development of health services and health human resources. Hall,[45] in his 'tool kit,' expanded on this model and provided the list of variables under the planning, production, and management components (Table 4). In addition, he developed guide-lines for conducting a situation analysis of HHRD, which include a policy review and determination of the perception of key stakeholders. However, a literature review did not reveal studies that have used Hall's tool kit or focused on perceptions of key stakeholders. These perceptions are considered extremely important because their values and beliefs play an important role in planning of health care, in making decisions, and formulating policies regarding HHRD.[45]

A study was, therefore, undertaken to explore key stakeholders' perceptions of the three components of NHRD in the Province of Sindh, Pakistan. Issues that provided impetus to this study were lack of reliable data on the various dimensions of human resource development in general and on Nursing Human Resource Development (NHRD) in Pakistan in particular, and the dearth of studies which address all components of HHRD. Health human resource development is a major challenge in any country, but more so in developing countries such as Pakistan which has specific characteristics such as a

Figure 1

COORDINATED HEALTH HUMAN RESOURCE
DEVELOPMENT (COHHRD) FRAMEWORK

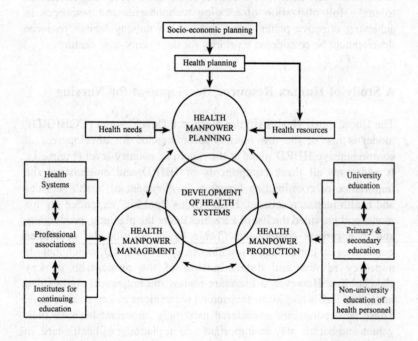

Source: World Health Organization (WHO) Study Group. 1990. *Coordinated health human resource development.* (Technical Report Series 801, p. 10.). Geneva: WHO.

Table 4

Variables in the Components: Planning, Production, and Management

Variables		
Planning	Production	Management
Demographic variables	Number of basic and post-basic schools	Conditions of work: full time, part time, private practice
Number of health workers by type, major areas of activity, level of care	Annual intake and output	Work schedules, duty rotations, staff coverage for health workers
Positions sanctioned, filled, vacant	Number of the faculty	Career advancement, pre-job orientation, clear job descriptions
Migration: inter-provincial, urban/rural	Curriculum	Existence of personnel policies
Health facilities survey (10-15%): distribution, size, capacity, productivity, staffing density, terms of employment, quality of care	Applicant, entrants, enrolments, and graduates	Procedures for staff recruitment, selection, placement, and promotion
		Salary scales, merit increases, monetary and non-monetary incentives, staff morale, apparent job satisfaction
		Qualification for practice, licensure, registration
		Shortages/surplus of personnel, equity of distribution of personnel, staff turnover

Source: Hall, T.L. 1995. *Guidelines for a human resource development study.* Geneva: WHO.

centralised bureaucratic system, gender disparity, financial constraints, absence of unions, and political instability.

The stakeholders whose perceptions were sought for this study consisted of active or retired government officials at federal, provincial and local levels. A total of nineteen nursing personnel and fifteen non-nursing officials participated in the study.

Since this study was dealing with the relatively unexplored phenomenon of nursing human resource development in Pakistan, a qualitative methodology, using a descriptive exploratory design, was chosen to capture the perceptions of key decision makers. A qualitative approach was used to obtain key insights into the phenomenon being explored, where face-to-face interaction was desired for holistic inquiry and for in-depth investigation of the complexities of a phenomenon.[46,47,48]

Perceptions of How Nursing Human Resource Development Works in Pakistan

Perceptions of the thirty-four study participants were recorded, interpreted and discussed. Their responses were organized into the three components of the COHHRD framework of health system development: Planning, Production and Management. It is critical to note that these components are not mutually exclusive and overlap is found among the components (see Figure 1).

The discussion is organized around those three components. Under Planning, three themes are considered: formulation of policies; planning and implementation gap; and supply-requirement imbalance. Under Production, the key theme is quality of education, encompassing: recruitment, integration of service and education, financial resources, and faculty complement. Under Management, the main theme is working conditions, which encompasses the issues of adequacy of resources, adequacy of the numbers of prepared nurses, respect and recognition, degree of satisfaction, salary and benefits, and quality of care.

Planning

Formulation of Policies: The theme, Formulation of Policies, incorporates both awareness of health policies and plans, and the process of planning and policy formulation.

In contrast to many countries which have not addressed HHRD at the macro level,[49] Pakistan, over the past twenty years, has incorporated the planning, production, and management dimensions of HHRD in its national health policies. Five year plans (FYPs) are regularly prepared. Additionally, in 1990; the Ministry of Health with assistance from the Asian Development Bank, developed a national Health Manpower and Training Plan (HMTP). That plan addressed all cadres of health care and used an effective-demand approach in estimating human resource requirements. Federal and provincial governments participated in development of the plan. The HMTP is comprehensive and congruent with the approach to HHRD advocated by Hall.[50]

The national health policies and the HMTP are indicators of the governments' awareness of the importance of HHRD. However, findings indicate that many of the key stakeholders, especially nursing personnel at the provincial and local levels, do not have awareness of the health policies and plans and/or of the processes by which they are formulated. None of the key stakeholders referred to the existence of the HMTP; all stated they believed that although there was a need for a comprehensive health human resource development plan, none existed. There was lack of clarity among stakeholders about the national health policies and five year plans. Some stakeholders viewed the FYPs as containing policies, whereas others viewed them as merely guidelines. The relationship between a policy and a plan was not clearly understood; some stakeholders were not clear as to whether plans were needed to formulate policies, or whether policies were needed to formulate plans. Findings are indicative of weaknesses in the process by which policies are formulated, plans developed, and information disseminated.

The FYPs were identified as being developed through a centralized process, not based on adequate information, and inaccessible to most health care professionals and the public. There was convergence in perceptions among most key stakeholders regarding current health planning in Pakistan in that they perceived planning to be defective, fragmented, and hierarchical in nature with a top-downward approach. The decision-making power is vested in a few individuals at a very senior level, such as the Chief of Planning Division, the Chief Minister of each province, and the Finance Minister. The overall structure is a carry-over from what existed pre-independence. This approach is characterized by an hierarchical structure of authority, often pyramidal in shape, with very little lateral communication or coordination.[51,52]

Although the process of planning FYPs occurs over a year and takes many 'human hours,' their development has not followed rational steps in the formulation of policies suggested in the literature. These steps are: definition of policies, weighing of alternative options, formulation of strategies, and preparation of a plan of action.[53,54,55,56,57,58] One of the key stakeholders reported that the process of FYP preparation process is lengthy. Working groups do a thorough job of studying issues, but problems arise when they present their reports. The presentation format is highly structured and there is rigid adherence to rules regarding length of the document, content, and language. Emphasis is often on projects that are donor driven and will allow access to development funds from external donors, which may not be based on requirements or needs of the sectors. Fragmentation occurs when donor groups support development of the infrastructure without human resource needs being addressed. Fragmentation in planning also occurs when a change in one sector has an impact on another sector, but no concomitant changes are planned for the second sector. For example, an increase in beds or services (planning) is not accompanied by a corresponding increase in nursing personnel (production).

The very nature of FYPs could be contributing to both the weaknesses of planning and the difficulty in implementation. Historically, a life cycle of FYPs was a norm for many countries, but these plans did not contain sufficient information or degree of detail that is needed for operation.[59] Recently, there has been increasing recognition that such a cycle is too long; according to today's context, where changes are occurring rapidly, planning cycles need to be short. Five year plans tend to quickly become out of date and out of touch with changing needs. Green[59] recommends that countries use three year rolling plans. Year One of the plan would contain the most detailed operational plans and Year Three would be a broad outline. Each year the plan would be rolled forward and prepared in a similarly detailed manner.

Although the strength of the policy formulation approach in Pakistan is such that, as recommended by Mazmanian and Sabatier,[60] it allows for the perspectives of decision makers at senior levels to be considered, it neglects other important players such as middle managers referred to by Lipsky[61] as 'street-level bureaucrats.' Middle level bureaucrats as the implementers require a thorough understanding of policies to ensure implementation. As pointed out by a key stakeholder, the top-down approach reinforces the belief that framers of policy decisions are the key decision makers and others are expected to follow instructions and 'obey their seniors.'

Pakistan is not unique with reference to health planning. For many countries the record on health planning has not been good.[62] These countries lack the planning culture, political will, resources, and expertise necessary for health planning.[59,62] As a result, health systems in many countries continue to have deficiencies and an imbalance of resources.

The literature is limited on policy formulation processes in developing countries such as Pakistan, characterized by chaotic, politically unstable conditions, rapid change in governments, and turnover of key officials. Research indicates that countries formulate policies in different ways, at different times, and for different purposes, and that the policy formulation process has to be tailored to the country's individual situation.[63] A number of political scientists and analysts have proposed macro and micro theories to describe important elements and constraints of a policy process in light of a country's social and economic circumstances. They have stressed influencing factors such as individual interests, beliefs, and values;[64,58] organization rules and procedures; the broader socio-economic environment in which political institutions operate; and the tendency for bureaucratic officials and interest group leaders to form relatively autonomous policy subsystems.[64,65,66] Understanding these factors in relation to Pakistan can assist in explaining the planning process.

Many of the decision makers and policy makers within the bureaucracy are political appointees and change as governments change or at the order of politicians and/or the Chief Minister. There is a rapid turnover of government officials. They seldom remain long enough in their positions to complete a cycle of formulation, implementation, and reformulation of policies. Therefore, their political commitment, responsibility, and accountability for formulation of policies is short lived. The political will, so necessary for any HHRD, is not present because officials often do not have a long-term commitment or may not be around to follow the process through to its implementation, monitoring and evaluation.

Bureaucratic systems require rules and regulations and adherence to those rules and regulations. Pakistan's systems have broken down under political pressures and the influence of powerful individuals. As aptly described by one stakeholder, the country is functioning on an informal process, whereby decisions are made on an *ad hoc* basis influenced by pressure groups and not in accordance with rules and regulations. This process is seen as providing band aid measures to maintain the status quo or avert disaster.

The key stakeholders identified that although input for the policy formulation process is obtained from selected provincial level government officials (e.g., Chief Ministers, Finance Ministers and Secretaries of Health), decisions are primarily influenced by members in a policy subsystem—selected bureaucrats and politicians, interest groups, and powerful feudal lords.[4,8] Baumann[67] reinforces that the policy subsystem influences policy formulation in situations where policy makers face constraints such as inadequate organizational resources, limited capacity to process information, irresoluble uncertainties, incomplete knowledge, and bureaucratic power struggles.[55] As indicated by key stakeholders, government officials in Pakistan face constraints such as lack of reliable information, breakdown of institutional rules and procedures in the country, and competing demands for limited resources. For instance, with 1 per cent of the GNP allocated to health and 1.6 per cent to education, Pakistan ranks as one of the lowest among developing countries. Janis[55] further explains that policy makers strive to obtain a comprehensive view of alternatives, recognizing and weighing trade-offs among competing values in making policy decisions. Pakistan ranks very low on the human development index (HDI) and very high for military spending.[68] The HDI ranking may be interpreted as reflecting the value given to health and women's development.

In contrast to government officials, the majority of nursing leaders were not aware of the policy formulation process and indicated they did not have influence on policy formulation and planning. Input of the predominantly female nursing personnel was seen as not comparable to that of their male counterparts. For instance, directorates for nursing in provincial governments do not have influence on policy formulation and decision making comparable to that of directorates of health led by male physicians. Bangladesh, another developing country, reported similar findings.[49] These findings could be attributed to nursing leaders being a predominantly female group in a society in which they have low status. O'Brien-Pallas and Hirschfeld et al.,[49] reported that WHO member countries such as Argentina and Colombia, 'argued that nurses by virtue of being a female-dominated group had low status and no place in policy development.' Some developing countries reported that professional associations had submitted policy recommendations to the Ministry of Health, but the recommendations were not given serious consideration.

In contrast to Pakistan, over half of the country respondents (54%) reported that nursing had, compared to other health professionals, influence on policy development at the national level. These countries perceived nurses' contributions as 'valuable and necessary for health service policy development'.[49, p. 60] Alternately, the perceived lack of influence in policy formulation by nursing personnel at provincial and local levels in Pakistan may not be discriminatory against nursing *per se*, but a reflection of the planning process itself in which those charged with implementing policies, regardless of gender and profession, are effectively excluded.

In Pakistan, emphasis has been on the formal process of planning, which has resulted in planning being seen as a bureaucratic function. WHO[62] states that if the planning does not incorporate production and management, then the document becomes only a paper document. Thus, planning the document is an end in itself and does not affect change. According to Green[59] such a plan ends up on the shelves of senior administrators and does not have any observable impact on the health status of the country. Findings indicate that this is occurring in Pakistan.

An example of policy not linked to planning in relation to the production component of HHRD was provided by one of the key stakeholders. A policy was formulated to address the shortage of nurses and an announcement made that enrolment of students in schools of nursing would be doubled. The policy was created by the federal government and provinces were directed to comply. A donor agency agreed to provide the development budget and the provinces agreed to pick up the operational or recurrent costs. In order to increase the enrolment, six new schools were opened in the districts of Sindh province. Overall enrolment of students in the province doubled. Although school buildings and limited equipment were provided through development funds, there was no corresponding increase in the overall number of positions for teachers, as funding of additional positions would need to come from the recurrent budget of the province. No recurrent budget funds were allocated for equipment or other teaching aids. Thus, the number of schools and student enrolment increased, but the quality of education remained poor as inadequate planning for implementation had been conducted.[69]

The development budget was committed at the federal level but provincial governments, although making a commitment to provide recurrent costs, did not follow through with that commitment. One could hypothesize that with respect to the issue of doubling enrolment, the decision makers did not want to: (1) antagonize the donor who may withdraw support; (2) jeopardize losing a larger project in which increasing enrolment of nursing students was a component; (3) antagonize senior provincial government officials such as the Chief Minister, who controls job promotions and transfers; or (4) transgress a cultural norm, that is, not disagree or confront seniors.

The health policy formulation process is complex in both industrial and developing countries. In a country such as Pakistan, the policy formulation process becomes more challenging and complex due to chaotic and unstable conditions, as well as political, economic, social, and cultural influences. Sabatier[70] argues that although beliefs of policy makers can change under unique conditions, it takes time. A decade or more is necessary for policy-oriented learning to take place. He further contends that coalitions, groups, and individuals or organizations can engage in a public debate about these beliefs and bring about changes. However, formation of coalitions and engaging in public debate is extremely difficult in a country marked by political and economic instability, with feudal lords exerting power, and in which an elitist culture, low literacy rate, and low status of women are prevalent. The high illiteracy rate and the fact that more than 30 per cent of the population lives under the poverty line, result in there being no voice of the people to demand their rights to the basic necessities of life.[71] The situation is further compounded by socio-cultural restrictions on females in a male-dominated society.

Planning-Implementation Gap: The theme, Planning-Implementation Gap, encompasses both the process of implementing health policies and nursing input into the process. The five year plans for 1978-1998 address all aspects of health human resource development.

The FYPs contain statements of targets to be achieved: for example, 'increase nurses to meet target of one nurse for five patient beds' (Sixth FYP) or 'award BSc degree to nurses' (Seventh FYP). However, NHRD issues are not analysed for feasibility of implementation nor in terms of need versus availability of resources. These policies are not followed by action plans, a subsequent essential step in policy implementation.[53,54,55,56,57,58] Views of key stakeholders converged on there not being an action plan for nursing. In comparison, the WHO study[49] reported that 38 per cent of respondent countries had a written action plan for nursing. The developed countries reported fewer written action plans for nursing but they indicated a more integrated approach to planning. Many of these countries such as Sweden, the United Kingdom, and the United States were currently monitoring the progress of the impact of previous activities to strengthen nursing practice, education, research, and policy. Fifty per cent of South-East Asian countries had a written national plan for nursing with a focus on improving delivery of services. In a number of these countries, educational programmes had been initiated to increase the number of caregivers and improve quality of services.[49]

The Ministry of Health in the federal government of Pakistan is responsible for health policy and senior government officials from the provinces have input. Implementation of policies, however, is primarily the responsibility of the less senior provincial government officials in the Department of Health—the Director-General Nursing and Director-General Health at the provincial level and medical superintendents and district health officers at the local level. The actual plans may not be received by many of these officials due to a lack of coordination among federal, provincial, and local levels. Among the stakeholders, nursing personnel at all levels and government officials at the local level reported that key documents such as FYPs are not readily accessible. Even if the information is transmitted, many of those responsible for implementation may not have the resources, expertise and/or financial or political clout required for implementation.

Key stakeholders in this study identified clearly the role of pressure groups and political instability in influencing implementation decisions. They identified other factors that impede implementation to be a lack of interest in nursing issues, presence of unrealistic plans, absence of follow up, lack of involvement at grassroots level, health not being a fiscal priority, policies regarding nursing being made by non-nurses, general apathy among the people, and deteriorating conditions of society.

Supply-Requirement Imbalance: The theme, Supply-Requirement Imbalance, includes the issues relating to supply and requirements, number of sanctioned posts for nurses, utilization of nurses, maldistribution of nurses, and labour substitution (use of student nurses in lieu of qualified nurses in delivery of services).

The fact that demands for nursing personnel outweigh the available supply of nurses has been consistently acknowledged in the FYPs. Actions for increasing the supply of adequately prepared nurses, such as increasing output and delinking services and education, have been contained in a number of FYPs. In Sindh, actions have been taken to increase the supply of nurses: for example, establishment of schools of nursing in rural areas. However, a shortage of nurses and a surplus of doctors were perceived by all stakeholders to be prevalent throughout Sindh and the rest of the country. Global trends indicate a general shortage of nursing personnel in the majority of WHO member countries. There were few countries where supply equaled demand. Shortages were generally related to factors such as poor utilization patterns, shortages in specific clinical areas, uneven distribution of nurses between rural and urban areas and between community and hospital care, supply-demand imbalances, inappropriate nurse-bed ratios, and poor status of nurses.[49] In Pakistan, the factors identified by key stakeholders as contributing to shortages were similar to the factors reported in the WHO study.

The shortage of nurses in the public sector in Pakistan is embedded in the socio-cultural, economic, and political milieu of the country as reflected in reasons given by the stakeholders—an inadequate number of sanctioned posts thus forcing the nurses into the private sector, a limited applicant pool, lack of security in student hostels and places of work, political unrest, and political pressures on the process of transfers and postings of nursing personnel. Findings revealed that the applicant pool was adversely affected by factors such as low status of women, low female literacy rate, family and cultural restriction, and inadequate understanding of work of nurses. A limited applicant pool resulted in vacancies in student seats which further exacerbated the shortage. These factors also impacted on the deployment of nurses to rural areas and other areas of need.

The situation regarding an inadequate number of sanctioned posts is complex and not well understood by key stakeholders. An inadequate number of positions in the public sector results in graduates of schools of nursing in the public sector seeking employment in the private sector. The governments bear the costs of educating the students but lose the benefits. The findings revealed that the real status of sanctioned positions (existing number, filled, vacant, and filled by non-nursing personnel) is not known by nursing leaders or others. The lack of a reliable database makes it difficult for strong arguments to be made for an increase in the number of positions.

Nursing respondents discussed the request process for additional posts. It is complex, and nursing personnel indicated that they are not involved in it. The request is initiated by a medical superintendent, then sent to the Director-General Health who forwards it to the Planning Division of the province. The Planning Division receives requests from all health units, reviews them and sends approved requests to the Finance Division which scrutinizes them and makes necessary changes based on the available budget. The requests are then sent to the federal Planning Chief who constitutes work groups to deliberate them. The working groups present their reports in a restricted number of pages to the Planning Chief who summarizes them. After approval from several levels, including Finance, Establishment and The Assembly, the summaries are incorporated in FYPs. The process includes the allocation of development funds at the federal level for the first year of the commitments and requires recurrent budget funds at the provincial level for the following years.

The rationale for the need for increased nursing positions may not even be presented. If government officials making the decisions perceive nurses to have low status and utility, budgets for these positions will be lost among other competing demands during the long process of approval. The fact that the number of nursing positions has increased only minimally since the establishment of institutions is an indication of the low priority given to nursing despite efforts of some government officials at the local level. For example, a key stakeholder at the local level remarked that a request for creation of additional posts had been submitted for the past ten years. Each year the answer was that the request could not be filled due to budgetary constraints, and that the request would be reviewed the next year. However, no new positions have been created.

The impact of poor quality of care, a theme that emerged from the data, may be associated with shortage of nurses. This situation has not been fully assessed, especially the impact on the costs of services, morbidity and mortality, or on the quality of life of the patient population. No research has been done in Pakistan on the relationship between quantity and quality of health care providers and health of the population. What is known is that Pakistan has one of the lowest nurse to patient ratios. Even with this knowledge, however, officials would have to possess the political will and finances to rectify the situation. There is no reliable information or data to make informed decisions on health human resources in general and nursing human resources in particular.

The impact of a shortage of nurses on working conditions, morale, and motivation of nurses is well documented in the literature.[72,73,39,74] Research has shown that a shortage of nurses results in role overlap between physician service and nurse service.[49] In Pakistan, the surplus of doctors has resulted in doctors performing many tasks ordinarily performed by nurses, such as taking blood pressure measurements and dressing wounds. That action leads to nurses being undervalued and low priority being given to creating additional sanctioned posts for them. The shortage leads to substitution of student labour for that of qualified nurses; that action contributes to poor quality education, which results in inadequately prepared graduates, and the justification for physicians performing what would normally be nursing tasks. This circular process illustrates the dynamic nature of the relationship among the components of planning, production, and management.

The Pakistan Nursing Council (PNC) has established a standard for determining the requirement for nurses, the international standard based on WHO guidelines of three nurses to ten beds. Government officials involved in planning were not aware of this standard. At the same time nursing leaders were not aware of the implications if the government decided to implement the standard. For example, are there sufficient numbers of nurses and/or will the educational capacity allow for adequate numbers of graduates. Standards are useful guidelines, but external standards should not be accepted until they are made country-specific. The situation in each country needs to be analysed and a plan of action developed to achieve those standards.

Production

Quality of Education: The theme, Quality of Education, encompasses the following issues: recruitment, integration of education and service, financial resources, relevancy and implementation of the curriculum, faculty sanctioned posts, and preparation of faculty.

Since its inception, Pakistan has addressed the need to develop its nursing educational capacity. Establishing schools of nursing (SONs) or increasing the capacity of existing SONs have been an integral part of FYPs. Concerns with the quality of education are also reflected in those plans; for example, separating nursing education from nursing service (Sixth Five Year Plan), and the need for competent faculty and adequate facilities (Seventh Five Year Plan). In the Province of Sindh, the office of Director of Nursing, established in 1991, was given overall responsibility for nursing service and nursing education.

There was consensus among all key stakeholders that improvement is needed in nursing education as the quality of basic education in nursing was unsatisfactory and not improving. Major factors identified as influencing the quality of education were a limited applicant pool and the low qualifications of applicants, integration of service and education, inadequate financial resources, relevancy of the curriculum and limited implementation of the approved curriculum, and inadequate numbers and preparation of faculty. The relationship among the factors was noted by the respondents. Nursing personnel stressed that with adequate resources, including operating budgets, a fully implemented curriculum, improved faculty-student ratios, and a separation of nursing services and education, improvement in the quality of education and the competency of graduates would occur.

Recruitment: The issue, Recruitment, addressed both the characteristics of the applicant pool and the selection of candidates to schools of nursing. Government officials identified the applicant pool as being limited as a result of the low literacy in the country, especially of females and in rural areas. In many instances, schools of nursing in the large urban centres would have more applicants than available student seats, while schools in the rural areas failed to meet their quotas. The limited number of young women from rural areas entering nursing was seen also as having implications for retaining graduates in rural areas. Women who are from a rural area have family ties which reinforce their retention in the area. Nursing personnel were optimistic regarding recruitment of local applicants as a means of increasing retention of graduate nurses in rural areas.

Another socio-cultural factor identified as influencing admissions to nursing schools is the nature of the work of nurses which requires them to have contact with non-family males such as doctors and other health care workers, patients and their relatives. Such contact is contrary to the socio-cultural norms in many sectors of Pakistani society which govern the behaviour of women. Studies have shown that this aspect of nursing contributes to its low social status.[75,76] There is a contradiction in Pakistan in that female doctors are free to transgress these social taboos; the high social status of medicine has a buffering effect.[43,77,15] The nature of nursing and its low social status combine to make it a less attractive occupational choice for young women and their families. In Pakistan, families play a decisive role in occupational choices of women.[76]

Students are paid stipends in the three year diploma programmes located in schools of nursing; the stipend is equivalent to the beginning salary of a staff nurse in the public sector. The provision of stipends was seen as having both positive and negative impacts on recruitment. Availability of stipends facilitated recruitment of applicants to nursing programmes, especially from lower income families. But stipends also contributed to recruitment of candidates more interested in economic incentives than nursing as a profession, and were seen by some respondents as reinforcing the low social status of nursing. Provision of stipends to students as recognition of their contribution to service is not unique to Pakistan. It was part of the apprenticeship model of nursing education in Canada prior to the movement of nursing education into educational institutions.[78]

The educational capacity, that is, the number of student seats, is controlled centrally by the provinces and is tied to the number of stipends available, but planning decisions at the federal level influence actions taken by the provincial governments. When Sindh established additional schools of nursing, government officials were generally supportive of this action which would result in more students to work on the wards. Nursing personnel were of the opinion that any increase in student seats should take place only if there is a corresponding increase in the number of faculty and in the number of positions for staff nurses so that new graduates will be employed.

Political interference was identified as another factor impacting negatively on the admission process and the quality of students being admitted. In some instances, admissions were not based on merit, but were the result of political pressures and resulted in less qualified applicants being admitted. Government officials recommended that consideration be given to raising the minimum entrance criteria from senior matriculation to intermediate with science. This may raise the standard of nursing education but it may also reduce the size of the applicant pool.

Academic qualifications of present applicants were associated with a deteriorating standard of general education. Urdu is the national language of the country and English is the language of instruction only at post-secondary educational institutions, including schools of nursing. Students entering nursing are from diverse backgrounds, with English being their third or fourth language, and many students enter with little or no proficiency in English. English as a subject is included in the nursing curriculum and most textbooks and other learning resources are in English. However, in many schools of nursing both students and faculty have limited ability in English and this is a major obstacle to learning.

Historically, admissions to schools of nursing were under the control of the medical superintendents of hospitals in which schools were located. Recently, a policy was introduced in the Province of Sindh that centralizes admission to all schools of nursing in the province under the office of the Director of Nursing, Sindh. The policy has the potential of ensuring that qualified applicants will be admitted on merit and quotas will be met by distributing the supply of applicants within the system. However, the creation of one central authority could make the admission process vulnerable to political pressure from higher officials, external groups, and individuals. This change in policy demonstrates that with policies which have no structural change, implications can be formulated and implemented by provinces if the political will exists.

Integration of Service and Education: Nursing respondents identified one of the major impacts on quality of education as the use of nursing students to provide service. The shortage of nursing personnel impacts on the production of nurses as the service needs take priority over education.

Students are considered to be integral members of the nursing service and both students and nurses are under the control of the nursing superintendent or chief nursing superintendent, who reports to the medical superintendent of the hospital. The Garsonnin[79] study provided evidence that nursing students are not supervised in the clinical area, posing a risk for patients, as well as being a comment on the state of nursing education. Historically, in many parts of the world including the industrialized countries, nursing education was developed within hospital training schools.[80,78] This practice, therefore, is not unique to Pakistan. In the apprentice model, considerable teaching-learning took place in the clinical setting, where the students were closely supervised.[81] However, in Pakistan that essential element of supervision of students in the clinical area was identified as being absent; this finding was supported by Garsonnin.[79]

The separation of service and education in nursing has been a global phenomenon, and in the United States and Canada the transfer of responsibility for diploma programmes from hospitals to educational institutions took place in the 1960s and 1970s.[78] In the United Kingdom, the transfer was being implemented as part of Project 2000. Kerr and MacPhail[78] identified that achieving the transfer of nursing education from hospitals to educational institutions required 'good communication, interaction, openness, objectivity, readiness to examine beliefs, attitudes and values, and willingness to accept that compromises are needed to move toward collaboration and joint accountability for practise, education and research' (p. 347). The United Kingdom experience is demonstrating that such a transfer is difficult. The findings indicate that in Pakistan, awareness of benefits of decreasing reliance on students for provision of nursing services, the concept of complete separation of education and service, has not permeated beyond nursing leaders. This is an interesting finding given that separation of education and service was a target in the Sixth Five Year Plan, 1983-1988. Inclusion of this target may be a reflection of a planning process which does not take into consideration the feasibility of implementation. Considerable planning and work with non-nursing government officials will be needed if changes in nursing education are to be accomplished.

Financial Resources: A major factor affecting the quality of education that was identified by nursing personnel was lack of a separate budget for nursing education. Apart from salaries of faculty and staff, no budgets are allocated for operation of the schools. A government official confirmed that the provincial government does not designate a separate budget for operational costs for nursing education; designated funds would be available to nursing only in instances in which problems were identified in the infrastructure such as repair of a building. Even when schools of nursing receive equipment that has been donated by an outside agency the equipment may not be used, as operational costs are not provided. The quality of nursing education is, therefore, negatively affected. Other than monies flowing to schools through hospitals, there is no other source of revenue. Tuition fees are not charged for nursing education in the public sector.

Curriculum: Government officials' and nursing leaders' perceptions diverged in their assessment of curriculum in basic nursing educational programmes. Government officials felt that the curriculum was based on the Western model and was not relevant to the needs of the country. Nursing personnel felt that the curriculum was relevant to the needs of the country, but was not being implemented fully. The current curriculum was revised in 1990 with assistance from a donor agency, including a consultant who worked with senior nurses for more than two years. Revision of the curriculum was well supported by the Ministry/Departments of Health at both federal and provincial levels. Government officials who participated in this endeavour have left their positions and current officials may not have the information on the revised curriculum.

Nursing personnel cited limited implementation of the approved curriculum for basic schools of nursing as being a factor contributing to the poor quality of education. Many schools do not have adequate resources for its implementation (e.g. teachers prepared in community health nursing, learning resources, transport). This issue is related to lack of financial resources, preparation of faculty, and number of sanctioned positions for faculty. It also illustrates limitations of the regulatory body, the Pakistan Nursing Council, which has responsibility for monitoring implementation and taking corrective action as well as approving curriculum. In addition, it demonstrates the need for ongoing monitoring and evaluation of schools of nursing by the office of the Director of Nursing, Sindh. Both the PNC and the office of the Director of Nursing, Sindh were identified by Morgan[63] as being in need of strengthening.

Faculty Complement: Perceptions of a majority of nursing personnel converged with those of government officials with respect to quantity of faculty in schools of nursing in the province, that is, the faculty-student ratio was inadequate. Government officials had limited knowledge of the quality of faculty. Nursing personnel discussed quality of faculty with respect to preparation of teachers, their workloads, number of sanctioned positions, and teacher-student ratios. There was consensus that faculty were generally inadequately prepared for their roles and that teaching loads were so heavy that teachers were not able to perform effectively. As noted by one of the nursing respondents, a teacher is expected to teach all courses to students in all three years of the diploma programme. The total number of students may be small (sometimes less than 100 in the entire programme), but the workload and the expectation that one teacher would have adequate preparation in all areas of the curriculum to teach all the courses are unrealistic.

A factor identified primarily by nursing personnel was that there were sufficient numbers of nurses with appropriate academic qualification, but that these individuals continued to work as staff nurses because they were not promoted to positions of teachers. One of the reasons for this situation was delay in departmental, provincial, and federal promotions which are dependent on Service Commissions. The Service Commissions appeared to have been delayed due to political instability and changes in governments. The delay in promotions is not unique to Pakistan, as Bangladesh in a study reported that there had been no promotions in the last fifteen years.[49]

Another factor identified as affecting the quality of teaching in schools of nursing was the very limited number of sanctioned positions for nursing faculty in relation to requirements. Nursing respondents at all levels indicated that faculty-student ratios varied across institutions with similar students enrolment; schools of nursing in rural areas had more inadequate ratios compared to those in urban areas. However, the majority of stakeholders felt that schools of nursing lacked competent faculty irrespective of the faculty-student ratio. The non-availability of accurate data on the number of sanctioned posts in both education and service, the extent to which they are filled and the qualifications of those in both education and service place nursing personnel in a difficult position to effect change.

Quality of teaching in schools of nursing may be associated with a deterioration in general education and a deterioration of standards in basic nursing education. This is compounded by weaknesses in the post-basic programmes offered at four Colleges of Nursing to prepare nurses for roles in nursing education. Although educational programmes at several of the colleges have improved, the need to revise curriculum to enhance its relevancy and improve the quality of teaching has been identified by nursing respondents and the governments as a priority in a CIDA-funded project.[20] Until recently, the Province of Sindh had been dependent upon federal Colleges of Nursing to prepare its future nursing teachers. A provincial College of Nursing Jamshoro is part of a larger project funded through the World Bank.[82] That programme includes preparation in community health nursing for future teachers. In addition, the province has been supportive of development of a post-diploma BScN programme in one of the colleges, a component of the CIDA developmental project,[20] and of nurses from Sindh receiving higher education through the BScN programme at the Aga Khan University.[20,82] These actions are an indication that the Government of Sindh, with support from external donors, is placing value on the need to improve the quality of nursing education through provision of improvements in teacher preparation and expansion of post-basic educational capacity,

Management

Working Conditions: The theme, Working Conditions, encompasses the issues of adequacy of resources, adequacy of the numbers of prepared nurses, respect and recognition, degree of satisfaction, salary and benefits, and quality of care.

There was convergence among key stakeholders that the working environment of nurses was poor. Factors identified as affecting work environment and job satisfaction included those in the immediate work environment, as well as in the socio-cultural, political, and administrative environments. Factors cited by both nursing personnel and government officials at all levels were lack of resources (finances, supplies, and equipment); lack of respect, low image, and low status of nursing; and political instability, political pressures, interference, and insecurity (personal safety). Other factors cited by some government officials and nursing personnel were long working hours, excessive workloads due to a shortage of nurses, no opportunities for further growth, lack of incentives and inadequate remuneration, inadequate benefits such as accommodation and transport, the working environment being male dominated, and lack of awareness by the general public of nurses' work. Additional factors identified only by nursing personnel were increased non-nursing and clerical duties, lack of teamwork, and lack of recognition for nurses' work.

Much has been written in the Western context[83,84] about factors necessary for quality work environments for nursing. Many factors identified by the respondents as affecting working environments and job satisfaction are reflective of problems experienced by nursing globally. In most regions of the world, working conditions of nursing are associated with a low status and that status is associated with the status of women.[85] Nursing in Pakistan is no exception to that global phenomenon.

The low status of nursing in Pakistan is reflected in the limited or non-involvement of nursing personnel in decision-making processes which impact on working conditions, as well as other dimensions of nursing human resource development. This situation is not unique to Pakistan. 'With so few nurses in key positions to influence policies regarding the employment of nurses, it is little wonder that, globally, nurses endure poor working and living conditions'.[85, p. 20]

A unique factor not identified in the literature, but prevalent in Pakistan, was the political influence on operational aspects of nurses' work. Findings indicate that political influences not only impact on what nurses will do, but which patients will receive care and where nurses will work. The structure of health services in Pakistan is very centralized. A small group of federal and provincial government officials make decisions regarding allocation of personnel to institutions.

Two indicators of working conditions cited in the literature[49] are increase in salaries and/or benefits and improvement in career opportunities. In Pakistan, nursing personnel are members of the public service system and salary and benefits for a grade are applied equally across cadres. This system is advantageous in that there is less room for discrimination. The majority of nurses are not in the officer classes, that is, BSP-17 and above. Senior nurses are in the officer category and some are at the very top of the scale. As members of the public service, nurses receive annual or periodic increments as provided for the entire public service in relation to job classification regardless of quality of performance. There is an annual increment amount fixed for each grade until the ceiling is reached for that particular grade. Although a number of respondents described salaries and benefits as inadequate, the situation is not nursing specific other than in relation to the starting grade for nursing personnel.

In the countries of the North and South, another factor in the workplace perceived by nursing personnel as affecting working conditions is discrimination on the basis of gender. In the North, nurses see this as being manifested in wage discrimination against women, job opportunity discrimination against men, and sexual harassment in the workplace.[86] In Pakistan, nursing respondents perceived sexual discrimination in the form of sexual harassment and in the delegation of power, authority, and decision making to men. The societal norm is for men to have power and authority in decision making in general and over women in particular.[87,88] Societal role expectations of men and women are being played out in the work environment of nurses. Women living or working outside the protection of their family are vulnerable targets for sexual harassment. Male health care workers, by virtue of being male and not just because they have a higher education or social status, exert control over nurses.[77]

SIMILARITIES AND DIFFERENCES

Similarities and differences were found across levels and between affiliations. Demographic profiles of key stakeholders showed similarities among respondents with respect to age, length of service and marital status, while differences were seen in gender between the affiliations and in educational qualifications. The majority of nursing personnel (89.5%) was female and government officials were male (93.3%). Findings demonstrated that key positions in government relating to health policy and decision making are gender specific. Issues and concerns of nursing may not be addressed adequately due to male domination in decision making and lack of knowledge and understanding of women's issues.[87]

Low prioritizing or not addressing nursing issues could reflect the socio-cultural and political environment prevailing in the country. Differences between nursing personnel and government officials with respect to planning may be seen as a reflection of nursing being a predominantly female occupation in a country in which women have low status. The finding that 89.5 per cent of nursing personnel were married is interesting in light of the commonly held belief that family constraints such as marriage lead to nurses dropping out of the work force. That belief was cited by government officials as a factor contributing to the nursing shortage.

All the government officials who participated in the study had obtained university degrees, whereas less than half of the nursing personnel had achieved that level of education. Government officials viewed HHRD from a broad societal perspective and had limited awareness or understanding of NHRD issues. At the same time, nursing personnel had a narrow perspective of HHRD. Although they exhibited an understanding of issues within nursing, they were focused on the micro picture at an operational level; they lacked an understanding of the government system, its structure as well as functions, and its influence on NHRD and the relationship of NHRD to health needs, health resources, and health research in Pakistan. The narrower perspective could be associated with the limited educational background of nursing leaders and their limited exposure to the government system and involvement (or non-involvement) with external groups. Furthermore, nursing leaders identified nurses as being socialized into performing tasks, rather than acquiring conceptual and strategic skills in problem identification and decision making.

The majority of government officials lacked awareness of some of the changes occurring in nursing education: for example, curriculum revision. They had limited knowledge regarding specifics of working conditions, whereas nursing personnel were informed regarding nursing education and management of nursing personnel. Differences may be associated with the degree of involvement in nursing. Findings demonstrate that officials at the local level who have more direct contact with nursing have more knowledge and understanding of issues related to NHRD. Officials at this level are involved in implementing policies impacting on nursing that are received from federal and provincial levels. Unfortunately, their input in policy formulation and decision making is minimal in the government's hierarchical system.

The key findings are interesting. Nursing personnel at all levels are not aware of many of the issues such as processes involved in development and implementation of five year plans. Senior government officials have a lack of awareness of critical issues, both environmental and professional, that face the nursing profession. However, there are many similarities between perceptions of nursing personnel and those of government officials. Both groups agree that there is a lack of resource data on which to base planning, and that needs assessments would provide necessary information. This mutual understanding is a strength on which future action could be built.

SUMMARY

This study explored the current situation of nursing human resource development (NHRD) in the Province of Sindh in Pakistan. Two main research questions were explored regarding: (la) The perceptions of key decision makers relating to planning, production, and management of NHRD; (1b) The differences and similarities that may exist, if any, between decision makers at various levels and of different affiliations; and (2) The issues identified regarding the current NHRD situation in relation to specific aspects of planning, production, and management of NHRD as perceived by the stakeholders.

Issues that provided impetus to this study were: (1) a dearth of studies which focus on all components of HHRD; (2) a limited number of studies on NHRD; and (3) the lack of reliable data on all aspects of HHRD, including NHRD, particularly in a developing country such as Pakistan. The study of a predominately female health profession in a developing country in which women have a low social status, and where development of the social sector has received low priority, provided an opportunity to investigate the impact of socio-cultural, economic, and political influences on HHRD in general and NHRD in particular.

Qualitative research methods were used for this study. The methodology was selected as NHRD is a relatively unexplored phenomenon in Pakistan, and the method allowed the richness and depth of the perceptions of key decision-makers to be captured through the use of semi-structured interviews focusing on the current NHRD situation. Key stakeholders were identified as government officials, nurses and non-nurses, in senior positions at the federal, provincial and local levels, and senior nurses in the regulatory body and/or professional associations at the national, provincial, and local levels.

The study used Hall's[45] expansion of the COHHRD model and guidelines for conducting a situation analysis of HHRD. A policy review of the five year plans (from 1978-1998) of the country was conducted to identify issues relating to NHRD.

The findings were organized under three components of HHRD: planning, production, and management. The analysis addressed the similarities and differences in the perceptions of the key stakeholders. The findings are summarized as follows:

Human Resource Planning

Planning was identified as being hierarchical in nature, with a top-down approach and ineffective. The nature of the process by which health policies were formulated, the absence of a comprehensive plan for HHRD, and the lack of a national approach to planning was identified as contributing to limited implementation of policies. There are no reliable data bases for decision making and planning was characterized by plans to increase the supply and add infrastructure based primarily on donor support. There was limited involvement of nursing leaders in planning; decision-makers operating with limited understanding of HHRD, low priority being given to nursing, and inadequate financial resources. The result was an inadequate supply of nurses in relation to needs, and a maldistribution in favour of urban areas and tertiary care services.

Human Resource Production

The production of nursing personnel was reported as not being coordinated with planning of nursing personnel. The quality of nursing education was deemed to be unsatisfactory and deteriorating, although there were differences of perception between nursing personnel and government officials as to why the situation is the way it is. The revised curriculum is not being implemented fully or effectively. Cultural barriers and societal pressures have an impact on the potential applicant pool for the nursing profession. Socio-cultural, economical, and political factors affect the quality of basic education in the country which in turn impacts on the quality of professional education. The increase in number of students has not resulted in an increase in faculty to provide the education. An example of the lack of integration of planning is that qualified teachers are under employed and are working as staff nurses due to a lack of sanctioned teaching positions in schools of nursing. Nursing education is administered by nursing service departments and hospital and service needs take precedence over students' educational or learning needs.

Human Resource Management

Management of nursing human resources is characterized by a poor working environment, job dissatisfaction, and inadequate salary and benefits of nursing personnel. Quality of nursing care in the hospitals is affected by the poor management of nursing personnel. Incentives are not provided to work in the rural areas. Lack of continuing education and a defined career ladder affect morale and motivation.

The factors affecting job satisfaction, working conditions, and reasons for a perceived shortage of nurses are interrelated and, in some instances, overlap. Most of these factors could be summarized under socio-cultural, economic, and political factors affecting nursing human resource management.

Conclusions

Findings from this study contributed to further understanding of the nursing human resource development in the Province of Sindh, Pakistan. Both the COHHRD model and Hall's[29] expansion of that model provided a framework for the study of the planning, production, and management components of HHRD. This study confirmed the value of the suggestion by Hall[29] that determining the perceptions of key stakeholders is an important initial step in HHRD. The study also reaffirmed the importance of interviewing key stakeholders at various levels and affiliations. Studying HHRD in Pakistan demonstrated clearly the influence of socio-cultural, economic, and political milieus on HHRD.

The current situation of nursing human resources development in Pakistan has deficiencies in areas of planning, production, and management. Although the nursing profession in Pakistan is organized and provides direction and leadership to its members, it would appear to have minimum impact on planning. The nursing shortage is a circular process in that poor quality of education and extensive use of students for nursing service results in inadequately prepared graduates and a lack of motivation to increase the number of sanctioned posts for qualified nurses. The inadequate number of sanctioned posts results in students being used for service, and poor quality of education. Although there were individual variations, as a group the key stakeholders, especially the nursing personnel, did not have an in-depth understanding of the policy formulation and planning process or of HHRD. NHRD was not related to the health problems and needs of the country. Changes such as a revised curriculum for basic schools of nursing have occurred, but knowledge of those changes and of difficulties nursing education is encountering are not known by government officials in decision-making positions.

Implications

The findings of this study have implications for the key stakeholders in relation to health human resource development in general and nursing human resource development in Pakistan in particular. It is important to note that Pakistan is not the only country facing problems with NHRD. Globally, countries in both the North and South are struggling with efficient and effective use of nursing human resources. The social and political structures that prevail in Pakistan are unique and associated with historical, political, religious, and cultural influences.

The perceptions of key stakeholders provided information on specific qualitative aspects of the NHRD situation and raised issues and questions that provide directions for intervention. The following implications arise from the study:

- A more in-depth understanding is needed by stakeholders (e.g. nursing leaders and government officials) of the policy formulation and the planning process, if they are to influence the process. NHRD should be related to health problems, health needs, health research, and health resources. In planning, the socio-cultural, economic, and political factors need to be taken into account. Key stakeholders need to acquire an understanding of the process by which policies are formulated and planning decisions made, and could be acquired through several strategies such as production of monographs, workshops, and other continuing education. Thus, these need to be concise, direct, and marketed in a way that will appeal to the stakeholders.
- Government officials have a lack of awareness of the issues at the hospital level in nursing. The nursing profession should

assist government officials to become aware of nursing issues and the value of a strong nursing service. There needs to be a focus on both data collection and synthesis, as well as effective dissemination to decision makers.

- The shortage of nurses and sanctioned posts need to be examined more closely. According to the stakeholders' responses and the policy review process, the demand for nursing personnel did not seem to be realistic or have a rational basis, for example, 'increase the nurses to have a target of one nurse to five beds.' The requirement for nursing personnel needs to be critically assessed for feasibility (financial, human resources, and material such as schools, equipment) and planned according to the realities of Pakistan within the socio-cultural, economic, and political milieu.

- One strategy for improving nursing education is to examine prototypes from other countries that transferred nursing education from hospitals to educational institutions. A complete separation of nursing education and service would take many years to accomplish and may not be preferable. A more immediate strategy may be to decrease the amount of time students spend in the provision of nursing service with the long-term goal being to remove them fully from nursing services. This strategy will require thorough planning involving key stakeholders and it would have to be done in a phased manner.

- The need for an assessment of curriculum for relevancy in relation to the health needs and health resources should be considered.

- The efficient and effective use of nursing human resources in terms of quantity and quality is an issue. Career ladders that recognize both education and experience need to be implemented.

- The nursing profession in Pakistan needs to explore strategies that would maximize its impact on all areas of NHRD. The infrastructure already exists in the form of a regulatory body and the professional association. The PNC has been given the legal authority and a clear mandate with respect to nursing education and standards of practice.[90,91] The PNC needs to enhance its credibility and capacity if it is to persuade the government to take the necessary action to improve nursing education and practice in the country.

- The PNC, the professional associations, and individual nurses in senior positions, need to review their goals and become politically active in lobbying the provincial and federal government. In addition to political skills such as lobbying, nursing leaders would need expertise in management and leadership.
- The PNC, in consultation with nursing superintendents and directorates of nursing needs to develop realistic standards for nursing education and strategies for implementation, monitoring, and evaluations.

Many issues are embedded in the socio-economic environment and administrative structure. However, further research will provide stronger data bases to assist decision makers to make more informed choices.

NOTES

1. World Health Organization (WHO) Study Group, *Coordinated Health Human Resource Development* (Technical Report Series 801), Geneva, 1990, p. 25.
2. UNICEF, *Situational Analysis of Children and Women in Pakistan*, Islamabad, Pakistan: Pictorial Printers, 1992.
3. S.A. Zaidi, *The political economy of health care in Pakistan*, Lahore, Pakistan: Vanguard Books Ltd., 1988.
4. A. Nasim, and A. Akhlaque, *Human Resource Development and Economic Policy: The case of Pakistan*, Lahore, Pakistan: Lahore University of Management Sciences, 1995.
5. Government of Pakistan (GOP), *Economic Survey, 1995-1996*, Islamabad: Economic Advisor Wing, Finance Division, 1996.
6. National Institute of Population Studies (NIPS), *Pakistan demographics and Health Survey 1990-1991*, USA: DHS IRD/Macro International Inc., 1992.
7. L.A. Delvoie, 'Development of Women Health Professionals,' Inaugural address, workshop on *Development of Women Health Professionals*, 4-7 December 1993, Bhurban, Pakistan: Ministry of Health, Government of Pakistan in collaboration with Canadian International Development Agency (CIDA), 1993.
8. United Nations Development Programme (UNDP), *Balanced Development: An approach to Social Action in Pakistan*, Summary Report, Islamabad, Pakistan, 1993.
9. United Nations Development Programme (UNDP), *Human Development Report*, New York: Oxford University Press, 1995.

10. Mahbub ul Haq, *Human Development Report in South Asia*, Karachi, Pakistan: Oxford University Press, 1997.
11. Government of Pakistan (GOP), *Health Sector: A Situational Report*, Islamabad: Planning Division.
12. M. Lockheed, *Improving Primary Education in Developing Countries*, Washington, DC: Oxford University Press (Published for World Bank), 1991.
13. J.E. Rosen and S.R. Conly, *Pakistan's Population Programme: the challenge ahead* (Country Study Series No. 5, p. 13), Washington, DC: Population Action International. 1996.
14. World Bank. *Staff Appraisal Report: Islamic Republic of Pakistan Social Action Programme Project* (Report No. 12588-PAK). Washington, DC: The World Bank, Population and Human Resource Division, Country Development III South Asia Region, 1994.
15. World Bank, *Staff Appraisal Report: Pakistan Second Family Health Project* (Report No. 11127-PAK), Washington, DC: The World Bank, Population and Human Resource Division, Country Development III South Asia Region, 1993.
16. F. Shaheed and K. Mumtaz, *Women's Economic Participation in Pakistan. A status report*, Islamabad, Pakistan: Shirkat Gah for UNICEF, 1990.
17. Government of Pakistan (GOP), *National manpower commission report*, Islamabad: National Manpower Commission, 1991.
18. L.L. Lim and C. Coenjaerts, *Creating the Enabling Environment of Women's Employment in Pakistan*, A report for the ILO mission for regional office for Asia and the Pacific Bangkok, Geneva: International Labour Office, November 1993.
19. A. Saeed, *Structural Issues in Women's Development in Pakistan*, Islamabad: UNICEF Pakistan, 1990.
20. Canadian International Development Agency (CIDA), *From Plan to Action. CIDA's Women in Development Programme in Pakistan*, Islamabad: Women's Development Fund, Pakistan, 1995.
21. World Bank, *Pakistan Towards a Health Sector Strategy*, May, Washington, DC: the World Bank, Population and Human Resource Division, Country Department I, South Asia Region, 1997.
22. S.J. Ward, *A review of Regulations and Incentives for Health Staff in Pakistan: With emphasis on female staff and rural areas*, Ottawa: Canadian International Development Agency, 1992.
23. Tariq Banuri, A.R. Kemal, and K. Mumtaz, 'Human resource development,' in Tariq Banuri, S.R. Khan, and M. Mahmood (eds.), *Just Development*, Karachi: Oxford University Press, 1997, pp. 45-60.
24. World Bank, *World Development Report 1996*, Washington, DC: Oxford University Press, 1996.
25. T.P. Schultz, *Women and Development: Objectives, Framework and Policy Intervention*, Princeton, NJ: Yale University, Department of Economics, 1989.
26. J. Leslie, *Weathering economic crises: The crucial role of women in health*, Washington, DC: International Centre for Research on Women, 1986.
27. A. Ghafoor, 'Development of human resource population manpower and employment policies in Pakistan,' *Pakistan's Occasional Paper*, Islamabad, Pakistan: Manpower Institute, 1984.
28. M.K. Bacchus, *Human resource development in a post-apartheid South Africa, report*, London: Commonwealth Secretariat, 1991.

29. T.L. Hall, *Human resource for health: Models for projecting workforce supply and requirements*, Geneva: WHO, 1993.

30. T.L. Hall and A. Mejia, *Health manpower planning: Principles, methods, issues*, Geneva: WHO, 1978.

31. S.E. French and P. Herberg, 'Capacity building: The challenge of strengthening the nursing system in Pakistan,' *Journal of Canada-Pakistan Cooperation*, 9, 1995, pp. 1-4.

32. A. Brihaye, *Nurses' pay: A vital factor in health care*, Geneva: International Labour Office, 1994.

33. M.E. Cowart and W.J. Serow (eds.), *Nurses in the workplace*, Newbury Park, CA: Sage Publications, 1992.

34. C. Hancock, 'Nurses and skill mix,' *Senior Nurse, 12*(5), 1992, pp. 9-12.

35. J. Reid, 'Computer individualized nursing care: Some implications,' *Journal of Clinical Nursing, 1*, 1992, pp. 7-12.

36. J. Stelling, 'Staff nurses' perception of nursing: Issues in a women's occupation,' in B.S. Bolaria H.D. Dickinson (eds.), *Health, illness, and health care in Canada* (2nd ed.), Toronto, Canada: Harcourt Brace, 1994.

37. J. Buchan and J. Ball, *Caring Costs: Nursing Costs and Benefits*, Brighton: Institute of Manpower Studies, 1991.

38. A. Tierney, 'Challenges for nursing research in an era dominated by health service reform and cost containment,' *Clinical Nursing Research*, 2(4), 1993, pp. 382-395.

39. H.P. McKenna, 'Nursing skill mix substitutions and quality of care: an exploration of assumptions from the research literature,' *Journal of Advanced Nursing*, 21, 1995, pp. 452-459.

40. International Council of Nurses, 'Worldwide survey of nursing issues,' *International Nursing Review*, 42(4), 1995, pp. 125-127.

41. Wazir Ali, 'Nursing services structure to be upgraded,' 7 December, *The Nation*, p. 3, Islamabad, 1993.

42. Ministry of Health (MOH), *Strengthening of human resources in nursing in Pakistan*, Executive action document, WHO Nursing Advisors Report, Pakistan, 1992.

43. Asian Development Bank (ADB), *Appraisal of the health care development project in Pakistan*, November, Islamabad, Pakistan, 1992.

44. F.G. Abdellah and E. Levine, *Preparing nursing research for the 21st century: Evolution, methodologies and challenges*, New York: Springer Publishing Company, 1994.

45. T.L. Hall, *Guidelines for a human resource development study*, Geneva: WHO, 1995.

46. P.A. Field and J.M. Morse, *Nursing research: The application of qualitative approaches*, London: Croom Helm, 1985.

47. C. Marshall and G.B. Rossman, *Designing qualitative research*, Newbury Park, CA: Sage Publications, 1989.

48. M.Q. Patton, *Qualitative evaluation and research methods,* (2nd ed.), Newbury Park, CA: Sage Publications, 1990.

49. L. O'Brien-Pallas, M. Hirshfeld, A. Baumann, J. Shamian, L. Bajnok, O. Adams et al., *A study to examine the strengthening of nursing and midwifery services:*

Phase 1. An examination of extent of implementation of resolution (WHA45.5), Ottawa: International Development Research Centre, 1997.

50. T.L. Hall, 'Guidelines for health workforce planners,' *World Health Forum, 8,* 1988, pp. 409-413.

51. Tariq Banuri, 'Just adjustment and just health,' in T. Banuri, S.R. Khan and M. Mahmood (eds.), *Just Development,* Karachi: Oxford University Press, 1997, pp. 3-15.

52. Charles Hank Kennedy, *Bureaucracy in Pakistan,* Karachi: Oxford University Press, 1987.

53. J. Cooksey R. Krieg, 'Metropolitan health policy development: Barriers to implementation,' *Journal of Public Health Policy,* 17(3), 1996, pp. 261-274.

54. M.L. Goggin, *Policy design and politics of implementation: The case of child health care in the America States,* Tennessee: University of Tennessee Press, 1987.

55. I. Janis, 'Causes and consequences of defective policy-making: A theoretical analysis,' in F. Heller (ed.), *Decision-making and leadership,* New York: Free Press, 1992.

56. P. Sabatier and D. Mazmanian, 'The condition of effective implementation: A guide to accomplishing policy objectives,' *Policy Analysis,* 5, 1979, pp. 481-504.

57. B. Walker, Jr., 'Impediments to the implementation of environmental policy,' *Journal of Public Health Services,* 15(2), 1994, pp. 186-202.

58. World Health Organization (WHO) Expert Committee, *Health manpower requirements for the achievement of health for all by the year 2000 through primary health care,* (Technical Report Series 717), Geneva, 1985.

59. A. Green, *An introduction to health planning in developing countries,* Oxford: Oxford University Press, 1995.

60. D.A. Mazmanian and P.A. Sabatier (eds.), *Effective policy implementation,* Lexington, MA: Lexington Books, 1989.

61. M. Lipsky, *Street-level bureaucracy: Dilemmas of the individual in public services,* New York: Russell Sage Foundation, 1980.

62. World Health Organization (WHO) Expert Committee, *Management of human resources for health,* (Technical Report Series 783) Geneva, 1989.

63. P. Morgan, *Development of Women Health Professionals: Institutional appraisal report,* unpublished report, Canadian International Development Agency, Ottawa, 1993.

64. J. Lomas, 'Making clinical policy explicit: Legislative policy-making and lessons for practice guideline development,' *International Journal of Technology Assessment in Health Care,* 9(1), 1993, pp. 11-25.

65. P.A. Sabatier, 'Knowledge, policy-oriented learning, and policy change,' *Knowledge: Creation, diffusion, utilization,* 8, 1987, pp. 649-92.

66. P.A. Sabatier, 'An advocacy coalition framework of policy change and the role of policy-oriented learning therein,' *Policy Science,* 21(2-3), 1988, pp. 129-168.

67. A. Baumann, *Global issues in health, labour and social policy,* paper presented at the International Council of Nurses Congress, Vancouver, BC, 18 June 1997.

68. United Nations Development Programme (UNDP), *Human Development Report 1994,* New York: Oxford University Press, 1994.

69. I. Moghul, Personal communication, June 1997.

70. P.A. Sabatier, 'Top-down and bottom-up approaches to implementation research: A critical analysis and suggested synthesis,' *Journal of Public Policy*, 6(1), 1990, pp. 21-48.

71. A.R. Kemal and M. Mahmood, 'Poverty and policy in Pakistan,' in T. Banuri, S.R. Khan and M. Mahmood (eds.), *Just Development*, Karachi: Oxford University Press, 1997, pp. 63-90.

72. S.M. Carlson and M.E. Cowart, *Shifts in supply and demand for nursing and other health care personnel in the 1980s: A review and evaluation of the literature*, Tallahassee: Florida State University, Institute on Aging, 1988.

73. J.C. McClosky, 'Two requirements for job contentment: Autonomy and social integration,' *IMAGE: Journal of Nursing Scholarship*, 22, 1990, pp. 140-143.

74. N.M. Meltz, *Sorry no care available due to nursing shortage*, Toronto: Registered Nurses' Association of Ontario, 1988.

75. Y. Amarsi and W.L. Holzemer, *Nursing at the Aga Khan University Medical Centre, Karachi*, unpublished report, Karachi, Pakistan: The Aga Khan University Medical Centre, 1990.

76. S. French, D. Watters and R. Matthews, 'Nursing as a career choice for women in Pakistan,' *Journal of Nursing Administration*, 19, 1994, pp. 140-151.

77. S. Siddiqui, 'Nursing—coming a long way,' *Dawn Tuesday Review*, 13 February 1995, pp. 2-8.

78. J. Kerr and J. MacPhail, *Canadian nursing: Issues and Perspectives*, St. Louis: Mosby Year Book, 1996.

79. J. Garsonnin, 'Human resource development in nursing,' *Management Plan Development of Women Health Professionals (DWHP): Nurses and Lady Health Visitors*, unpublished report, Hamilton, Canada: McMaster University School of Nursing and Karachi, Pakistan: The Aga Khan University School of Nursing, 1994.

80. A. Baumgart and J. Larson, *Canadian nursing faces the future,* (2nd ed.), Toronto: C.V. Mosby Company, 1992.

81. O. Hughes, B. Wade, and M. Peters, 'The effects of a synthesis of nursing practice course on senior nursing students' self-concept and role perception,' *Journal of Nursing Education*, 30(2), 1991, pp. 69-72.

82. World Bank, *Islamic Republic of Pakistan health sector study: Key concerns and solutions,* (Report No. 10391-PAK), Washington, DC: The World Bank Population and Human Resource Division, Country Development III South Asia Region, 1993.

83. L. O'Brien-Pallas and A. Baumann, 'Quality of nursing work life issues: A unifying framework,' *Canadian Journal of Nursing Administration*, 5(2), 1992, pp. 12-16.

84. L. O'Brien-Pallas, A. Baumann, and M.J. Villenueve, 'The quality of nursing work life,' in J. Hibberd and M.E. Kyle (eds.), *Nursing Management in Canada*, Toronto: W.B. Saunders Company, 1994, pp. 391-409.

85. World Health Organization (WHO), December, *Nursing practice around the world*, Geneva, 1997.

86. J.R. Ellis and C.L. Hartley, *Nursing in today's world. Challenges, issues, and trends* (6th ed.), Philadelphia: Lippincott-Raven Publishers, 1998.

87. N.S. Khan and A.S. Zia (eds.), *Unveiling the Issues*, Lahore, Pakistan: ASR Press, 1995.

88. A.S. Zia, *Sex crimes in the Islamic context*, Lahore, Pakistan: ASR Publication, 1994.

89. C. Attridge and M. Callahan, 'Women in women's work: Nurses, stress, and power,' *Recent Advances in Nursing*, 25, 1989, pp. 41-69.

90. S.E. French, *Assessment of the Capacity of the Government Institutions*, unpublished report, Contribution to Development of Women in Pakistan Institutional Appraisal Report, Ottawa, Canada: Canadian International Development Agency, 1993.

91. Pakistan Nursing Council (PNC), *Act No. XXVI of 1973: Passed by the National Assembly of Pakistan*, Islamabad, 1973.

10

Reporting from Bangladesh

Rahima Jamal Akhter, Ira Dibra, Nancy H. Bryant
and *Janet James*

REPORTING FROM BANGLADESH

Nursing in Bangladesh developed in a pattern similar to that of nursing in other Asian countries after the establishment of independence. A small number of nurses endeavoured to maintain standards developed by departing British Matrons and Sisters. They attempted to overcome a severe shortage of nurses by recruiting local girls and women, particularly Muslim girls, many of whom were not educationally prepared to enter schools of nursing.

In fact, the history of professional nursing in Bangladesh is linked to the political history of the country. Developments before 1947 are associated with the common origin of nursing from Great Britain along with the rest of the Indian Subcontinent. Advances between 1947 and 1971 are linked to developments in Medical and Nursing fields in combined Pakistan, while those after 1971 (when Pakistan was divided) are associated with the new national policies and programmes of Bangladesh.

The nursing profession had progressed before 1977 through the leadership of the Superintendent of Nursing Services and the Directorate of Health Services under the auspices of the Ministry of Health. That was the year the Directorate of Nursing Service was established, and it has provided leadership for the profession until now.

The College of Nursing was established in 1970 and then affiliated with Dhaka University in 1977. The Bangladesh Nursing Council (BNC) was recognized as a regulatory body by an ordinance of government in 1983.

Over the years, the World Health Organization and other international donor organizations helped in the development of nursing education and services in Bangladesh.

The profession, however, has suffered from lack of higher education opportunities for nursing faculty and leaders, from lack of resources to enable the profession to move ahead, from lack of recognition of the skilled nurses to take advantage of modern technology, educational methods and from lack of leadership skills to enable nurses to take challenges of new advances in clinical nursing, education, primary health care and research. Besides these limitations nursing and nurses work are seen as low prestigious and low valued jobs in the society, which builds a negative image for the profession.

In addition, Bangladesh's financial resources were not adequate to meet the demands or requirements of the health needs of the people. The organization and resources of the Directorate of Nursing Services in regard to nursing human resources were not enough to provide adequate nursing service and education countrywide. Nursing leaders also felt left out of the policy and decision-making process affecting their own profession.

This was the situation when, in 1993, the Strengthening Nursing Education and Services (SNES) Project began its work. The SNES Project was a bilaterally funded initiative between the Government of Bangladesh, the Department for International Development in Britain and the International Development Agency. It was conceived as a process of collaboration through which knowledge, skills and experience would be shared in order to strengthen nursing education and service in Bangladesh. The ultimate aim of the project was to improve the quality of care for patients in the government health sector. The project has worked towards empowering and motivating nurses to take control of, and responsibility for, their own profession. They have begun to identify the standards of practice, management and education which are required, and the control and regulatory mechanisms which are prerequisites for improving the quality of care for patients.

SNES's primary objectives were to develop nurse's skills in policy making and planning, and to improve operational management of nursing services and the quality of basic and post-basic nurse education. These were to be achieved through the development of a demonstration area to provide examples of good practice in education and management, revision of the BSc curriculum at the college of nursing, strengthening the capacity of the Bangladesh Nursing Council and staff training and development. The construction of four divisional continuing education centres, two rural teaching centres and an extension to the College of Nursing were to be planned. A newsletter was to be published in order to disseminate information and generate debate. Accordingly, at the beginning of the SNES project in 1994, a mini size SNES newsletter was published.

From an outsider's perspective (NHB), a major accomplishment of the SNES project is the establishment and publication of a national Nursing Newsletter. The newsletter, published quarterly since 1996, contains articles by nurses, project staff and consultants on a great variety of topics. Much of the success of the newsletter can be credited to the editor, Rahima Jamal Akhtar and three co-editors, Ira Dibra, Salma Khatun and Saleha Khatun. Carol Chamberlain who, as the Nurse Educator to the project, supported and guided the National Consultants to produce the newsletter.

A careful review of the newsletters documents the work of the SNES project through reports on workshops, training programmes, educational tours, the project demonstration area, continuing education centres and so forth. The newsletters also contain information that is helpful to practicing nurses regarding various clinical conditions and the appropriate nursing care for patients with these conditions.

Articles about ongoing policy issues, and the functions of the Bangladesh Nursing Council (BNC) and the Directorate of Nursing Services (DNS), often present problems and dilemmas that these organizations and individuals frequently face.

Of particular interest are the articles that reveal the difficulties, hardships and often humiliation that nurses at all levels face due to the continued low status and image of nursing in Bangladesh.

One purpose of the newsletter has been to generate debate among nurses in the country about the profession. What follows in this chapter are articles or excerpts of articles that have appeared in the Nursing Newsletter, which cover topics such as teacher training and curriculum development, management and supervisory skills, status and image of women and nursing, reproductive health and so forth.

Most telling of the newsletter articles are those that deal with the status and image of women and nursing in a patriarchal and male dominated society, despite the fact that Bangladesh has had two women

Prime Ministers since 1991. Articles by Salma Khatun and Ms Ferdousi describe the current situation.

Nurse-'giri' or Nurse-'ing': Fair Attention is Required
by Salma Khatun, NNC, SNESP, October 1998

Unfortunately, the nursing profession is not getting its due respect in Bangladesh. The media has put the profession in a worse position by portraying a very negative image of nurses and presenting wrong and misleading information regarding nursing and nurses. Due to the low profile and status that society gives nursing, nurses are frustrated, which in turn causes demotivation and low self-esteem.

The success of health services depends mostly on the quality of care required for the nation. Health personnel like Family Welfare Visitors, Family Welfare Assistants and Health Assistants can help in preventive care and can advise the sick to access curative care. In Bangladesh, nurses represent a major work force in the field of curative care. Available information shows that up until 1994 there were 26,000 sanctioned hospital beds, 6,057 nurses and 8,749 doctors in Bangladesh (The Nursing Task Force, 1994). That means one nurse was available for approximately every four patients, and one doctor for every three patients.

The health of a nation is related to the strength and effectiveness of the nursing profession and the quality of nursing care. Unfortunately, the Health Authority in Bangladesh has created a sharp division between medical and nursing professionals. Medical professionals are given the opportunity to prepare themselves to deal with new dimensions of medical science, but nurses are not. In both emergency and specialised care areas, nurses need to update knowledge and skills in order to develop and implement nursing care plans and become familiar with rapidly advancing medical technology.

In the case of salary pensions, nurses are also viewed differently. For example, other diploma holders like medical technologists are given a higher scale than nurses. This is hardly surprising since the majority of nurses are women and women nationwide are subordinate in terms of monthly salary and daily wages. Culturally, the status of Bangladeshi workers or officials depends mostly on their monthly salary. The status of nurses is therefore affected badly by the low payscales. These factors affect nurses' confidence and behaviour towards patient care. Consequently, the quality of nursing services is deteriorating day by day.

No initiative has been taken by policy makers to overcome this problem.

It appears that the male-dominated society and the health structure are pushing the profession backwards in Bangladesh. Society as well as policy makers have a crucial role to play in identifying the root causes of the poor status accorded to nurses and possible solutions for increasing the image of nurses in society. Beside this, nurses themselves also have the prime duty to enhance the respect and prestige of the profession by maintaining a high standard of work, which will help to get a respectable place for the profession in society.

To acquire this, nurses need to have a strong mechanism for establishing nurses' rights by formulating a national nursing policy, preparing a national code of practice, setting standards and controlling the quality of nursing education and services. But without due attention from the Health Services and policy makers, it will not be possible to do.

PROBLEMS FOR FEMALE NURSES: NURSING SERVICES AND ACCOMMODATION

by Ms Ferdousi, BSc in Nursing, MSS (Pol. Science), LLE. Senior Staff Nurse, IPGM&R, Dhaka, January 1997

We nurses are government service holders, and undergo expensive and long (four years) training. After completion of training, Registered Nurses are supposed to be posted throughout the country. These nurses, however, face many problems, and the accommodation problem is one which needs attention.

At the Thana level, a nurse's dormitory is available within the boundary of Thana Health Complexes to accommodate 'single' nurses. Though there are government quarters, these are mainly provided to the office staff. Nurses' demands regarding accommodation are usually neglected.

At the District level, at least twenty-five Registered Nurses are working but the existing capacity of the nurses' dormitory/hostel is not enough to accommodate them, as there are no fixed government quarters for nurses.

The accommodation problem is more acute at the Division level and in the large cities. Due to limited hostel facilities some nurses have occupied students' hostels, which creates another problem. Others need to make their own arrangements within their limited salary. To reduce the transport cost and save time, most nurses try to rent houses near the hospital. In this way they may spend almost all of their salary on rent which affects their economic and family health. Due to non-availability of suitable houses many nurses have rented houses far from their working places. In this situation they need to get up early in the morning to get transport. For the evening and night shift they need to wait a long time for a bus etc. Even to get transport home they need to leave their work place early, which affects patients' care. The ultimate result is that nurses become lethargic, which leads to an unsatisfactory work situation.

To provide high quality care a nurse needs to keep herself free from tensions and anxieties such as how she will get transport or when she will get home, etc. But in reality most nurses in large cities are totally unable to detach themselves from such tensions.

The Nursing Superintendent of the related hospital should be responsible for nurses' accommodations because it is clearly mentioned in her job description. But the fact is that nursing superintendents of large hospitals always push this issue aside.

For instance, in the IPGM&R Hospital, the nurses' issue of residential accommodation is not an undue demand, because 450 crore Taka has been sanctioned and transferred to the hospital authority for development of the IPGM&R Hospital including accommodation of hospital staff. However, nothing has been done to solve the accommodation problem.

I hope that all nursing superintendents of large hospitals and other related authorities will come forward to take the initiative so that all nurses will be properly accommodated. We expect the intervention of the Director of Nursing Services for realisation of this issue. It is not only for the nurses' benefit; it is for the public's too.

* * *

A recent WHO report noted that nurses worldwide lack training in policy and management skills and as a result are not included in the decision making process of their country's health care system. This is certainly the case in Bangladesh and as a result, the SNESP focused on ways of improving management and supervisory skills of nurses who are presently holding management positions. Numerous training programmes, workshops, and study tours have been conducted since 1993 to bring modern management theories and examples of practice to a large number of Bangladeshi nurses. These activities and their results are described in the following articles.

THE CHITTAGONG EXPERIENCE
by Mina Prova Biswas, Ward Manager & Biva Kanungoe, Nursing Supervisor, Ward No. 17, CMCH, October 1998

We work in Ward 17 of the Chittagong Medical College Hospital which is a busy surgical ward. The number of sanctioned beds is 60; however, the total patients vary from 80 to 100. The ward has three admission days per week.

We participated in the Middle Management Course for Nurses. The main subject areas were planning and time management, communication, delegation, supervision and discipline, use of procedural guidelines, problem solving and decision making.

We hoped to apply our new knowledge through improving the ward systems, priority setting, and better managment of our duty time. We also hoped to improve communication between various staff in the ward. Although in recent weeks we have seen some achievements, we have faced many constraints in applying our knowledge into practice.

- What difficulties have we faced? We have experienced a lack of cooperation from senior medical staff, who are unwilling to support any change. They also allow junior medical staff to misbehave. The lack of control over admissions to the ward makes planning difficult. Like many of the wards in CMCH, we have a shortage of water and essential supplies. We have also had very few nurses on the ward. This problem has eased slightly now since the newly appointed nurses joined the hospital, but they are not familiar with the new activities of the ward.
- How are we trying to overcome some of these constraints? We continue to communicate with the medical staff so that they are aware of what we are trying to achieve. We also communicate with the supporting staff (MLSS) about changes we want to make. We

have established better liaison with the linen and general stores to ensure supplies. We have also made personal efforts to improve the ward by buying paper ourselves and purchasing a white board on which to record and display information. Patients and company representatives have also helped us regarding purchasing.

- What improvements have we made on the ward since the Management Course and the evaluation by Dr Ian Yaxley? The ward is much cleaner than before and this is being maintained. We have established a better control of visitors. We have developed a written hand-over system to ensure that important patient information is communicated between shifts. We have prepared a post-operative block on each side of the ward (male and female) and have improved the nursing management of these patients.
- What are our plans for the future improvement of the ward? We will continue the work which we have started, especially with the post-operative patients.

EVALUATION OF THE MIDDLE MANAGERS TRAINING, MAY 1998
by Ian Yaxley, Lecturer, QMC, Edinburgh, July 1998

As part of the SNES Project, 15 Middle Managers received management training at the Continuing Education Centre, Chittagong, during July to October 1997. Most of those managers were staff nurses and in May 1998 the outcome of their training was evaluated by Dr Ian Yaxley, Ira Dibra and Saleha Khatun.

The participants came from three Medical College Hospitals— Sylhet, Barisal and Chittagong. In Sylhet, the Nursing Supervisors of Ward 4 were actively initiating management principles and changing the ward through time management and patient charts. This ward has become a calm and pleasant place for nurses to practice nursing. In Barisal similar changes were made. The nursing instructor from the Nursing Institute had also implemented changes. Importantly, the library was open and the instructor had developed a method to control and register the loan of books to students. This change indicated that students were now borrowing more books. Also, the instructor had introduced participatory seminar where students exchange views and learn amongst themselves instead of being lectured to by instructors.

For all those teachers who want to see what it is possible to achieve, you should visit Barisal.

In Chittagong some very positive changes had occurred in Wards 19, 20 and 13. These wards were being assisted by James and Beryl Green. The changes in these wards since October 1997 are amongst the most effective that anyone will see in Bangladesh. There are clean floors, no patients on the floor, control of visitors, and admittance and discharge procedures. The staff nurse had become a ward manager and was in full control of the ward. Nurses were fully occupied nursing patients and patients were happy to be receiving care. These wards are an example of what nurses can achieve in Bangladesh by applying basic management if they have the support of the doctors.

For all those nurses who say we cannot make changes, we cannot do things for ourselves—go and see these wards and when you do, compare them with other wards. Then ask yourself, where would you prefer to work?

Review of the Nursing Supervisors' Training
by Ira Dibra, National Nurse Consultant, SNES Project

The first workshop for a group of Nursing Supervisors of Thana Health Complexes (THC) was held at the Divisional Continuing Education Centre (CEC), Chittagong from 22nd to 31st March 1998...Ten nursing supervisors attended...These nursing supervisors are newly posted in the THCS. They have neither any written job description nor have they received any training course after completion of their Diploma in Nursing and Midwifery, except the District Public Health Nurse (DPHN).

The aim of the workshop was to assist nursing supervisors to identify their roles and responsibilities in THCs and to develop knowledge and skills in supervision and management related to the local policy of health service delivered by the THCS.

The workshop was mainly focused on the aims and functions of THCs in which nursing supervisors can take part in achieving the goal of THCS. During the course they were asked to tell why they are posted and what roles and responsibilities they have in the health complexes. Along with supervisory tasks, nursing supervisors need to deal with management tasks, communicate with other staff and manage all nursing and supportive staff of THCS. The management process was discussed. Methods of time management at work and in personal life were also addressed. Participants discussed in groups the proportion of their time spent on their tasks, considering the priority in their workplaces. They were encouraged to look at the ways by which they could use their time and energy more usefully and effectively.

The importance and the process of planning were discussed in detail. The participants were divided into groups and the planning procedure was practiced. On the last day of the workshop nursing supervisors were asked individually to make a systematic plan to introduce the specific nursing procedures in THCS. Monitoring was also emphasized because it is an important part of effective supervision. So, nursing supervisors should know why it is important to achieve the goal, and how they will monitor nursing activities performed by nurses and other staff, and how they could improve their own performance. They were also asked to discuss how they could measure whether the activities of staff are being effective or not.

The workshop also stressed the main elements of effective supervision. These are: management tasks, administrative tasks, direct teaching, professional development activities and direct clinical work.

Some basic procedural guidelines were developed for some common tasks of THCs, taking into consideration the availability of local resources. These are the steps and rationale of hand washing, wound dressing, care of intravenous fluid, nasal feeding and catharization. Participants committed to introduce these procedures in their respective areas. They were asked to identify resistance and supporting factors for the introduction of the developed procedures in the THCS. They were also asked to identify ways of overcoming resistance and of maximizing support.

Due to lack of job descriptions and opportunities for in-service education and training, they were not confident in performing their jobs...

Through a detailed discussion of Maslow's Motivation Hierarchy, participants were encouraged to deal with their staff in such a way that they may get respect and cooperation from the staff, as well as to take initiative for staff and professional development. They were also given a self-evaluation checklist and asked to develop suggestions regarding how they could deal with their existing weaknesses as a nursing supervisor.

Throughout the workshop all participants were enthusiastic ...although initially they were reluctant to respond to the class lecture and were inactive in group tasks. But within a few days, it was observed that they became involved in assigned tasks and actively participated in group presentations. Consequently, at the end of the workshop the participants stated that this kind of workshop is essential for all nursing supervisors for gaining knowledge and skills to improve the quality of supervision and management. I would like to mention here that to encourage the effort to implement participants' knowledge and experiences in their workplaces, they should be followed up by the senior nursing managers from the district, division and central levels.

It can be said that the in-service training for nursing supervisors of Thana level is really an appropriate and timely step. However, many nursing personnel are deprived of such programmes. By providing in-service education and training for the nursing personnel, the activities of THCs could be strengthened in achieving the goal of health policy at Thana and community levels in Bangladesh.

* * *

An important health area for nursing input and consideration in every country is Women's Reproductive Health. It is especially important in developing countries and particularly in many Islamic societies, where women often do not have the autonomy to seek health care when needed and only want to receive care from female health workers. Several articles in the Newsletters deal with these issues in an open and constructive way.

REPRODUCTIVE HEALTH ISSUES
An Editorial, April 1997

It has been acknowledged that healthy and educated women are the key to a healthy nation. However, women in our society are neglected in various ways, and their rights are also ignored. The reproductive health of this generation has an implication on the health of the next generation and this is vitally important for socioeconomic development. The magnitude of reproductive health problems of women is demonstrated by the maternal death figure which is 600/100,000 live births per year in our country. In the global context, this high mortality rate requires special attention...because of its traumatic consequences on the family and the community as a whole.

In fact, reproductive health of both women and men in Bangladesh is deliberately overlooked by their families and society from the very beginning of their childhood. Reproductive health care can be defined as the incorporation of means and procedures, techniques and services that contribute particularly to reproductive health and the well-being of people, through preventing and solving reproductive health problems.

- As health professionals what can nurses do to improve the reproductive health situation?
- How can nurses involve themselves to make the family and the community more aware of reproductive health factors?

These questions need to be addressed:

There are currently no nurses represented on the following national bodies related to reproductive health: HIV/AIDS, STD, EOC, Family Planning and Population Control, Maternal Health Committees and Sub-Committees. This situation prevents nurses from contributing to the improvement of reproductive health. It would be possible if nurses are recognised by the Government as health care providers...this issue calls for Government attention towards appropriate training and utilisation of nurses in the field of reproductive health.

NURSE-MIDWIVES' ROLES IN THE PROMOTION OF REPRODUCTIVE HEALTH
by Shamim Akhter, MSc, Senior Staff Nurse, NIO, Dhaka, April 1997

According to the World Health Organization (WHO), 'Reproductive health is a condition in which reproduction is accomplished in a state of complete physical, mental and social well being and not merely the absence of diseases or disorders of the reproductive process.'

When discussing women's reproductive health it is necessary to include reproductive rights and freedom, women's status in the society, development and empowerment. The basic elements covered by reproductive health can be grouped as follows:

- Safe Motherhood
- Family Planning
- Infant and Child care
- Adolescent Reproductive Health
- Male Participation and Responsible Behaviour
- Infertility
- Reproductive Tract Infections (RTIS) and Sexually Transmitted Diseases (STDS)
- HIV / AIDS
- Cancers of Reproductive Tract and Organs
- Safe Abortion Facilities
- Reproductive Health Needs of Disabled.

According to the 1991 census, the number of currently married women of reproductive age (15-49 years) is 22 million and there is a prediction that it will rise to 31 million in 2005. These women will require proper care regarding reproductive health.

In Bangladesh, according to a 1995 UNICEF report, only 5 per cent of deliveries are conducted by trained personnel and the maternal mortality rate is 600 per 100,000 live births. These figures could be higher, inasmuch as reporting systems are inadequate.

Women die during childbirth because of:

- lack of antenatal, intra-natal and post-natal care.
- having too many children.
- not wanting to go to hospital or health centre.
- non-availability of, or inability to afford transportation.
- lack of the provision of Emergency Obstetric Care (EOC).
- lack of knowledge about pregnancy-related complications which could be treated.
- superstitions and beliefs related to labour and reproductive health.
- delivery usually attended by non-trained Dai or without attendant.
- distance to health care facilities
- illegal abortions.

Maternal mortality and morbidity could be prevented to a certain extent by proper utilisation of well-trained and well-equipped nurse-midwives. This concept is strongly supported by WHO (1995) which states that where 75 per cent or more of all deliveries are performed by midwives, maternal mortality is reduced.

The community-based study at Matlab, Bangladesh established that when nurse-midwives had access to delivery; provided the ante-, intra- and post-natal care; and also made arrangements for referral to the district hospital, the maternal mortality rate fell from 3.8 to 1.4 per cent per 1000 live births. In reality, nurse-midwives are under-utilized in the provision of health care services in Bangladesh. They do not have the opportunity to provide care to pregnant women as they are not involved in the national maternity and child health programme. However, motivated and well-trained nurse-midwives could work together with other health personnel in various areas of reproductive health as educators, counselors and care providers. They could help to reduce the magnitude of reproductive health problems in Bangladesh if there was a national and political commitment to do so.

* * *

An issue that arises frequently in many countries, both developed and developing, is the working relationships between nurses and doctors. In Bangladesh, as in other countries where patriarchy is strong, clashes often occur when nurses (mostly female) move into a more independent manner of functioning. Doctors (mostly male) often resent this change and conflict occurs. This situation is one that needs to be discussed in an atmosphere where each party's concerns can be addressed. Such was the workshop held in Edinburgh by SNESP and reported on in the January 1997 newsletter.

PROMOTING COLLABORATION BETWEEN THE MEDICAL AND NURSING PROFESSIONS IN BANGLADESH
by Mairi Telford Jammeh, Lecturer, Centre for International Health QMC, Edinburgh, UK, January 1997

In May 1996, a one-day workshop was held in Queen Margaret College, Edinburgh to consider how collaboration between the medical and nursing professions in Bangladesh could be promoted. This workshop linked up the nurse managers funded through the Strengthening Nurse Education and Services (SNES) Project studying in Queen Margaret College, Edinburgh with the doctors funded by the Further Improvement of Medical Colleges (FIMC) Project studying in Dundee.

The workshop used a participatory approach and those attending were involved in discussions, presentations and 'brainstorming' sessions. They began by identifying the meaning of the terms 'team' and 'collaboration.' The participants then conducted discussions in small groups to consider what roles nurses and doctors take when working together in teams in Bangladesh. It was agreed that nurses are the first point of contact for patients and while the doctors diagnose and prescribe, the nurses implement 'doctors orders.' The doctors are the leaders while the nurses were described as the coordinators of care. It was felt that doctors and nurses had very different social statuses, with doctors rated as being high status and nurses as low. It was agreed that the roles of doctors and nurses in Bangladesh are influenced by differing sets of values and priorities and that this affects the agenda for health care which is by and large determined by doctors. Some of the doctors studying in Dundee gave presentations on promoting collaboration between the two professions.

The most useful part of the day, however, was when the two professions worked in mixed groups to identify how collaboration could be promoted in Bangladesh. These proposals were categorised into professional, political, education and management issues and are summarised below:

Professional:
• developing common policies
• promoting the status of nursing
• ensuring a raised entry level for nurse training
• promoting nursing publications
• developing a common ethics group
• encouraging nursing research

Political:
• seeking support from the Government and other organizations
• posting nurses to strategic positions
• increasing the number of nursing posts in Bangladesh

Education:
• utilising a curriculum with a community focus
• developing a core curriculum for nurses and doctors
• improving the status of nurses by increasing academic training both in length and breadth

- holding joint seminars and workshops
- enabling nurses to attend foundation training for administration within the Government of Bangladesh programme

Management:
- introducing job descriptions in appropriate posts
- developing a team approach to problem solving
- organizing team training
- improving communication between the two professions
- having regular clinical meetings
- employing clerks for administrative tasks

The workshop was very positively evaluated by those taking part. It was felt that this was a useful 'first' which would be well worth repeating in Bangladesh. It is heartening to know that many of the proposals to promote inter-professional collaboration put forward by the workshop participants are already being addressed by the SNES project team including those producing this newsletter. Congratulations and keep up the good work!

* * *

Issues that relate to nurses' positions, ranks and promotions are also addressed in the Newsletter. The following articles about seniority and promotion policies for nurses in Bangladesh deal with important and sensitive topics that are common in most Middle Eastern and South Asian cultures.

Promotion Policy in Nursing
by Major (Rtd) Datia Hossain, Principal, JM4CH & JINTI, Bajitpur, Kishorgonj, January/April 1999

With much interest I read Rahima Jamal Akhtar's article in the October 1998 issue of 'Focus on Nursing.' The article explained the complexity of postings in the higher positions. In that same edition I read about a workshop of the Bangladesh Masters Graduates Nurses Forum. Both of these articles made me feel that the time is right to express my own thoughts and ideas about the Posting and Promotion Policy in Nursing, in Bangladesh. The hope is that it will stimulate other people to think and take action on this matter as well.

The Strengthening Nursing Education and Services Project finished its activities after five years in November 1998. The SNES Project aimed partly to strengthen nursing services in Bangladesh. The project achieved some of its objectives, and certainly there are things which have changed for the better; for instance, we read 'Focus on Nursing.' However, what has stayed untouched in these last five years, is the policy of posting and promotion. This complicated and essential part of the service remains the same as before.

I believe that, besides the experiences we gather by the passing of years, training and practice raises the potential of people. I regret to observe that many professionals in nursing, having higher qualifications and experiences, work for twenty years in an 'acting' function, which means without proper responsibility and possibilities for further development. They seem to have no influence to create a function or role which both suits their qualifications and experience and stimulates them to further professional growth.

In the present situation, senior positions in nursing are occupied by the most senior persons. There are no rules and regulations for circulation or regulated job-flow in these positions, which results in an 'obstructed market.'

In my professional life, I worked in different places like Medical College Hospital in Dhaka, Rangpur and Rajshahi, Modernised Hospital Bogra, Air Force, Army and last of all JIMCH and JINTI. At all the different places I had various experiences...As a result I have collected different views on nursing...and would like to present my ideas for everyone to consider:

a. Transfer from one post to another is often undesirable, but if promotion accompanies the transfer, it may be acceptable for all, regardless of the present level in nursing service.
b. The maximum time to occupy a senior post should be three years. This could be extended for another three years if performance is satisfactory and...approved by a Posting and Promotion Board. This will stimulate job-flow and offer opportunities to younger but qualified nursing officers to function according to their ability. It may also stimulate nursing officers to develop themselves.
c. Retired elderly officers should not hold places in autonomous bodies but give the opportunity to younger qualified officers.

d. The Nursing Directorate should select an independent Posting and Promotion Board. That board should be responsible for the allocation of appropriate people to the appropriate posts.

e. Promotion and posting should not be based on seniority alone. For selection, the following three (or more) criteria could be used: seniority, qualification and past service record...

SENIORITY AND NURSES IN BANGLADESH

by Minati Mazumder, Nursing Instructor, Divisional CEC, Barisal, October 1998

In the context of subcontinental culture there is a strong belief of 'respect for seniority.' This is followed strictly in nursing services, especially in Bangladesh.

If we look at the dictionary, the word 'seniority' means 'being senior over age or in rank'. Over my past twenty-one years in nursing I have seen that the vast majority of nurses consider the term 'seniority' as nothing but the length of service, and to them, this is the norm for getting higher ranks. However, the length of service sometimes does nothing to enhance the quality of services.

While striving to attain goals for nursing, we need to think strongly about quality rather than longevity. Along with work experiences (not including seniority) it is important to consider the following for the improvement of nursing services:

- professional and academic qualifications, as quality of education can have a great impact on services;
- competence, and
- most importantly, love of work.

Generally speaking, in the case of promotion in nursing, the length of service is basically followed. At different levels, we have some praiseworthy experienced and qualified nurses with a substantial length of service. Unfortunately, many of these efficient nurses are serving either in 'acting' positions or in inappropriate places.

One of the reasons for this is the inadequate promotion policy which exists in nursing. As a result of this, nurses have very little or no opportunity to utilize their acquired knowledge and experience. For these reasons, they are frustrated, have no accountability for their actions, and no job satisfaction. This ultimately leads to a poor outcome in relation to nursing services.

In order to minimise these problems and strengthen nursing services as a whole, it is crucial to reduce the convoluted process of the promotion policy and use the right persons in the right places. Nurses can then contribute to the sustainable development of nursing services by using their knowledge and experience.

* * *

Articles that describe Teacher Training and Curriculum Workshops point out the desperate need for nurse educators in Bangladesh to be brought up-to-date with modern and varied teaching methods as well as changes in health care. These should be reflected in the nursing schools' curricula.

TEACHERS TRAINING WORKSHOP—CHITTAGONG
by Mazeda Akhter, Principal, Chittagong NI, July 1998

In this workshop a range of interactive teaching methodologies was discussed, e.g., interactive lecture, group discussion, case-presentation, role play, debate, snow-balling and experiential learning. Though some of the methods were known to us, we had never practiced them before.

The lecture method of instruction is not as effective as role play, group discussion, case presentation and snow-balling. In group discussions, students get the chance to expound on their views and share knowledge and ideas. Role play is another effective method where students can take part individually and act out some roles themselves. They get the chance to develop the correct attitudes and communication skills. For case presentation, students need to know many things. So they need to observe patients and their relatives closely, study many books, and work hard to fulfil the patients' needs. During case presentation, students get a chance to talk in front of teachers and other students, so they also develop presentation skills. In debating, students can learn to speak fluently and to explore appropriate points that are relevant to the topic. This encourages students to study hard and read more books to extend their horizon of knowledge. The snow-balling method is very good for learning because it encourages students to think and develop appropriate answers for the questions.

It appears from the workshop that students may obtain information and gain basic knowledge from lectures but they can develop different skills from using other methodologies. Students will therefore gain more knowledge that helps them provide proper patient care.

TEACHERS TRAINING WORKSHOP-CHITTIGONG
by Ms Mathanu, Rangamati NI & Aloka Sarker, Chandraghona NI, July 1998

In the Teachers Training Workshop at Chittagong different methods of teaching and learning were discussed. Amongst them some were quite new and interesting. We were also introduced to teaching resources which help to make teaching attractive and more effective. We also gathered knowledge on 'Clinical Teaching.' Clinical teaching may be knowledge, skills and attitude based. Facilitator C.C. Stuart introduced us to the several steps of clinical teaching and assessment of students performance.

We were introduced to and became familiar with the use of a 'learning diary.' It is a very important part of the learning process because the student can recall and keep in mind ideas from the day's teaching. We also learnt that a proper classroom setting makes the learner more comfortable and receptive to the teaching. This workshop also helped us to set up the classroom according to the needs of the learners as well as the teaching method...

* * *

Who develops and implements policies that affect nurses in Bangladesh? Several articles appearing in the Newsletter deal with the workings of the directorate of Nursing Services (DNS), the Bangladesh Nursing Council (BNC) and the National Nursing Policy and Planning Committee (NNPPC), all of whom are responsible for nursing in Bangladesh.

HUMAN RESOURCES FOR HEALTH
by Lori Harloe, WHO Nursing Adviser, Dhaka, January/April 1999

Nurses in Bangladesh do not seem to have job satisfaction. Years of development of human resources for health have had little effect in building the capacity of the health service to provide an acceptable system within which nurses can work.

There is no team approach to health care, nor is there any apparent dedication to service. Under the Health and Population Sector Programme (BPSP) a whole new focus has been developed—behavioural change communication. It is an attempt to refocus care providers on the real reason for their existence, that is, to give service to the people of Bangladesh. The services include illness prevention, health care and family planning.

Donors and technical assistance can do a lot to assist in the development of health services. Under various projects and programmes, foreigners can and do offer suggestions, advise, guide and work alongside local people. But ultimately a well functioning system of healthcare is Bangladesh's responsibility and local attempts should not be overshadowed by outside influences.

The current system for transfer and posting is an area which cries out for a local Bangladeshi solution. Instead of the health sector being characterised by ineptitude, lack of service, poor quality, failure of patients/clients to be treated as human, lack of team work and uncoordinated services, there is hope that each and every person working in the health and family welfare system can make a difference, working together and in teams.

Arbitrary transfer and postings are one example of the powerlessness of health workers. A lack of career planning is also a disincentive for health workers to strive for excellence. The outdated colonial strategy of ruling from a distance and posting and transferring to keep control is no longer working as Bangladesh strives to be democratic. This can be changed if nurses become involved in policy making and planning and if they play an active role in the decentralisation process under HPSP.

It is well known that a successful human resources plan must have three key strategies:

- Health workers must not be posted arbitrarily.
- Positions must be created and filled by pre-determined selection criteria and by interviewing candidates, with selection based on merit (relevant education, experience and ability to do the job).
- Job satisfaction must be considered.

Once the health workforce (especially nursing) recognises its importance and acts accordingly, a behavioural change is assured. The result will be a well motivated and committed health workforce, delivering excellent nursing and health care.

From the Team Leader, SNES Project
by Janet James October 1998

Dear Colleague,
We are almost at the end of the five year SNES Project. As you have read through this issue of the Newsletter you will have seen many articles on progress in different fields.

These give you a summary of achievements along the long and challenging road towards strengthening nursing in Bangladesh.

The main focus of our work has been:

- developing a demonstration area, to provide examples of good practice in nursing education and services.
- improving operational management of nursing services and education.
- revising the BSc curriculum at the College of Nursing.
- strengthening the capacity of the Bangladesh Nursing Council to regulate nursing.
- constructing four Divisional Continuing Education Centres, two Rural Teaching Centres and an extension to the College of Nursing.
- publishing the Nursing in Focus newsletter to disseminate information and generate debate among nurses.

Many nurses should be proud of their individual contributions to the development of nursing over the last five years. Often, changes and improvements have been made by nurses with few resources but a lot of determination.

If I were asked to highlight the most important factor in developing nursing in Bangladesh I would say it was not any specific action but the development of a positive and assertive attitude. Nurses must take themselves and their responsibilities seriously and realise that only through their own efforts, will standards of practice be improved. It is useless to wait for the motivation or resources to come from outside. There has been a positive change in attitude over the last five years. At the moment it is confined to a relatively small number of individuals and groups. The challenge for the Directorate of Nursing and for the next project is to help it to spread much wider, through all levels and all areas of nursing, so that nurses can stand together as a united professional group and be a strong force for change. That way they will convince each other, the public, medical colleagues, Ministry officials and politicians that they have a voice which must be heard. If this is not achieved, internal arguments and divisions will always be a weakness which opponents can easily exploit. The other important function of the project will be to provide encouragement and support when the process of change is hard, as it inevitably will be. I hope that many of you will feel that you have gained from the collaboration, exchange of ideas and professional support which the SNES team has offered.

11

Women and the Nursing Profession in Saudi Arabia

Nagat El-Sanabary

'Women constitute the key resource for attaining the goal of health for all by the year 2000,' maintains a report by The World Health Organization.[1] Achieving this goal requires massive efforts including (1) the training of women health care professionals; and (2) the nonformal health education of women, the primary health care providers to their families and communities. This study focuses on the first area, specifically on the education of women nurses in Saudi Arabia, where traditional attitudes persist against the intermingling of the genders and in respect to the treatment of women by men. It examines the progress and problems encountered in recruiting Saudi women for nursing education and practice; describes the evolution of nursing education programmes; and analyzes the obstacles to women's participation in these programmes and in the nursing profession. The work concludes with recommendations to address the problem, increase women's participation, and contribute to that country's health development.

BACKGROUND

The Problem and Related Literature

Research on women's work in Islamic countries suggests that acceptance of women's participation in an occupation rests upon identifying it as appropriate for Muslim women.[2] This is generally true and helps explain the acceptability of teaching as a profession at all levels, and the generally high levels of women's participation in the medical profession in most Muslim countries. But how can we explain the low participation rate of women in a 'culturally appropriate' female occupation such as nursing? In this study I argue that deeming an occupation culturally appropriate is not enough to harness popular support and guarantee women's participation in it. Other factors, such as prestige, class-association, general reputation, and the potential moral and social risks of women's occupational involvement are implicated. By focusing on nursing, this study explains the dynamics of women's educational and occupational choices, and identifies the opportunities and challenges facing the development and utilization of health 'womanpower' in Islamic countries.

In most Western nations, nursing is a female occupation while the prestigious medical profession is predominantly male. The situation differs in Islamic countries where women's participation is low in nursing and high in medicine. This disparity is paradoxical considering that these countries consider both nursing and medicine culturally appropriate female professions. Nonetheless, medicine is the most acceptable and prestigious profession for Muslim women, whereas nursing remains a low-status occupation shunned by both women and men. Consequently, despite the national need for female doctors and nurses, popular demand is high for medicine but low for nursing. This discrepancy has created a major problem for traditional, gender-segregated Saudi Arabia for over thirty years. Ironically, the same factors that promote women's participation in nursing mitigate against it. Popular attitudes toward nursing keep women from getting the training they need, or utilizing their skills after graduation. This problem has obstructed Saudi Arabia's efforts to solve its nursing shortage by recruiting women for this 'culturally appropriate' occupation.

This problem is not unique to Saudi Arabia but is found, at different levels of intensity, in all Arab countries,[3] especially the rich. In a 1973 article, Khoury, noted that nursing was not fully appreciated as a career for young Kuwaiti women, a situation which led them to seek prestige in other professions.[4] Similarly, in 1980, Meleis and Hassan argued that a crisis confronted the nursing profession in the Persian Gulf countries, threatening 'not only the quality of nursing care available to the people who live in the area, but the very future of nursing itself.'[5] Kronfol and Affara also maintain that, in Bahrain and the Gulf in general, 'the shortage of nurses constitutes the primary limiting factor to the effective provision of health care'.[6]

In .1990, the crisis is more intense in oil-wealthy Saudi Arabia, where after thirty years of establishing the first nursing education programme, popular demand for nursing education is low, and the numbers of female students and graduates are too small to meet the national need. Consequently, nursing education has failed to make a dent in the nursing shortage in that country, and reliance on foreign nurses continues. Although a shortage of the indigenous health labour force has existed for decades, the situation is more serious in nursing and has significant implications for the status and employment of Saudi women, and for health development in general. In a study of health manpower in Saudi Arabia, Alawi and Mujahid, two faculty members at King Saud University, noted that the numbers of Saudi men and women entering the nursing and medical professions is far below the national need, and that the rate is declining, leaving the Kingdom dependent on foreigners well into the year 2000.[7] This is one of the most difficult problems facing Saudi planners and educators.

This work examines this problem by tracing the development of female nursing education programmes in Saudi Arabia, and analyzing the problems encountered and the contradictions that hamper the full utilization of Saudi women in that profession. This analysis should add to the existing body of knowledge about the education and workforce participation of Muslim women, and the constraints on the educational and occupational options of women in Saudi Arabia and elsewhere. The study is divided into five parts: the first part provides an introduction to the problem and its Saudi Arabian context; the second discusses the development of nursing education programmes; the third analyzes the difficulties and constraints affecting nursing education and practice; the fourth outlines the limited contribution of Saudi women nurses to health development; and the fifth offers recommendations and outlines some measures to increase Saudi women's participation in nursing.

Popular Western literature about Saudi women focuses primarily on their veiling, gender segregation, and limited options. It fails to recognize that these women are caught in the grip of vast social changes, that they face difficult choices, and have indeed made major progress in various spheres of life over a relatively short time. Scholarly research has documented the changes. Altorky revealed the major progress in the lives and opportunities of elite urban Saudi women[8] as well as women in smaller towns.[9] Parssinen,[10] Gerner,[11] El-Sanabary,[12,13] and Ramazani[14] described major changes in the educational, personal, and occupational situations of Saudi women over the past three decades, although they also noted certain persistent problems and constraints. Sudden oil wealth provided great opportunities for development, but traditional cultural and religious attitudes, as well as the country's educational and employment policies, have been a major constraining factor. The changes that have swept over the country affected people unevenly, having a greater impact on economic than social infrastructures. These uneven changes are evident in the evolving situation of Saudi women, and their generally low labour force participation.

Three development areas underscore Saudi Arabia's need for female health care professionals in the midst of rapid socio-economic change: (1) the vast expansion of female education and the desire to provide culturally and female-appropriate occupations; (2) the astronomical expansion of health care facilities and government's commitment to train needed health workers, and (3) the heavy reliance on expatriate health personnel and the desire to replace them with Saudis.

Saudi Arabia, formerly a poor nomadic tribal country, was catapulted into the twentieth century by the oil wealth of recent decades, which made it a middle-income country.[15] Its new-found wealth dramatically changed all spheres of society, especially the educational and health sectors. Beginning in the early 1960s, the government embarked upon a massive development programme facilitated by systematic planning and financed by oil revenues. Despite the unprecedented changes, the Saudi government has maintained a determination to modernize without deviating from traditional social and religious values,[16] especially those pertaining to women. Accordingly, the genders are separated in education and employment, and veiling in public is mandatory. Major educational and economic changes have occurred within this traditional framework, the most dramatic of which has been the vast expansion of female education, and the increase in women's employment especially in teaching, and to lesser extent, in social work, nursing, medicine, and a few occupations.

Expansion of Female Education and Women's Employment

Prior to 1960, Saudi Arabia had no public schools for girls, and no women were employed outside the home. During that year, the government opened its first primary schools for girls, under the auspices of a separate agency, the General Presidency of Girls Education (GPGE), thereby marking the beginning of a new era for Saudi women. Gradually, a separate, full-fledged system of girls' education emerged that now provides free schooling from the primary to the doctoral level. In 1988, more than one million girls and young women were enroled in Saudi schools and colleges: 770,370 in primary education, 308,700 in intermediate and secondary education, and 50,430 in higher education. Females made up 45 per cent of the enrolment at the primary level, 42 per cent at intermediate and upper secondary levels, and 39 per cent at the college and university levels.[17]

The increase in female education led to a gradual and steady rise in women's participation in occupations designated suitable for Muslim women. According to Saudi government policy issued in 1970, the two main objectives of girls' education are to prepare them for their roles as mothers, and 'to perform those jobs which suit their nature like teaching, nursing and medicine'.[18] These occupations are an extension of women's qualities of caring, nurturing, and service to others. They are also deemed culturally and religiously appropriate because they help maintain gender-segregation through women's work with other women in segregated work environments. This condition applies easily to education but not to the health sector. Therefore, teaching and school administration are the most widely held occupations by Saudi women, particularly at the primary and secondary levels. In 1986, 44,653 Saudi women were employed as school teachers and administrators by the GPGE, having replaced Egyptian and other Arab women. Another 1273 were working in the universities. According to the Civil Service Bureau, over 88 per cent of Saudis working in the non-agricultural sector, were employed by the GPGE and the Universities (85.9 and 2.4% respectively) as compared to only 7.4 per cent employed by the Ministry of Health (MOH).[19]

Vast Expansion of Medical Facilities

Since the 1950s, the goal of official government policy has been to provide health care for all citizens free or at nominal cost. Oil wealth has prompted astronomical growth in health-care facilities and personnel. Since 1980, the MOH emphasized preventive health measures: a massive vaccination programme, environmental health and hygiene, health education, early screening, primary care, and maternity and child care.[20] The number of public and private hospitals, dispensaries and primary care centres has skyrocketed. By the 1980s, Saudi Arabia had established some of the most advanced and best equipped hospitals in the Middle East. At King Faisal Specialty Hospital in Riyadh—which receives patients from various countries in the region—European, American, Saudi and Arab doctors perform such intricate operations as open-heart surgery, and kidney and cornea transplants. The country also boasts the best eye clinic in the Middle East. By 1989, 1650 primary health care centres (PHC) were operating throughout the country.

To staff its expanding health facilities, the Saudi government recruited vast numbers of foreign health care providers. Between 1970 and 1980, the number of doctors increased 4.5 times, and the number of nurses tripled. The country needed to expand its own supply of Saudi health professionals. The Third Development Plan (1980-85), emphasized health manpower. It stressed the necessity 'to increase the public awareness of the need for and utilization of health training programmes especially nursing education for girls'.[21] In the meantime, the MOH forged ahead with the expansion of facilities and personnel. During the Fourth Development Plan (1986-1990), it expected to add 45,500 new positions in the health sector. The ratio of physicians and other health care providers to the population increased dramatically. For instance, the number of physicians per 10,000 inhabitants rose from 3.8 in 1975 to 6.7 in 1980. The target during the Fifth Development Plan (1990-95) is one physician per 500 inhabitants and one nurse and health technician per 225 inhabitants.[22] Achieving this ambitious objective required the training of 4200 physicians, 565 specialist physicians, 5880 nurses, and 7560 health technicians.[23] The numbers are almost overwhelming and only a small fraction can be trained by Saudi medical and nursing colleges, especially the latter due to various factors outlined later in this chapter.

NURSING EDUCATION IN SAUDI ARABIA

The history of female nursing education in Saudi Arabia dates back to the early 1960s. As in other Arab and developing countries, it began with a lower high school programme then advanced to higher levels. In the mid-1970s, a new college-level nursing programme was introduced to upgrade the training of nurses, and to improve the status and image of nursing. Since then, Saudi Arabia has provided two types of nursing education for women: at the secondary-level health institutes,[24] and at the post-secondary nursing colleges.[25]

The Health Institutes

In 1958, under a five-year agreement with the World Health Organization (WHO), the Saudi MOH established three secondary-level health institutes for males. In 1961, under a similar agreement with WHO, it opened two institutes for girls, one in the capital, Riyadh, the other in Jeddah, Saudi Arabia's largest seaport and commercial centre.[26] At that time, the institutes admitted girls who had completed six years of primary education, mostly at private schools. Soad H. Hassan, an Egyptian consultant to the WHO, was involved in planning and implementing the first health institutes. She indicated that the first nurse-aide programme for elementary school graduates initially met with objections from parents and students as well as the Saudi government itself. She and her Egyptian-educated Saudi colleague, Lutfiyyah al-Khateeb, gave speeches, made public appearances, and wrote articles for radio and newspapers to promote nursing and encourage an interest in it. The MOH decided to promote the programme as a viable educational option for women only after it was agreed that students would remain veiled, would provide care to female patients only, and would not be expected to work with male physicians. They were not to work afternoon or night shifts either.[5]

As female education progressed, nursing training was extended to admit only students with nine years of education for a three-year course. The MOH has been adding new institutes for women and men in various Saudi towns throughout the country. By 1990, it had a total of seventeen health institutes for female and sixteen for males.[27,28] To attract and retain students, the MOH provides free meals, lab uniforms, and transportation. Upon admission to the institutes, students are hired by the MOH at grade II and provided, according to 1987 rates, a monthly salary of SR. 1825 ($490.00). Upon graduation, they receive a certificate in technical nursing, are appointed to hospitals or dispensaries, and are guaranteed a job at grade V (one level below university graduates) at a monthly salary of SR. 3590 ($965.00).[29]

The female institutes offer a limited nursing programme which has recently been expanded in some institutes according to need, to include programmes in gynecology and obstetric nursing, pediatrics, x-ray, and physical therapy.[27] By contrast, the institutes for males provide a more diverse educational programme in eleven specialties to train nurses, health inspectors, pharmacy assistants, and technicians in the following specialties: health and vital statistics, nutrition, laboratory work, X-ray, surgery, anesthesia, and physical therapy.[28] The reforms continue in both the institutes and new specialties are being added to the female institutes. MOH has also initiated curriculum reforms to improve curriculum content and teaching methods, and has introduced clinical nursing practice during the summer months to supplement classroom learning. Additionally, all graduates have to undergo a 20-week period of condensed practical training as a prerequisite for employment.[27]

The health institutes have opened new educational and employment opportunities for Saudi women, but have not gained the acceptance anticipated by their planners. Their students and graduates have been much fewer than expected or required to meet the national need for Saudi nurses, despite the slow and fluctuating rise in enrolment over their 30-year history. In 1969/70, 112 female students were enroled in three health institutes as compared with 977 enroled in ten institutes in 1982. Enrolment declined to 757 in 1983/84 to rise again steadily between 1985 and 1990, when it doubled reaching 2520 in 1990. While this increase indicates a growing interest in nursing, it is still far below the country's need for women nurses. Despite the growing number of institutes, their wide geographic distribution, and the available pool of middle school graduates eligible for admission, female enrolment in the seventeen female institutes in 1990 was slightly over half of the male enrolment of 4342.[27]

The total number of female graduates has also increased over the years, from thirteen in 1964/65 to 270 in 1985/86, to 476 in 1990. Yet, the increase in graduates has been very modest in some institutes, while it has actually declined in others. This is mainly because few of those who enrol persist until graduation, as indicated by Saudi faculty and others affiliated with the health field. Additionally, graduation statistics reveal a wide gender gap. About half as many females as males graduate from the health institutes annually, 467 as compared to 915 in 1990.[27] Between 1961/62 and 1982/83, only 758 females had graduated as compared to 1798 males. The gender gap widened between 1985/56 and 1990 when about three times as many males as females graduated: 4668 as compared to 1642. This discrepancy indicates that the female institutes are both inefficient and ineffective in meeting the ever-growing national need for female nurses.

Nursing Colleges

To stimulate the demand for nursing and improve its image, the Saudi government followed the proverbial advice to 'raise the status of nursing by requiring a high educational standard for entry and making courses more and more academically demanding'.[30] It thus decided to start a nursing programme under the auspices of the existing women's medical colleges at King Abdelaziz University in Jeddah and King Saud University in Riyadh. The first was opened in 1976 and the second in 1980.[31] To avoid the use of the term nursing, with its negative connotation, these were designated as colleges of medical sciences. Because both nursing and medicine are undergraduate college programmes admitting high school graduates from the scientific track, students in both colleges share the same classes in the first preparatory year.

When the first nursing college was opened, the Ministry of Health then needed 20,000 male and female nurses: 2000 with college degrees, and 18,000 with secondary-level diplomas in nursing, hoping they would be trained by the nursing institutes and colleges. But, contrary to expectations, the nursing colleges did not raise the public demand for nursing education, and the discrepancy between supply and demand persisted. Few qualified high school graduates wish to pursue nursing education, instead, most want to become doctors. These colleges have been struggling for survival as a result of low enrolment and high attrition.[32] For instance, in 1989, only 80 female students were enroled in the college of allied medical sciences (nursing) at King Abdelaziz University, as compared with 455 in medicine. In four years, between 1979/80 and 1986/87, a total of 56 women had graduated from nursing as compared to 245 from medicine. Annual graduation figures in nursing are only a small fraction of those in medicine.[33] Although definitive statistics on attrition are not readily available, faculty members report that few of those who enrol complete their studies. Lack of interest in nursing persists despite the incentives provided to all students: free tuition, textbooks, lab uniforms, a monthly stipend of

1000 Saudi Riyals ($269) per month, and free boarding facilities for those who need them.

Furthermore, not all graduates practice the profession. As Abel-Smith noted for many developing countries 'the most qualified nurses tend to be supervisors rather than practitioners of nursing',[30] thus leaving the actual day-to-day nursing operations to less skilled people. Hussein Alawi and Ghazi Mujahid[7] arrived at a similar conclusion based on a study of health human resources development in Saudi Arabia. They noted, 'after completing their studies, many qualified Saudi females prefer either to stay home or to take an administrative job because it is comfortable, convenient and more rewarding. In some cases, the career shift is imposed by the husband as a condition for a stable marriage'.[7]

CONSTRAINTS ON WOMEN'S PARTICIPATION IN NURSING

As noted above, Saudi officials, writers, and religious leaders sanction nursing as a suitable occupation for Muslim women. So, what are the constraints on Saudi women's participation in nursing education and practice? They are numerous and complex.

The first pertains to women's work generally. In Saudi Arabia and elsewhere, gender-role expectations and female socialization are a major obstacle to women's entry into the workforce. The prevailing view is that a woman's place is in the home and that outside employment is justified only when necessary. The pressure to get married, and to stay at home and care for their families compels many young women to either forgo employment completely or to choose an occupation such as teaching, which is easy to integrate with family responsibilities. Very few are willing to venture into a demanding education and career, unless it has the prestige that justifies the sacrifice, such as medicine. Saudi society has not fully accepted the idea of women's work outside the home, despite the thousands of employed Saudi women, most of whom are in the education sector. The ongoing debate about women's role in the family and society and the perceived potential threats to the family from women's employment has not abated. Several conservative Saudi and other Muslim writers continue to write extensively on women's work and its potential effects on society. Books as well as pamphlets are issued regularly debating the issue of women's roles in society. The following book titles are revealing: 'Remain in Your Place and Be Grateful,' 'Women's Work in the Balance,' 'The March of Saudi Women, To Where?' Such books speak at length about woman's primary role in the family, oppose women's work, and warn of the anticipated breakdown of the Saudi family as a result of women's employment. They cite perceived ills of Western societies: 'moral deterioration,' the 'collapse of family values,' and 'the loss of children' blaming them all on women's work outside the home. They contrast this situation with 'ideal Islamic society and values,' extol the virtues of motherhood, and exaggerate the dangers of women's work. They do, however, sanction teaching, medicine, nursing, and social work as culturally and religiously appropriate feminine occupations. Their writings convey a conflicting message to Saudi women by telling them in one breath that it is their duty to serve their country in appropriate occupations, and in the other that their place is in the home. Only teaching gets the full endorsement of these writers because of its congruency with women's traditional roles and its fully segregated work environment. The following are just a few samples of their writings.

Suhaila Zein El-Abedeen, an influential conservative Saudi woman journalist, opposes women's employment outside teaching. She argues, however, that nursing education should be made compulsory at all stages of female education starting with intermediate schools to ensure that women have the nursing knowledge they need to perform their duties as mothers in peace time, and to shoulder their responsibilities toward their country in case of war.[34] Another Saudi writer, a Western-educated physician, Mohammad Ali el-Bar, a staunch opponent of women's work, concurs. He points out that the role of women in nursing the wounded and sick, and serving the soldiers by providing them with food and water, is an important role in the battlefields, a role played by the mothers of the Muslims and pioneering women in the early Islamic period. He mentions Rufaida, a Muslim woman who nursed the wounded in the battle of al-Ahzab, and other women who practiced medicine in various periods of Islamic history.[35] Yet, he stresses that these duties are only required in times of emergency and he exhorts contemporary Saudi women to stay at home because of alleged dangers of women's work and the 'unavoidable' moral corruption that results from the intermingling of the genders.

Ahmad Mohammad Jamal, another staunch opponent of women's work, has written extensively about the pernicious effects of women's work, especially where men and women work together. He recognizes women's right to work as 'a teacher, physician, nurse, or a midwife in female environments only where there is no intermingling of the genders, and no fear of the corrupting influence of such intermingling'.[36] Jamal argues that Saudi women, by virtue of their Arab Islamic society, do not need to compete with men for jobs except those that are fit for them such as needlework, sewing, and teaching girls. He adds that some Saudi women actually perform these kinds of quiet occupations that suit women's abilities and her domain. They are the teachers, school administrators, and physicians, who educate and treat other women.[36] He cites the example of courageous Muslim women nurses during the early Islamic period. But he affirms that he mentions them only to demonstrate their courage, and not to encourage contemporary Saudi women to follow their example in the battle fields since 'military warfare has advanced and no longer needs women to satisfy the thirst of the warriors, or care for the wounded or the sick'.[36] These writers also oppose support systems that enable married women to work and care for their families. Child care is a concern, especially for women who cannot afford live-in nannies or who have no extended-family members to care for their children. But these writers reject childcare centres for the alleged harmful effects on children. Their writings reflect the attitudes of a broad segment of traditional Saudi society, not the younger generations of educated men and women, who have read and traveled widely and recognize the need for Saudi women to assume new roles and contribute to national development.

In addition to the general resistance to women's employment among the traditional strata of Saudi society, several other reasons specific to nursing discourage women's entry into the profession. The first is a negative image and a deep-seated prejudice against nursing. This is not peculiar to Saudi Arabia but is found in other countries as well. The image of the nurse as a doctor's helpmate is a worldwide stereotype that has persisted for decades. Negative images of nurses are found in Western literature as reported in studies by Hughes,[37] Kalisch et al.,[38] Kalisch and Kalisch;[39] and Austin et al.[40] In most Arab and Islamic countries, a stereotype of the nurse as a subservient uneducated female hospital worker discourages many Arab women from entering nursing. A WHO report indicates that 'the public image of the nurse appears to be particularly negative in countries where strong cultural traditions severely restrict the participation of women in paid occupations outside the home. As a result, nursing functions in these countries are performed by women of the lowest social class—a situation reminiscent of the earliest days of nursing'.[1] Therefore, few young women study nursing by choice but only as a last resort when their grades do not qualify them for more prestigious fields of study.[1]

For instance, Meleis argues that, in Kuwait, nursing is viewed with suspicion, and considered a profession for educationally or economically disadvantaged women.[41] A Saudi woman professor, Samira Islam, a former dean of the colleges of medicine and medical sciences at King Abdelaziz University and a consultant to the World Health Organization, spoke about the negative image of nursing in Saudi Arabia. Citing evidence from her professional experience, she reported that the general public and members of the health team, especially physicians, lack an understanding of the nature of the nursing profession. Negative perceptions often pop up in professional discussions, she said, and medical educators consider nursing students less intelligent and less capable. In her view, physicians have a 'superiority complex' and consider anyone else in the medical team inferior to them. They view the physician as the boss and the rest as 'apprentices or laborers.' She stated 'people like to look up, they like power and prestige.' She noted that even women physicians who spent their freshman year in the same classes with nursing students still look down on nurses and consider them inferior to them. She added, 'the problem is not just with the girls who like power, fame, and glory by having a medical degree or being a physician, but also with the medical team...we try to convince the physicians that the nurses and other paramedical personnel are colleagues not servants....'[42]

Work conditions are another problem that hampers women's participation in nursing but less so in medicine. First is the difficulty to integrate nursing with women's family responsibilities because hospital work involves long hours and night shifts. This is especially a burden in view of women's restricted mobility and lack of autonomy. The Saudi governments' ban on driving by women makes it very difficult for them to commute to their jobs. Furthermore, parental opposition to women living away from home prevents them from accepting positions in the villages that need their services the most. The second is a more formidable obstacle: the intermingling of the genders in hospitals. Women nurses must interact with Saudi male physicians and patients, as well as with non-Saudi physicians and other health care providers. It is generally believed that such intermingling in the workplace, which is unavoidable in hospitals although prohibited by Saudi law, promotes immorality. Thus, contrary to Western literature that associates nursing with such characteristics as virtue and purity, the taint of immorality associated with nursing in Saudi Arabia and some other Arab countries is the most damaging to the profession and to the peace of mind of the women who want to pursue it. The concern over a woman's reputation and honour limits women's access to and persistence in nursing. In their aforementioned study, Alawi and Mujahid found that many Saudi families do not consider nursing an 'honourable profession.' They argue that 'this attitude rests on the belief that nursing forces a girl to mix with men, to stay long hours away from home and to work night shifts: a job condition that is socially unacceptable and runs contrary to deep rooted beliefs of what is permissible for a girl to do....'[7] My interviews with Saudi nursing students, as well as those who have transferred from the nursing colleges, confirmed that most parents oppose their daughters' desire to become nurses. Likewise, some men interviewed for Saudi newspapers have stated their objection to their sisters', daughters', or wives' entry into nursing due to the moral 'hazards' involved. Sadly, some practicing Saudi nurses refer to harassment, or 'annoyances,' on the job which impel some nurses to quit. Those who persist often risk their reputation and pay a high personal price: possibly forfeiting marriage altogether. Some practicing Saudi nurses, and others, hint at sexual harassment on the job. One of the earliest graduates of the health institutes stated that should she marry and have a daughter she would never allow her to become a nurse so as to spare her what she herself has endured.

Ironically, while sharing the same working conditions, medicine has not been stigmatized like nursing, but enjoys high prestige and status, which makes it the most favoured and prestigious educational and occupational option for Saudi and Muslim women in general.

In contrast to nursing, the demand for medical education is so high that every year, more than four times as many women apply for admission to medical schools as those accepted.[43] The opposing images of the two professions prompt women to gravitate toward medicine and shy away from nursing. The symbolic opposition between the two professions, discussed by Ohnuki-Tierney and Susan Orpett Long for Japan, applies equally to Saudi Arabia. 'Physicians are 'educated', 'scientific', 'mental' labourers, 'clean', and male. Nurses are their symbolic opposites: uneducated, emotionally responsive, manual labourers, who do the 'dirty' work of medical care'.[44] In Saudi Arabia, as in the other Gulf states, the association of nursing with menial work requiring no intelligence or education, relegates it to those occupations below the dignity of most Saudis, male and female, and are better left to foreigners. The low educational association relates to the history of nursing education in Saudi Arabia, where it evolved as a vocational education programme. As such, it suffers from the general stigma of being the catch-basin for the lower classes and those who cannot make it academically.[45]

Class is a related problem. As with women in most Third World countries, women's socio-economic background has a major influence on their educational and career choices. The wealthy and more advantaged groups are more likely to enter prestigious occupations and professions than the socially and economically disadvantaged who are less likely to pursue higher education. In wealthy Saudi Arabia, despite democratization efforts and free education, the majority of the females who graduate from high schools and enter colleges come from middle and upper-class backgrounds. As with other Islamic countries, women of the social elite choose the prestigious field of medicine.[46] For these women, education is a status symbol. Very few, if any, are willing to risk their social prestige by entering low-class associated nursing.

Popular literature contributes to the tarnished image of nursing and intensifies people's concerns. The above-quoted Saudi writers enumerate the horrors and moral corruption resulting from male doctors and female nurses working together on the graveyard shift. They consider nurses easy prey for male doctors and patients. For instance, Ali el-Barr,[35] cites examples of sexual harassment of working women in the West and in some Muslim countries, using nursing as a prime example of moral corruption. He laments the degradation of the reputation of nurses in an Arab country, placing the blame, not on the women nurses, but 'on the systems which compel a young budding girl to spend the night shift with a young unmarried and recently graduated doctor'.[35] He argues that it is impossible for young people working together at night not to fall victim to sexual desires. He delivers the final blow to nursing suggesting that, 'hospital wards are witnesses to what happens between interns or the doctor on duty and the nurse working the night shift, when they spend the whole night in one place. After only few hours, the nurse gives sleeping pills to the patients to enjoy the desired solitude...'.[35] Such statements reinforce a common belief that some foreign female nurses enjoy sexual freedoms morally unacceptable to mainstream Saudi society, and help taint the nursing image further.

These stereotypes and the apprehensions they evoke are common threads in most discussions about women and nursing in Saudi Arabia. As with the 'backlash' against the feminist movement in the US, these writings play upon women's underlying fears and anxieties during a time of unprecedented social change and uncertainties. Educated Saudi women who read and hear about the stereotypes feel tremendous pressure, and they fear the potential effects of a choice of nursing education and work on their personal lives. The women interviewed for this study, and for several newspaper and magazine articles, voice the dilemmas facing Saudi women. They recognize the need for Saudi women to replace non-Saudi nurses who do not fully understand the Saudi culture and cannot communicate well with Saudi patients and their families. Many of them need to work to help support themselves and their families, but are unwilling to take the risks to their reputation and personal lives.

SAUDI WOMEN NURSES AND HEALTH DEVELOPMENT

These attitudes have discouraged many Saudi women from entering nursing, thus helping exacerbate the existing nursing shortage. Those who have entered the profession remain underdogs: their status is low, and their power limited. They are maligned by the stereotypes and negative propaganda. Consequently, the nursing profession in Saudi Arabia is female and foreign. The latest available figures indicate that the proportion of female Saudi to non-Saudi nurses was only 6.5 per cent (1388 Saudis and 21,269 non-Saudis), comparative figures for males were 1431 Saudis and 4178 non-Saudis, at a ratio of 34 per cent.[49]

Despite the problems and dilemmas, Saudi women who have entered nursing, although small in number, have contributed to health development in their country as individuals and professionals. The greatest contribution is credited to the first Saudi nurse-midwife, Mrs Lutfiyyah al-Khateeb who received a nursing diploma from Cairo, Egypt, in 1941. Upon her return to Saudi Arabia, she dedicated her life to uplifting the educational and health condition of Saudi women. She lobbied for female education, nursing and medicine, was instrumental in establishing the health institutes, and became the first director of the institute in Jeddah. Her efforts on behalf of Saudi women—which are recorded in her memoirs,[47] and acknowledged by those who knew her—are a testimony to the commitment, resilience and courage of women in the face of seemingly unsurmountable obstacles. By championing the cause of female education and health, she laid the foundation for Saudi women's empowerment. As a pioneer and social reformer, she was the driving force behind the founding of government education for girls and health care facilities for women and children. During her fifteen years of practice as a midwife, she campaigned for girls' education and was a driving force behind the founding of government schools for girls. She also laid the foundation for the first health education programme in the country. Single-handedly, she taught women about care during pregnancy and delivery, proper child-care, nutrition, sanitation, and the risks of childbirth. Under the motto 'Prevention is better than the cure' she called for massive immunization against contagious diseases such as diphtheria, whooping cough, tuberculosis, polio, typhoid, cholera, tetanus, typhus, and the plague, and for improved sanitation practices. She believed, like Dr Elizabeth Blackwell before her, that 'sanitation is the supreme goal of medicine, its foundation and its crown'.[48] She called upon every citizen to urge pregnant women to make full use of primary health care centres and hospitals for pre-natal care and safe deliveries. Her campaign for the establishment of a specialized maternity and obstetrics hospital succeeded in persuading the government to convert a newly established eye clinic into a maternity hospital staffed by Arab physicians. She won the support of the Saudi leadership and the common people for her ideas, mission, and her common sense views on education, nutrition, sanitation and clothing. Her success was largely due to the fact that she worked within the framework of the prevailing traditional cultural and religious values.

Pharmacology professor Samira Islam has been an advocate of nursing for almost twenty years, promoting it as part of her work as a faculty member of the colleges of medicine and medical sciences, a member of the Gulf health committee,[49] and as a consultant to WHO on health human resources in the Mediterranean region. In addition to her newspaper articles, lectures, and radio talks, she sometimes calls parents on the telephone to urge them to consider nursing for their daughters who could not get into the medical college at King Abdelaziz University. Similarly, the directors of the health institutes often give newspaper and radio interviews in which they stress the importance of nursing for Saudi society, and the role of nurses 'as angels of mercy since the time of the Prophet, in peace and war times,' and argue that nursing is as important as medicine and complements it.[29] These female nursing educators appeal to parental concerns by stressing that Saudi nurses in hospitals are assigned only to women's sections, maternity wards, or children's hospitals; and that nurses meet men only during family visiting hours when veiling is observed. This publicity aims at helping ease parental worries, silencing the critics of nursing, and removing the stigma attached to hospital work.

Saudi Arabia has come a long way since the pioneering work of Lutfiyyah al-Khateeb. The country has changed and women have assumed new roles. Either by necessity or choice, hundreds of Saudi women have disregarded the prevailing stereotypes and restrictions by taking advantage of the available opportunities to train for and practice nursing. In 1989, according to government statistics, 1398 female Saudi nurses were working in hospitals, dispensaries and primary health centres run by the Saudi Ministry of Health.[50] Many others are employed in the military hospitals run by the Ministry of Defence; in clinics for female students and staff operated by the General Presidency of Girls' Education; and in numerous private hospitals and clinics in the main Saudi cities. Whether they choose nursing because it is their only option, to take advantage of the stipend, to obtain a needed job, or to alleviate human suffering, these women are providing essential health services and contributing to the welfare of their families, communities and wider society. One hopes that they will ultimately succeed in changing the public's attitudes toward women and their role in society, and help pave the way for other women making educational and career choices.

Currently, the number of these women is too small to make a dent in the existing nursing shortages. This situation limits their role in alleviating the numerous health problems that still afflict the country and require the attention of Saudi nurses and other health care providers. These include a relatively high infant mortality rate (72 per 1000 females and 87 for males); and a high maternal mortality rate also (52 per 100,000);[15] high incidence of infectious and deficiency diseases; endemic diseases such as malaria and bilharzia in certain regions; and high occurrence of trachoma—a sanitation-related disease that often leads to blindness—among a large proportion of school-age children in certain communities, and very high occurrence of intestinal parasites among children under five years of age in some poor areas.[51]

The country is also experiencing an alarming increase in disabilities among children and youth, some are a result of consanguineous marriages, others are caused by driving accidents. These health problems underscore the need for health care and education of women, the primary health care providers, and an urgent need for Saudi female health professionals and health educators.

These health problems cannot be effectively solved by foreigners, but need Saudi health care providers, especially women, cognizant of local conditions, and sensitive to Saudi women's needs and concerns. Continued dependence on foreign health care providers interferes with the proper delivery of health care to the Saudis, specially women, because of the communication problems resulting from differences in language and culture between the health care providers and patients. As one report noted, 'the effectiveness of non-Saudi, often non-Arabic-speaking health personnel [is] limited by their inadequate understanding of the Saudi environment and culture. Patient communication has suffered because of the cultural gulf'.[51] The same problem exists in other Gulf states. In Kuwait, for instance, Meleis noted that 'visiting health care professionals who are there only on a limited permit, no sooner having adjusted to their clients and the clients to them, find that it is time for them to leave. Therefore, health care clients have to continuously adjust to new workers ignorant of the culture and system'.[52] Hence, the goal of Saudization, or achievement of some balance between the numbers of Saudi and foreign health care providers, is not just a matter of national pride, but also of practical necessity.

This is a daunting challenge for Saudi planners. Both the fourth and fifth national development plans (1985-90 and 1990-95) note the discrepancy between the number of health graduates, especially nurses, and the continued need to utilize foreign personnel at all levels of the health sector.[21,23] They emphasize the 'need for further educational initiatives and incentives designed to draw Saudi students into careers as health professionals.... Ultimately, the Kingdom's health services rely upon the success of the universities, medical and nursing colleges, health institutes, and intermediate polytechnic health colleges to produce sufficient numbers of graduates to provide these services'.[23] Stressing the need to increase the country's human resources in health, the planners argue for expanded training programmes and incentives for students entering the health profession, especially primary health care.[23]

CONCLUSION AND RECOMMENDATIONS

The preceding discussion highlights some progress but also major constraints on nursing education and practice in Saudi Arabia. Despite the Saudi government's endorsement of nursing as a culturally appropriate female occupation, its financial support, and its commitment to providing nursing education and employment for women, popular demand for nursing remains far below national need. The female health institutes and nursing colleges, which provide alternative career options for Saudi women, remain under-utilized. Government officials, Saudi writers, and the general public are aware of the national need for Saudi female nurses to serve the health needs of women and children, but few are willing to provide moral support for the women wishing to enter the profession. Hesitancy and apprehension on the part of the government, and misconception among the general public about nursing and nurses, and about women's work in general, have curtailed the development and utilization of the potential of women in this 'culturally appropriate' female profession. Thousands of Saudi women want to work, but few are willing to pursue the training that qualifies them to fill thousands of nursing jobs occupied by foreign women.

What can be done to solve this problem? It certainly cannot be solved by piecemeal cosmetic solutions, but rather, it calls for innovative and far-reaching solutions requiring hard work, determination, and courage on the part of nurses, nursing educators, and policy makers. Increasing the popular demand for nursing and enhancing women's participation in the profession are necessary to achieving the long-term objective of providing quality health care for all citizens. This requires a comprehensive strategy which includes education and training; health education; support systems, action to change people's attitudes toward women; employment policies and opportunities, and infrastructure development.[1] The following are some tried and some suggested solutions.

First, it is important to change public attitudes and improve the nursing image. Changing attitudes toward women and their role in society is beyond the scope of this study. Change is already underway, and is bound to accelerate with increased female education and workforce participation. I focus here on current measures and recommendations aimed at enhancing women's participation in nursing.

The first relates to the image problem. As Meleis and Hassan note, the key to solving the nursing crisis in the Gulf, is not a matter of which education model to adopt, but 'a much-needed and drastic change in the image and status of nursing itself'.[5] This can be done in many ways. Public education campaigns are necessary to improve the image of nursing among the general public and health care providers. The aim is to remove the stigma attached to nursing and to promote it as an honourable profession. Meleis reports on a similar campaign in Kuwait in the 1970s, where 'extensive public image modifiers' were used to glorify nursing as a women's domain, with roles congruent with those of wife, mother, and as a service-oriented field where women can be of service to humanity.[41] Similarly, Alawi and Mujahid recommend campaigns to promote nursing as an honourable profession for women that contributes to the well-being of Saudi Society.[7] So far, Saudi Arabia has not launched such campaigns. Instead, the matter has been left to the individual efforts of leading Saudi women educators such as Lutfiyyah al-Khateeb in the 1950s and early 1960s, and Samira Islam since the 1970s. Their efforts, however, are limited without official support and a political commitment. Needed is a government-sponsored national campaign targeting public school students, parents, and the general public. Such a national campaign requires the collaboration of the Ministry of Health; the Ministry of Education; the General Presidency of Girls' Education; the Ministry of Information; and the women's welfare associations that exist in various Saudi cities and towns. Changing the attitudes of physicians and other health care providers toward nurses may be an equally formidable task. Samira Islam emphasizes that physicians need to be sensitized to the importance and value of nursing, and to the need to develop a true team spirit. She adds, 'If there is anything in nursing that elevates it to the level of medicine, people will accept it'.[42] That magic formula is yet to be found.

Another measure is to improve the standard and level of nursing education. Saudi Arabia and other Arab countries have done this by introducing university-level nursing programmes hoping that this would move nursing into the general stream of education, enhance the nursing image, elevate its status in the eyes of young women, increase nursing enrolment and provide a high caliber of nurses.[4,40,29] But this strategy has not been effective in increasing the enrolment or persistence of women in nursing education programmes. For instance, after the opening of a nursing college at King Abdelaziz University in

Jeddah, nursing educators were disappointed by the low applicant pool. Nonetheless, efforts in this direction continue. In 1987, discussion was underway to allow top graduates of the health institutes to enter the colleges of medical sciences but the colleges feared this would dilute their academic standards. Another effort aims at establishing a Master's Degree programme in nursing, mostly to prepare top female graduates for teaching in the nursing college. These are cosmetic solutions to a deep rooted educational and social problem. A more effective approach may be to broaden the focus of nursing education.

As with many other Third World countries, Saudi Arabia has adopted the clinical model geared toward hospital care. This focus needs to be broadened to encompass preventive health in accordance with the government's health policy emphasizing primary health care. Ample employment opportunities for women exist in the 1650 PHCs around the country. Daytime work in the PHCs is comparable with women's family responsibilities and is bound to gain wider acceptance. Similarly, a programme for training school health nurses may also be effective in increasing women's interest in nursing and contributing to health development in the country. Thousands of nurses can be trained to meet the primary health needs of over a million girls enroled in primary and secondary schools, thus making a substantial contribution to health development. Kuwait tried a junior-college programme to train 'health inspectors,' but it was short lived. This does not mean that a similar programme may not work in Saudi Arabia, a much more conservative and restrictive country than Kuwait. The specialization 'health supervisor' and several other health specializations are available in the health institutes for males and should be made available for females as well.

A programme to prepare nurses for work as 'health educators' or 'public health nurses' could also prove highly successful in attracting women into nursing and in meeting the health education needs of all Saudi citizens. The ongoing health education programme sponsored by the GPGE in the girls' schools in Jeddah is a step in the right direction. This multifaceted and comprehensive programme is orchestrated by Dr Laila Al-Zubair, an Egyptian-educated Saudi physician and director of the health clinic of the GPGE in Jeddah. She has instituted a health record-keeping system for all female students, provides immunization to students, and health education to the girls and their mothers. The programme is currently conducted by the GPGE clinic in Jeddah and draws upon resources of their staff and volunteer women doctors and nurses from various hospitals and clinics in Jeddah. Extending such a programme to all girls schools throughout the country, a long-term goal of the GPGE, requires vast numbers of school nurses and health educators. This can only be accomplished through collaboration between the MOH and the GPGE in both the educational and employment arenas. A collaborative school nursing education programme, sponsored by both the MOH and the GPGE, could solve much of the recruitment problems of nursing education and practice and help meet the health needs of the country.

Women health educators continue to seek innovative solutions to the problem. Women faculty and administrators at the women's college of allied health sciences at King Abdelaziz University proposed, in 1986, to introduce a new medical technology programme focusing on nutrition. It aimed at preparing nutritionists for hospitals in an effort to increase women's participation in a female-appropriate specialty. This is in contrast to the men's college of allied health sciences at the same university which offers specializations in various medical technology fields, many of which should be made available to women also. The existing gender-role stereotypes which limit women's curriculum options must be re-evaluated, and medical specialties should be seriously considered to determine those most acceptable to women and to society at this stage of its development.

Another measure believed to increase women's participation in health occupations generally is the founding of women's hospitals. This is one way of dealing with the problem of intermingling of the genders by modifying the work environment. The first women's hospital was founded in Jeddah, in 1983, by a woman physician, Dr Saddiqa Pasha, as an 'exclusive medical facility managed and run by women to serve women—in keeping with Islamic principles,' states the hospital brochure. Although many health educators and planners do not accept the idea of such exclusive medical facilities, women's hospitals provide a viable model of health care delivery to women that is bound to gain wide acceptance among patients and health care providers. It is only one of many alternative solutions to a complex problem.

Finally, systems and infrastructures are also needed to help women juggle their work and family responsibilities. The option of part-time is available but the difference in pay is often too great to warrant the sacrifice. Saudi Arabia also provides generous maternity benefits to all female civil employees.[53] Yet some working women are demanding an extended maternity leave of upto two years, such as that available in Egypt. Also needed are infrastructures such as child care centres; transportation services; and boarding facilities in villages and small towns for female nurses living away from home. For many married women, the best solution is to have reliable quality child care, provided by the employer. Such support systems and infrastructures should help ease women's burden and enhance their participation in nursing and other professions.

These measures should help increase women's participation in nursing education and practice, and ensure that 'all women receive education, training and/or orientation that will enable them to provide health care for themselves, their families, and other members of the community'.[1] This is the best way to bring the country closer to achieving the goal of 'Health for All by the Year 2000.'

NOTES

1. World Health Organization, *Women as Providers of Health Care*, World Health Organization, Geneva, 1987.
2. N.H. Youssef, *Women and Work in Developing Societies*, University of California, Berkeley, Population Monograph Series No. 15, Berkeley, CA, 1974.
3. M. Jansen, 'Nursing in the Arab East,' ARAMCO Wld Mag., April-May 1974, pp. 14-23.
4. J.F. Khoury, 'Nursing in Kuwait,' *Int. Nurs.* Rev. 20, 1973, pp. 12-21.
5. A.I. Meleis and H.H. Soad, 'Oil rich, nurse poor: the nursing crisis in the Persian Gulf,' *Nurs. Outlook* 28, April 1980, pp. 238-243.
6. N.M. Kronfol, 'Nursing education in the Arabian Gulf: the Bahrain model,' *Int. J. Nurs. Stud.* 19, 1982, pp. 89-98.
7. H. Alawi and M. Ghazi, 'Skilled Health Manpower Requirements for the Kingdom of Saudi Arabia (1980-1990),' (Riyadh: King Saud University Press, 1982, quoted in J.W. Viola, *Human Resources Development in Saudi Arabia: Multinationals and Saudization*, International Human Resources Development Corporation, Boston, MA, 1986).
8. S. Altorky, *Women in Saudi Arabia: Ideology and Behavior Among the Elite*, New York: Columbia University Press, 1986.
9. S. Altorky and D.P. Cole, *Arabian Oasis City: The Transformation of Unayzah*, Austin, Texas: University of Texas Press, 1989.
10. C. Parssinen, 'The changing role of women,' in A. Beling (ed.), *King Faisal and the Modernization of Saudi Arabia*, London: Croom Helm, 1980, pp. 145-170.
11. D.J. Gerner, 'Roles in transition: the evolving position of women in Arab-Islamic countries,' in F. Hussain (ed.), *Muslim Women*, New York: St. Martin's Press, 1984, pp. 71-99.

12. N. El-Sanabary, 'Educating the second sex: Saudi Arabia's educational policy for women and its implications,' *Western Regional Conference of the Comparative and International Education Society*, Sacramento, California, 1988.

13. N. El-Sanabary, 'Higher education for women in Saudi Arabia, the paradox of educational reform,' *Annual Conference of the Comparative and International Education Society*, Pittsburgh, PA, 1991.

14. N. Ramazani, 'Arab women of the Gulf,' *Middle East J.*, 39, 1985, pp. 258-276.

15. According to the World Bank *World Development Report*, p. 219. Washington, DC, 1992; although the GNP/capita fluctuates from year to year depending on oil prices.

16. This point is emphasized in all literature about Saudi Arabian development.

17. UNESCO, *Statistical Yearbook*, UNESCO, Paris, 1991.

18. Kingdom of Saudi Arabia, *Educational Policy of the Kingdom of Saudi Arabia*, Riyadh: Ministry of Education, 1979.

19. Kingdom of Saudi Arabia, Civil Service Bureau, 1987, mimeographed.

20. R. El Mallakh, *Saudi Arabia, Rush to Development*, Baltimore: The Johns Hopkins University Press, 1982, p. 243.

21. Kingdom of Saudi Arabia, *The Third National Development Plan: 1980-1985*, Riyadh, Ministry of National Planning, 1980, (in Arabic), pp. 83, 355.

22. Nurses and health technicians are trained either in the health institutes or the colleges of allied health sciences.

23. Kingdom of Saudi Arabia, *The Fifth National Development Plan: 1990-1995*, Riyadh: Ministry of National Planning, 1990, pp. 309-313.

24. Known also as the nursing institutes.

25. Known as the colleges of allied medical sciences.

26. Kingdom of Saudi Arabia, Ministry of Education, Centre for Statistical Data and Educational Documentation, *Educational Statistics in the Kingdom of Saudi Arabia*, 1981/82, 15th Issue.

27. Kingdom of Saudi Arabia, Ministry of Health, *Annual Health Report*, 1990, pp. 335, 338.

28. Kingdom of Saudi Arabia, Ministry of Health, *Annual Health Report*, 1985.

29. Interviews with the directors of the health institutes in Riyadh and Taef, *al-Riyadh Daily Newspaper*, 9 April 1986 and 12 January 1987.

30. B. Abel-Smith, 'The world economic crisis, Part 2: Health manpower out of balance,' *Hlth Policy Plan*, 1, 1986, pp. 309-316.

31. Arab Bureau of Education in the Gulf States, *Directory of Higher and University Education in the Arab Gulf States*, Riyadh, 1983; and King Abdelaziz University, *The Yearly Graduation Book*, 1987, (in Arabic).

32. Information received in personal interviews with women faculty, Spring 1987.

33. King Abdelaziz University, *The Annual Graduation Book*, 1989.

34. S. Zein el-Abedeen, *Maseerat al-Mar'ah al Saudiyyah ela Ayn?* (The March of Saudi Women: To Where?), 2nd edn., Jeddah: The Saudi House for Publishing and Distribution, 1983, p. 99.

35. M.A. el-Bar, *Amal el-Mar'ah fil Meezan* (Women's Work in the Balance), Jeddah: The Saudi House for Publishing and Distribution, 1987 (in Arabic), pp. 203, 219-220.

36. M.A. Jamal, *Makanek Tuhmadi* (Keep to Your Place, Thank You), Beirut, Lebanon: Dar Ihyaa al-Uloum, 1986. The book was first published in 1964, pp. 131-132, 199, 247.
37. L. Hughes, 'The public image of the nurse,' *Adv. Nurs. Sci.* 2, 1980, pp. 55-72.
38. P.A. Kalisch, B.J. Kalisch and E. Livesay, 'The angel of death, the anatomy of 1980s major news story about nursing,' *Nurs. Forum* XIX, 1980, pp. 212-241.
39. P.A. Kalisch and B.J. Kalisch, 'Nurses on prime time television,' *Am. J. Nurs.*, 82, 1982, pp. 264-270.
40. J.K. Austin et al., 'Cross-cultural comparison on nursing image,' *Int. J. Nurs. Stud.*, 22, 1985, pp. 231-238.
41. A.I. Meleis, 'International issues in nursing education: the case of Kuwait,' *Int. Nurs. Rev.*, 26, 1979, pp. 107-110.
42. Personal interview, July 1987.
43. Saudi women are 42 per cent of medical students and practicing Saudi physicians.
44. Long S. Orpett, 'Roles, careers and femininity in biomedicine: women physicians and nurses in Japan,' *Soc. Sci. Med.*, 22, 1986, pp. 81-90.
45. N. El-Sanabary, 'Vocational and technical education for women in the Arab countries,' in N. El-Sanabary (ed.), *Women and Work in the Third World: The Impact of Industrialization and Global Economic Interdependence*, pp. 253-264. Centre for the Study, Education and Advancement of Women, University of California, Berkeley, CA, 1983.
46. A survey of Saudi medical students in the early 1980s by Semin Saedi Wong, showed that the majority of females came from upper- and middle-class background.
47. Reported in al-Khateeb memoirs and the author's personal interview with her daughter.
48. G. Marks and W.K. Beatty, *Women in White*, New York: Charles Scribner's, 1972.
49. That health committee was founded in 1978 by 'A General Secretariat composed of the Ministers of Health in the Gulf States,' see note (5, p. 240).
50. Kingdom of Saudi Arabia, Ministry of Health, *Annual Health Report*, Riyadh: Ministry of Health, 1989, p. 18.
51. R.F. Nyrop, *Saudi Arabia A Country Study*, 4th edn., Foreign Area Studies, The American University, Washington, DC, 1984, p. 131.
52. A.I. Meleis, 'A model for establishment of educational programmes in developing countries: the nurse paradoxes in Kuwait,' *J. Adv. Nurs.*, 5, 1980, pp. 285-300.
53. Six weeks paid maternity leave which may be combined with a six month sick leave upon the recommendation of a physician.

Reprinted from Social Science and Medicine, Vol. 37, Nagat El-Sanabary, 'The Education and Contribution of Women Health Care Professionals in Saudi Arabia: The Case of Nursing', pp. 1331-1343, 1993, with permission from Elsevier Science.

12

The Malaysian Example

Nancy H. Bryant

INTRODUCTION AND BACKGROUND

The information in this report draws from the findings of several reports prepared for the World Health Organization Regional Office for the Western Pacific and interviews of several Malaysian nurse educators and practitioners whom I met while on a short trip to Kuala Lumpur, Malaysia in February 1995.

This was not meant to be an exhaustive report on Nursing in Malaysia; instead, the purpose was to try and compare the status and roles of nursing and nursing education in Malaysia with that of other Islamic countries. A helpful supplement and background reading for this report is a chapter I wrote on 'Progress and Constraints of Nursing and Nursing Education in Islamic Societies,' in *Global Perspectives on Health Care*, Prentice Hall, 1995. The chapter is based on my own experience of eight years in nursing education and administration at the Aga Khan University, Karachi, Pakistan and on a literature review of nursing roles and women's issues in other Islamic societies.

I went to Kuala Lumpur with a list of questions that I hoped would encourage dialogue about the status and image of nursing—how nursing is perceived as a career for young women, especially Muslim women; how nursing relates to the culture and traditions of today's Muslim society; and how government policies affect the development of nursing and nursing education.

In the amount of time available and because of the Eid holiday, I was able to obtain only a brief impression of nursing in Malaysia and make a few preliminary comparisons with other Islamic countries.

Malaysia is a country in South-East Asia with a population of about 20 million people mixed religiously and racially with 51 per cent Malay (Muslim), 39 per cent Chinese (Confucian, Buddhist,

Muslim and Christian) and 11 per cent Indian (Hindu and Christian). The most striking aspects of Malaysian society (especially Kuala Lumpur) for a visitor are the apparent congenial mix of numerous cultures, varied forms of dress, and freedom of movement of men and women, both together and alone.

STATUS AND IMAGE OF NURSING

There was general agreement among the nurses I spoke to that nursing had a low status. The public still saw it not as a profession but as a menial job. In fact, one educator indicated that many present nurses and doctors would not encourage their daughters to go into nursing. One point of interest was that doctors held nurses in higher regard than did the public. This situation of low status and image needed to be worked on, and some felt that the current nursing leadership was not doing much to change the situation.

The problem regarding status and image of nurses is wide-spread in many Islamic countries and in some other countries also. The roles of women in a particular society also play a large part in how certain professions are perceived and accepted. It appears that Malaysian society does not differ much from other Islamic societies in its attitude toward the status and image of nursing. Low pay, lesser educational qualifications, compulsory bonding and poor working conditions also add to the low image of the nursing profession.

CULTURE AND TRADITION

From several conversations with nursing officials and educators, it seems that despite its low status, Malaysian society has adjusted to nursing as a career choice for young women. Issues that have emerged as problems in other countries concerning women in nursing are: allowing women to be educated beyond the minimum level; women out and about on the streets and in the work force; close association with male coworkers and patients; wearing inappropriate dress; living away from home as students; and the rotating shifts that require evening and night work. Similar issues are seen as problems in Malaysia.

One nurse educator explained how positive changes have occurred over the past two decades. When she entered nursing it was not considered an acceptable profession for a Muslim girl. Her parents tried to encourage her to go to university, but because they were not as conservative as other parents they permitted her to enter nursing school. At that time, Muslim religious leaders were still saying it was not proper for young women to care for men and work with male physicians. Also, under the British system, nursing students wore Western uniforms with relatively short skirts, tight belts, and caps. Most of the young women entering nursing were non-Muslim Chinese; very few were Malays. Gradually, however, more moderate religious teachers made a case for the care of sick people being an important and honourable job that should not be seen as unworthy. Instances of women nursing sick and wounded soldiers during the Prophet Muhammad's (PBUH) time were used as examples to make this point.

Although one educator remarked that the practice of Islam is in the heart, not in the dress, another educator felt that nursing received a big boost when the Nursing Board allowed students and RNs to wear pant suits as uniforms instead of the usual skirt. Previously, parents feared that if their daughters as student nurses wore short skirts at school and work, they would gradually change over and want to wear Western type clothing at home and in their social life. Today in Malaysia, nurses are free to wear skirts or pant suits. Caps are always worn by students. Head scarves are permitted but required in only one conservative private hospital in Kuala Lumpur. The educator also felt that now most students entering nursing are Malay and Muslim or Indian. Young Chinese women are increasingly going to Singapore for their education.

NURSING EDUCATION AND LEADERSHIP

As reported by a WHO consultant in 1993, the educational requirements of a graduate nurse fall below those for a university degree. In fact, until 1992, schools of nursing issued only certificates instead of diplomas in nursing. Programmes in nursing are patterned after the British system, but, as one consultant reported, 'They seem to be in a holding pattern.' Just within the last few years, however, several important changes have taken place. Most important has been the upgrading from a certificate to a diploma for the three-year basic programme in nursing. Students enter between the ages of 17-28 years after eleven years of schooling. As in some other countries, students must be single and are required to live in dormitories. I was told that teaching in Malay is not required and classes can now be held in English.

The problems and constraints in nursing that were pointed out to me by several nurse educators are ones that also occur in other Islamic countries. For example, beginning the basic nursing programme just one or two years short of secondary school graduation relegates nursing to a technical rather than a professional school and puts graduates at a severe disadvantage for obtaining higher education. Advanced nursing programmes such as public health, teaching, administration and midwifery award diplomas on completion. Only in 1993, when the first BScN programme began at the University of Malaysia, was there an opportunity to receive a degree in nursing. Unless talented nurses are sent abroad for higher degrees, the nursing leadership does not reach the higher levels of administration and policy making that other professions do.

Requirements of students being single and living in dormitories, and five years of bonding discourages bright, independent young women from entering nursing. Many of these requirements are changing in other Muslim countries. For instance, the Pakistan Nursing Council no longer requires students to live in hostels, married women can be admitted, the maximum age has been relaxed to thirty-five years and preference is given to students who have completed intermediate education (the same requirement as for university admission). Bonding continues to be a thorny issue in many countries, and only when students pay tuition and other expenses will institutions and governments feel that students should not repay the nursing service for their free or almost free education. In Malaysia, bonding appears to be at the maximum with five years required for a three-year basic programme and two years for each one-year post-basic diploma programme.

Another sometimes explosive issue regarding education is the language medium. My understanding is that previously in Malaysia, English was the medium of instruction in nursing. Then, all instruction was changed to the national language. Now, one educator informed me, English is again allowed as the medium of instruction in nursing schools. Since secondary education is in the national language, most nursing schools will need to offer classes in English for students who otherwise cannot cope with the English textbooks and journals. Language also presents problems and barriers between doctors and nurses working together, when doctors communicate in English and nurses are fluent only in Malay.

The ability to read English medical and nursing textbooks cannot be overemphasized when preparing nurses for the numerous and fast moving changes in technology and standards of care. Very few countries translate these textbooks into their national language, and relying on instructors to give the information through lectures does not develop the problem-solving, self-learning capabilities that enable nurses to become life time learners.

Raising the educational level of nursing in Malaysia has been a long and difficult task. It took from 1981 to September 1993 to convince university officials that a degree programme in nursing should be started. The concern then and now is finding enough academically qualified nurses to teach and administer the programme. The BScN programme is part of the new Department of Allied Health Sciences, headed by a physician. The acting head of the programme at the time of my visit was a nurse who received her Master's in Education from Manchester University, UK and has been encouraged to obtain her PhD abroad in order to be fully qualified for her position.

Malaysia, like many other countries with a colonial tie to Great Britain, has maintained the three-year diploma programme for basic nursing education along with one to two-year certificate courses in midwifery, administration, teaching and public health. While adding greatly to the professional capabilities and qualifications of the nurses, these courses have been difficult to equate with university standards and credits. Therefore, while other countries, such as Thailand, have moved their basic nursing programmes into the university setting, nurses in Malaysia and some other countries are blocked from pursuing higher education. Even Great Britain has changed much of its nursing education to make it university-based.

My impression of the BScN programme at the University of Malaysia is that it is innovative, creative and fair. It gives credit for previous work experience and post-basic courses, so nurses do not have to repeat courses, but can add to their present store of knowledge and skills. Receiving credit for post-basic courses that can be applied to the BScN degree is possible, however, because of the high standards maintained in these courses over the years. From my brief visit, the BScN programme looks good, but more nursing faculty need to be prepared at the masters and doctoral levels to build a strong academic department which will provide future leadership to the profession. For the time being, graduate programmes in the UK, Australia, Canada and the US should be used to prepare future faculty members. Sending nurses to different universities and countries will help broaden the scope and depth of the BScN programme. In addition, a faculty appointment plan that allows nurse faculty members to be a part of the university faculty should be developed and put in place as soon as possible. We accomplished this at the Aga Khan University in Karachi, Pakistan without any dilution to the quality of the medical faculty. This plan can be made available on request.

The BScN programme is over-subscribed and in urgent need of more qualified nursing faculty. Many older nurses will want to take advantage of this programme and it is flexible enough to make it realistic for them to do so. Long range plans should address the possibility of adding a generic BScN programme where students enter directly after secondary school completion and receive their BScN degree in four years. This would save a considerable amount of time for young women who want a career but who also do not want to delay marriage until they complete their university education. It would also permit the university to select students with high academic standards.

PRIMARY HEALTH CARE

The characteristic that sets Malaysia apart from other countries of the South is its well-developed primary health care system. It covers the population through health centres and basic health units which serve populations of 15,000-20,000 and 2,000-4,000 respectively and are spread throughout the thirteen states—eleven in Peninsular Malaya and two in the Island of Borneo (Sabah and Sarawak). I was told that the PHC system works well outside the larger cities. PHC in the cities, however, is still lacking and this needs to be developed. A portion of the population in the cities is not covered by the government or private doctors and hospitals.

Public Health nurses who are RNs with one additional year of midwifery and one year of public health form part of the staff at the health centres. Their responsibilities include MCH clinics, child health, school health, health and nutrition education, and supervision of auxiliary staff, among other duties. They supervise the community nurses in the basic health units which are about five kilometers from the health centre. Community nurses are not RNs. They are auxiliary midwives who have completed the Midwifery II course and the MCH course.

An Assistant Principal Matron at the Ministry of Health, Division of Nursing reviewed the structure of the country's health system for me and noted that Malaysia has been training public health nurses and community nurses to fill roles in the health centres and basic units for many years.

Apparently it is not a problem to get these community nurses to stay in the rural areas since they have housing provided for themselves and their families. Most are married women. They don't usually want to be moved and it is sometimes difficult to get them to come to the big centres for additional training. One educator noted that community nurses need considerably more training in assessment skills. Some community nurses are single women but that does not seem to present any security problem. They are well respected and can move about the community to do their work without fear of harassment. The freedom of movement for women outside the home is quite different from some other conservative societies. It presents a much easier task for government policy makers and nursing administrators when trying to distribute health personnel throughout the system.

In many Islamic societies it has been extremely difficult to recruit young women for work in rural areas and for work in cities or rural areas that requires home visiting or community activities. Mobility of these workers is hindered by their requiring escorts and/or vehicles. The safety of female workers is a major issue in some work places and providing secure living quarters can present numerous problems. The health care system in Malaysia also differs greatly from some other countries where nurses have not even been trained in public health and therefore, no government career posts exist for them.

GOVERNMENT AND PRIVATE HEALTH SYSTEMS

Government officials, WHO and other agencies are aware of the need to upgrade nursing education in Malaysia and have taken specific steps to do so. As mentioned, a new curriculum for the basic programme was designed and implemented in 1992. Upon completion of three years of study, students receive a diploma in nursing instead of a certificate. For many years, because of the limited opportunities for higher education, senior nurses have been awarded scholarships to study abroad, mostly in the UK, Australia and Canada, with a few going to the US. Nurses have also been sponsored to attend workshops, conferences and seminars as a form of continuing education.

Obtaining a higher degree abroad, however, does not guarantee a place in the nursing leadership of Malaysia. This same situation prevails in other countries where senior nurses with many years of experience are strongly entrenched in top government nursing jobs. Nurses returning with more education and expertise are seen as a threat and are not given the responsible positions and opportunities to upgrade and improve nursing nationwide. They either become discouraged and gradually slip back into the old system or they move to the private sector where their skills are lost to the government system, or they leave nursing altogether.

Another factor affecting nursing in Malaysia is the migration of nurses to work in other countries such as Saudi Arabia and Brunei where they can make enough money so they do not need to worry about the loss of their government pensions. As a result, Malaysia is recruiting nurses from other countries to make up for the shortage.

There has been a tremendous growth in the number of private hospitals in Malaysia, and more and more nurses are leaving government service and taking jobs in the private sector. The pay is higher than in government service and private hospitals are willing to pay off graduate nurses' bonds just to recruit them. I had an interesting and informative visit to the Puteri Nursing College (PNC) where I learned more about the education of nurses in a private health system.

PNC admits forty new students each semester. Science, math and 'O' level examinations are required for admission. I was told by school officials that top students, however, usually do not choose nursing, since they can get a better education or job elsewhere. Nor are all who apply qualified for admission. English language capability is especially important at PNC since most of the clients speak English. The college offers English classes to students who need them.

PNC uses its own hospitals for clinical experiences and government health centres for community health. Government hospitals are also used for some specialty clinical experience such as mental health, pediatrics, and eye, ear, nose and throat. At PNC, the student uniform is a pant-suit with a cap while graduates can choose to wear skirts or pants. I'm told that most Malays wear pants and most Chinese and Indian young women wear skirts.

Hospitals of the KPJ Healthcare system sponsor students to attend Puteri Nursing College. The hospital pays PNC for the education of the students and provides a stipend for them. The student is then bonded for work in the system for five years. She can be moved to another hospital within the system on request. This system has hospitals in all but two states. They also plan to expand their hospitals into Indonesia in the future. PNC also provides in-service education to nurses within the system. They offer 'top off' courses for trained nurses who wish to return to nursing after 10-20 years absence. The college provides two clinical instructors at each hospital for student's clinical experience, but they are often short of instructors. PNC uses numerous consultants from Australia and elsewhere to conduct short courses of one to three months in critical care, nursing management and neo-natal intensive care, especially for its post-basic programmes.

The college has made concerted efforts in career guidance to promote nursing in schools of general education. As in most programmes, single girls are preferred. Students live in hostels because of transportation problems. This problem was solved in our school in Karachi by providing private buses to pick up students who lived within a reasonable distance and allowing students from other parts of the country to live in the hostel.

Nursing Board

As in many other countries, the Nursing Board controls, regulates and sets standards for the nursing and midwifery professions in Malaysia. With only limited time at the Nursing Board, I concentrated on several issues that reflect nursing control over its profession and methods used to solve nursing shortages.

One issue has to do with the methods used to develop and conduct national examinations for RNs and midwives. The Assistant Principal Matron explained that a panel of nurse educators develops the questions used in the written exams and the practical exam is conducted as an OSCE (Objective Structured Clinical Examination) by senior nurses. Only one OB-GYN doctor is used in the midwifery practical. This system differs from and is an improvement over the method formerly used in Pakistan, where most of the practical RN exams were conducted by doctors. Using doctors to determine the nursing skills required for graduates had been very unsatisfactory and relinquishes control over the profession to physicians.

The Nursing Board is also attempting to update skills of the 2000 plus traditional birth attendants (TBA). Their numbers are gradually decreasing as more women have babies at the health centres or hospitals with trained midwives in attendance. This action, however, also increases the requirement for more nurses and midwives in the Primary Health Care system.

The Assistant Principal Matron noted that Malaysia is suffering from a shortage of nurses and it is often difficult to adequately staff the hospitals and health centres, which is done through the Nursing Board. As mentioned, many nurses are leaving government service to work in private hospitals or in other countries such as Brunei or the Middle East where the pay is higher. The bond that each nurse must repay (five years for RNs and two years for each additional one-year diploma) has recently been increased in monetary value in an effort to stop this exodus. The RN bond was M$10,000, but is now M$35,000. Still, private hospitals and other countries will pay the bond in order to recruit nurses. As a result, some foreign nurses have been recruited by the Health Ministry to help relieve the nursing shortage. Their registrations must be approved by the Nursing Board. In addition, the Ministry has increased the in-take of students to 1800 per year in the schools of nursing.

SUMMARY

When comparing nursing and nursing education in Malaysia with nursing in other Islamic countries, one notes many similarities and some striking differences. It is similar, unfortunately, in some of the following ways:

- it has a low status and image among the general public;
- educational requirements for entry are still below secondary school graduation;
- the pay is low and the working conditions and hours have many disadvantages;
- advances into higher education for the profession have been slow; and

- nursing education and service have not changed with the British systems from which they were copied.

In some ways, nursing in Malaysia enjoys some advantages over other Islamic countries. For instance, the less restricted life style encourages more women to be employed outside the home. The ability of women to move about in the community permits nurses to be an integral and important part of the country's health care system, especially in areas of public health. This is extremely important as the health care systems for the future will be increasingly designed to provide more care outside the hospital, and nurses will be given more responsible leadership roles.

Nursing in Malaysia also enjoys continued support from government, WHO, and NGOs for continuing education programmes and post-basic courses which have helped to upgrade the qualifications of individual nurses and enhance the level of the profession generally.

What appears to be lacking is a major commitment or drive to move nursing into the twenty-first Century regarding education for the leaders, practitioners and researchers. Until nursing can provide professional opportunities at the university level for education, service and research, other fields that do so will attract the best and the brightest of the young women seeking careers. A step in this direction would be a substantial investment in educational preparation of nursing faculty at the masters and doctoral levels to strengthen the new post-basic BScN programme in the Department of Allied Health Sciences, University of Malaysia.

ACKNOWLEDGEMENTS

The author is grateful for the information provided by the following persons about nursing in Malaysia: Cik Nik Safiah Nik Ismail, Universiti Kebangsaan Malaysia; Puan Chee Chong Hwai, Office of the Director General of Health; Dr L.R.L. Verstuyft, WHO Representative; Ms Nik, Puteri Nursing College; Puan Siti Aizah Zahari, Allied Health Science, University of Malaysia.

13

Nursing in Iraq

Joyceen S. Boyle and *Khlood Salman*

Professional nursing in Iraq has been profoundly influenced by changes in social, political and economic systems. The early history of professional nursing and nursing education is an account of how a developing Islamic country successfully created a professional system of nursing. During the 1980s, Iraq was a leader among Persian Gulf countries in nursing education and service. However, after the Gulf War the sanctions imposed by the United Nations had drastic repercussions on all aspects of Iraqi life, including the disintegration of the health care system. This chapter will discuss the development of professional nursing in Iraq and describe the unique barriers and difficulties that have faced the profession of nursing in the country.

For purposes of clarity, it is easier to separate a discussion of professional nursing in Iraq into two eras; the first is that period of time when professional nursing education was firmly established within an academic environment and began to flourish. The second time period started with the end of the Iraq-Iran war in 1988, continuing through the Gulf war up to the present time.

THE ESTABLISHMENT OF PROFESSIONAL NURSING

Undoubtedly, nursing existed in some form in early Islamic society as there are historical accounts of women organizing to care for the sick and wounded on battlefields.[1] Western missionaries reintroduced these activities during the latter part of the nineteenth century and the introduction of modern nursing, as we know it, was established when Iraq was placed under the control of the British in 1917.

The first formal nursing programme in Iraq was established in 1933 in Baghdad. The school admitted only women who had finished their primary education (six years) and after completion of the three-year programme, graduates received a certificate and were appointed to staff positions in various hospitals in Baghdad. In 1936, only ten women graduated from the school as the development and growth of nursing in Iraq, as in other Persian Gulf countries, has always been tied to the status of women in Islamic societies. Health officials in Iraq, as in other Islamic societies, attempted to cover the shortage in nursing by importing nurses from all over the world, offering high salaries and providing free accommodations and paid vacations. Of course, this was not a satisfactory solution as most foreign nurses had difficulties due to the language and the social barriers faced by women. As Bryant[1] observed, more than almost any other group of women, those of the Islamic faith have been bound by customs and traditions and have had to overcome significant obstacles in order to progress and develop. This has been obvious in the development of Iraqi nursing.

Nursing and the Role of Women

While nurses in Europe, the United States, and elsewhere have been hampered by the restrictions placed on women, the development of professional nursing in Islamic societies has been curtailed by traditional customs and norms related to the role of women. These conservative customs and traditions have perpetuated rules and regulations restraining the activities of women. Islamic nurses, primarily women, have had to struggle against considerable odds to overcome many social barriers to advance their career and professional status. Chief among them is that in Islam, the 'natural' progression or development for women is tied to marriage and their families. This includes the major responsibilities for the care of children and the household with little help from male spouses. Historically, Muslim women have never been the passive creatures that the Western world has imagined them to be. However, women were active only within very limited parameters. Although Abu Gharbich and Suliman[2] referred specifically to nursing in Jordan, their concerns apply to Iraqi nursing as well. They questioned if a woman who is dependent upon, and subordinate to, male family members, can be expected to initiate change, exercise independent judgement, and develop collegial relationships with primarily male physicians. Closely related to these norms in restraining the development of nursing is that anything related exclusively to women is of lower status and social prestige. Traditionally, it has been difficult to attract bright, well-educated men and women to professional nursing in Islamic societies. In addition, the twenty-four-hour responsibility of nursing to patient care results in a dilemma as women in traditional families are not allowed to be away from their home at night regardless of the reason. Women do not drive cars; they do not go out alone and they do not interact with men outside of their own family members.

Further compounding these difficulties, as in some other countries, is that the control of Iraqi nursing has never rested within the profession itself: government controls and directives from within the ministries of health and education have dictated the role and place of professional nursing and the educational system that produced it. Professional organizations have remained in a nascent state, unable to provide leadership for change. Even when Iraqi nurses achieved some level of education, they were never in a position to effect significant changes in either nursing education or practice.

Influence of Social and Economic Changes on Iraqi Nursing

In the 1960s, Iraq like other Gulf countries achieved some degree of independence and began to expand social and economic opportunities for all citizens, including women. Saddam Hussein came to power in 1968 and set his country on a course of modern development. Of considerable importance was the oil wealth that provided the economic resources to finance the priorities of development.[3,4] At the same time, other important social and political changes taking place in Iraqi society enhanced the transition of nursing into a professional institution.

Improving health status of the population and increasing the educational level of all citizens were important priorities for the new government. The expansion of the health care system and the emphasis on improving the country's health status increased the need for well-prepared physicians and nurses. As educational institutions expanded, formal education was made available for women. In 1975, the Free Educational Law was enacted promoting access to education for both men and women.[3] While this law increased the access of all women to a basic and higher education, specifically, it promoted access to education for rural women and encouraged their admission to universities. Financial support was provided to selected students to study abroad. A number of nurses continued their nursing education, some of them received both bachelors and masters degrees in nursing from universities in England and the United States. Later, a few nursing leaders obtained advanced degrees from Egyptian universities when universities in the Middle East established graduate programmes in nursing. The majority of nurses with higher degrees became teachers in schools of nursing or went into nursing administration positions.

Nursing in the Academic Setting

In 1962, the College of Nursing was established at the University of Baghdad.[5] For the first two formative years, the World Health Organization (WHO) in conjunction with the Iraqi Ministry of Health administered the College. In 1964, administrative responsibilities were transferred to Baghdad University. Primary objectives in establishing the nursing programme were to prepare well-educated nurses who could provide and supervise high quality care and to prepare nursing administrators and instructors for other schools of nursing.

There were problems in the nursing education programme from the beginning. The first dean of the College was a female physician who had no prior knowledge about nursing. The faculty were from different countries and were assigned by WHO, thus many of them had no prior knowledge about the social restrictions on women in Iraq, nor did they understand the unique problems faced by nursing in that particular society.

However, despite the difficulties the policies of the Iraqi government and the aspirations of nursing coincided in the desire to advance professional nursing through opportunities in advanced education with the establishment of a masters programme in nursing at the University of Baghdad in 1986. At that point in time, professional nursing education in Iraq had reached a point where it served as a model and incentive to other Persian Gulf countries. However, there were still long standing problems. Nurses, regardless of their educational background, were paid the same salary. Professional standards for practice were non-existent and nurses, by default, became responsible for supplies, housekeeping duties and other non-professional tasks. Because nurses were women, they faced disrespect and censure from other health professionals, administrators and often patients as well. Baccalaureate graduates were assigned to different institutions to cover the nursing shortage without consideration of job descriptions, personal interests, experiences skills, and abilities. Job satisfaction and morale were routinely low.

The lack of standards of practice and position descriptions created a confusing situation in the workplace. All nurses from different educational backgrounds practiced without licensure or certification. There were no mechanisms for evaluation of job performance or outcome criteria for patient care. Different levels and titles of nurses created confusion. For example, there were baccalaureate (BSN) graduates who were prepared to assume leadership responsibilities, but often were assigned to staff duties. Technical nurses were those women who had graduated from three-year programmes following a primary education of six years. Skilled nurses also completed three-year programmes but their basic education was completed at the level of intermediate school. Technical or practical nurses completed two-year programmes of training.

According to information gathered by K. Salman[6] the total number of all nurses from different levels of preparation in 1989 reached a total of 12,687 nurses with 5,932 holding the baccalaureate degree. After 1990, several new universities were established throughout Iraq to meet the demands for higher education. Several of these institutions have established BSN nursing programmes. The latest statistical information available indicated there were approximately 56,800 nurses throughout the country with about 22,800 holding a baccalaureate degree. Nursing in Iraq still suffers from the lack of standards, as well as lack of agreement regarding minimum educational preparation for the profession.

Table 1 shows the numbers of graduating nurses in Iraq from 1978-1997. Although information from the Iraqi Ministry of Health should always be interpreted with caution, there are several interesting trends in these data. The Iran-Iraq war began in 1980 and by its end in 1987, the number of nurses graduating from all levels of nursing programmes had more than doubled. Secondly, there was obviously a tremendous effort during the years of the economic sanctions (from 1990 to the present) to produce adequate numbers of nurses to meet the health needs of the country. In part, this was a response on the part of the Iraqi government to demonstrate that Iraqi society was still able to maintain educational and health programmes in spite of the sanctions

Table 1
Number of graduating trained nurses (all levels)
from 1978-1997*

Year	1978	1979	1980	1981	1982	1983	1984
Nurses	96	69	209	180	370	403	500

Year	1985	1986	1987	1988	1989	1990	1991
Nurses	700	560	900	1015	880	1600	1200

Year	1992	1993	1994	1995	1996	1997
Nurses	2100	3600	4000	3000	3500	3800

*Information supplied by Ministry of Health, Baghdad, Iraq.

and ensuing economic hardships. In addition, many well educated nurses fled the country during the sanctions and the total numbers of nurses must have been seriously depleted. It can be assumed, given the rapid increase in numbers of graduating nurses, that the majority are from the technical, skilled or practical levels of nursing rather than baccalaureate programmes.

THE NURSING CURRICULUM AT THE UNIVERSITY OF BAGHDAD

It is instructive to examine the nursing curriculum leading to a baccalaureate degree.[5] Changes or revisions in course offerings and underlying philosophy frequently reflected the social changes within Iraqi society as a whole. For example, Table 2 shows the four-year nursing curriculum, 1962-1966. In 1962, four years of course work were required with two semesters per year. Similar to early baccalaureate programmes in the United States, the curriculum consisted primarily of 'required' courses (few, if any electives) and a substantial number of clinical hours each week. Courses in Arabic society and Islamic culture reflected the pan-Arabism that was sweeping the Middle East. Nursing courses reflected the medical model, for example—medical and surgical nursing, pediatric nursing, obstetrics and gynecology, and so on. There was a continual struggle

Table 2

Curriculum 1962-1966, University of Baghdad, College of Nursing B.Sc. in Nursing

First Year 1962-1963 Courses	Credit	Theory Hrs.	Lab Hrs.	Clinical Hrs.	Weeks
Anatomy	3	2	2	–	15
Chemistry	3	2	2	–	15
English	3	3	–	–	15
Fundamentals of Nursing	6	2	2	–	30
General Psychology	2	2	–	–	15
Microbiology	3	2	2	–	15
Parasitology	3	2	2	–	15
Physiology	3	2	2	–	15

Second Year 1963-1964	Credit	Theory Hrs.	Lab Hrs.	Clinical Hrs.	Weeks
Arabic Society	3	3	–	–	15
English Language	6	3	–	–	30
Fundamentals of Nursing	8	4	8	–	15
Introduction to Statistics	3	3	–	–	15
Medical Surgical nursing	9	4	–	20	15
Microbiology	2	2	–	–	15
Nutrition	2	2	–	–	15
Psychology	2	2	–	–	15

Third Year 1964-1965 Courses	Credit	Theory Hrs.	Lab Hrs.	Clinical Hrs.	Weeks
English Literature	3	3	–	–	15
Fundamentals and Methods of Teaching	3	2	2	–	15
Medical Surgical Nursing	9	4	–	20	15
Medicine	1	1	–	–	15
Surgery	1	1	–	–	15
Pediatrics Nursing	9	4	–	20	15
Pharmacology	2	2	–	–	15
Surgery	1	1	–	–	15

Fourth Year 1965-1966	Credit	Theory Hrs.	Lab Hrs.	Clinical Hrs.	Weeks
Administration and Human Relations	3	3	–	–	15
Administration & Organization in Public Health	3	3	–	–	15
History of Education	3	3	–	–	15
Islamic Culture	3	3	–	–	15
Maternal & Child Health Nursing	9	4	–	20	15
Mental Hygiene & Psychiatry	3	3	–	–	15
Obstetrics & Gynecology	2	2	–	–	15
Public Health Nursing	9	4	–	20	15

1 credit = 1 theory hour or 2 lab. hours or 4 clinical hours.

Source: Curriculum 1962-1987. Republic of Iraq. Ministry of Higher Education and Scientific Research. University of Baghdad. College of Nursing

Table 3
Curriculum 1986-1987

Fourth Year 1986-1987 Courses	Credit	Theory Hrs.	Lab Hrs.	Clinical Hrs.	Weeks
Community Health Nursing	10	4	–	18	15
Epidemiology	2	2	–	–	15
Introduction to Research	2	2	–	–	15
Nursing Administration	4	2	–	6	15
Principles & Methods of Teaching	4	2	4	–	15
Psychiatric and Mental Health Nursing	10	4	–	18	15
Social & National Education I	2	2	–	–	15
Social & National Education II	2	2	–	–	15

1 credit = 1 theory hours
       2 lab. hours
       4 clinical hours

Source: Curriculum 1962-1987. Republic of Iraq. Ministry of Higher Education and Scientific Research. University of Baghdad. College of Nursing.

on the part of early nursing educators to move away from the model established by diploma programmes as well as the control of physicians.

By 1986, new courses had been added to the curriculum, including community health nursing, military nursing, and sociology and human relations. Table 3 shows only the fourth year of the nursing curriculum in 1986. Along with military nursing, the addition of courses in social and national education I and II reflected the major societal changes in Iraq, primarily the eight-year war with Iran and the consolidation of political power by Saddam Hussein.

The addition of community health nursing and epidemiology prepared nurses to function in community-based settings focusing on nationally targeted programmes of public health, maternal and infant health, the eradication of infectious diseases, as well as improved sanitary measures. Content in ethics and computers was also included. As a result of the thousands of soldiers wounded in the Iran-Iraq war, rehabilitation content was added to medical-surgical nursing. Faculty were beginning to integrate concepts such as 'self care' and 'continuity of care' throughout the curriculum. The curriculum in 1986 certainly prepared nurses within a university context, with a background of professional knowledge and clinical skills. Yet an emphasis on developing leadership skills was notably lacking.

The newly established masters programme offered clinical specialties in areas of medical-surgical nursing, psychiatric nursing, public health and obstetric and pediatric nursing. The two-year graduate curriculum had courses common to each clinical specialty during the first year. An emphasis was placed on research and theory within each clinical specialty during the second year; a thesis was required for graduation from the programme. By 1987, each clinical specialty had three to five masters students enroled.

By 1988, there were a total of 406 undergraduate students; approximately 100 of these students were diploma graduates returning for a baccalaureate degree. Upon completion of the programme of study, all graduates completed a year of 'residency' in an institution assigned by the Ministry of Health. After completion of the residency, professional nurses were assigned (by the Ministry of Health) to either teaching or service, depending on identified needs. Again, it is instructive to note governmental control over the profession.

THE ACADEMIC FACULTY

By the late 1980s, the College of Nursing had a competent, well-educated faculty. The majority were masters prepared (many of them from Boston University or University of Pittsburgh in the US). Two or three faculty members held doctoral preparation; several others were on educational leave in the United States completing doctoral work in institutions such as the University of California at San Francisco and the University of Arizona. The College had adequate overall resources. In particular, the holdings in the health science library were superb, equal or better than many similar institutions in the US.

SOCIAL AND POLITICAL TRENDS INFLUENCING NURSING

It is of interest to examine the structure of the College of Nursing, the curriculum, as well as the faculty and students in relation to what was occurring politically and socially in Iraqi society. The emphasis on access to education for women continued and nurses took advantage of opportunities to pursue further education, including doctoral degrees. Yet the College of Nursing reflected the general norms and values of the wider society, a society where men controlled the workplace and women were relegated to subordinate positions. Nursing still was primarily a women's profession and continued to suffer from a negative image and low status. All nurse members of the faculty were female, the majority holding masters degrees. Faculty reported that one male faculty member was on leave pursuing doctoral study in the US. The dean of the College was a male and a non-nurse, a pharmacist who represented the College of Nursing to the wider university. He was respected and well liked by the female faculty although several of them privately regretted that the dean of the College was male and a non-nurse. It was acknowledged by the faculty that a female, regardless of her educational credentials, would never be as respected within academic circles as males were. Even though modernization polices encouraged education for women and the advancement of professional nursing, nursing leaders still did not have ready access to sources of power or any role in policy making. Their influence was contained within the limited educational sphere of the College of Nursing and did not extend to university levels or national health care policies.

The 'natural' role of women within Iraqi and the wider Islamic society has always been inexplicitly bound to marriage and family. Educated working women, including nursing faculty, struggled constantly with the responsibilities of child care and household duties. The war with Iran dragged on for a total of eight long grueling years, finally ending in 1987. Although it is difficult to obtain exact numbers, it is estimated that 200,000 Iraqi soldiers died in that conflict, a staggering number in a nation of only 16 million people.[7] The war had a profound and personal impact on nearly all Iraqis as fathers and sons went to war, leaving women with the primary responsibility for their families. Women who were faculty members were not exceptions; they too had husbands and sons at war and they were left to work full time and manage the children and household responsibilities on their own. Many of them were caring for aging parents as well.

THE WAR WITH IRAN

The Iran-Iraq war was fought over fierce desert terrain, often involving tank warfare. This led to specific kinds of traumatic injuries, especially head and spinal cord trauma as well as amputations and other crushing injuries. The addition of rehabilitation nursing to the baccalaureate curriculum was viewed by the faculty as a necessary and important addition to the curriculum. Psychological conditions, in both returning war veterans and the civilian population influenced course content and clinical practice. Faculty research as well as several masters' theses focused on the impact of war on children as well as other family members.

A course on military nursing was added to the third year of the programme and was taught by an army officer who was also a physician. Prior to the Iran-Iraq war, nursing was almost exclusively a women's profession. Even though nurses and other women worked outside the home and a substantial number had university educations, nurses' and other women's roles were still restricted by traditional norms. It was simply unthinkable that a woman (even a professional nurse) be sent to the front to care for the injured. The unique solution in this Islamic society was to admit men into nursing via career assignments made through university admission policies. At the height of the Iran-Iraq war, nearly 75 per cent of the students in the College of Nursing were men who went directly into the military services upon graduation. Many of them reportedly would have preferred engineering, or other typically 'male' occupations. While this solution addressed the supply of military nurses, it only increased the shortage of nurses in the domestic health care system. Baccalaureate nursing graduates were prepared to fill leadership positions in nursing throughout the country and a shortage of female graduates diluted the leadership and limited the contributions of professional nursing throughout the health care system. Lay volunteers were assigned to 'hospital duty' to assist with the nursing shortage. These volunteers were young college graduates, usually women, who were required to perform a limited amount of time in 'volunteer service' prior to employment in the public sector. Since nearly all employment for educated females was in the public sector, there were adequate numbers of volunteers. The shortage of nurses in leadership and management positions along with the deprofessionalization of nursing through the volunteer programme further decreased the power, prestige and professional growth of nursing.

The end of the Iran-Iraq war did not bring noticeable improvements or support for professional nursing. In August 1988, the Minister of Education met with the University of Baghdad nursing faculty to inform them that the baccalaureate programme would be phased out. The official reasons were related to the current political and economic situation following the war. Baccalaureate programmes in nursing are expensive in terms of numbers of faculty and require four years of academic study. Iraqi government officials had decided that it would be economically more feasible to 'train' technically oriented nurses in hospital settings.[3] Of course, the nursing faculty protested these plans, arguing that the overwhelming health care needs, including those of returning veterans, required professional nursing. No students were admitted to the nursing programme in the fall of 1988 and some faculty were assigned to other positions in service or in hospital training programmes.

When professional nursing is closely tied to traditional norms that view women and nursing as occupying an inferior status, the profession occupies a very precarious position within any system. While modernization policies in Iraq encouraged advanced education for women and thus facilitated the advance and development of nursing, nursing leaders did not have ready access to power, decision-making, or control over their own profession. Apparently after one year, in 1989, government officials re-evaluated the decision to close the College of Nursing. Students were admitted and classes continued. However, morale among nursing faculty was at an all time low as the faculty members realized how vulnerable and precarious the future of professional nursing was and how little control nurses were able to exert on the future of their profession.

THE GULF WAR AND PROFESSIONAL NURSING

The Gulf War and the ensuing economic sanctions have had devastating effects on the economy and social fabic of Iraq. It is difficult to overestimate the horrific impact that the sanctions have had on individual lives. Since embargos affect the entire population and because they continue over long periods of time, their relative impact on civilian institutions is severe. When coupled with political oppression, the impact of economic severity including the scarcity of food, medicine and other life-sustaining resources on women and their families and by extension on professional nursing has been crippling. Information about professional nursing as a whole has been hard to come by, but the authors have had intermittent, fragmentary, yet consistent reports about individual faculty members and the situation of the College of Nursing. Tentative conclusions can be drawn about professional nursing in Iraq based on our information as well as what we know about the status of women after the war, the poignant impoverishment of most Iraqis, and the deteriorating social situation.

THE EFFECTS OF THE WAR AND SANCTIONS ON IRAQI WOMEN

The majority of nurses in Iraq, including those with professional education are women and they have always had the primary responsibility for domestic tasks and the care of children. Iraqi women, including nurses regardless of their educational backgrounds, have suffered immensely from the effects of the two wars—the Iran-Iraq war and later the Gulf war and continuing economic sanctions. During the Gulf war, civilian infrastructures were destroyed during the bombing campaign; these included, but were not limited to, hospitals, electrical power plants, and sewer and water treatment facilities. Health and well-being of the Iraqi people, especially women and children, have suffered and the difficulties, frustrations and disappointments faced by women and their families have worsened. All of this adds up to a rather bleak portrayal of the effect of the ongoing sanctions on Iraqi society.

As the economic and social situation became worse due to the deteriorating effect of the sanctions, women picked up the slack. Food was scarce, medicine was not readily available and survival became a full time occupation. Compounding this situation, many men, often returning veterans, were unemployed, without any income and unable to provide economically for their families. This has increased the responsibility of women. Rising unemployment in the 1990s has particularly affected women. With declining public sector employment, many more women than men have lost jobs.[8] The repercussions, while somewhat improved after the Oil for Food Programme was initiated by the United Nations, still continue from the shortages of food and medicine, the spread of illnesses, malnutrition, and the lack of sanitation. The psychological effects of war and sanctions on women and their families have been devastating.

Taken all together, war and militarism have had catastrophic effects on the lives of individual Iraqis, their effects have destroyed homes, communities and families as well as portions of minority populations. Iraqi women have been invisible casualties in the aftermath of the fighting.[9] Embargoes such as the one imposed on Iraq affect the entire population and because they go on for relatively long periods of time, their relative impact on civilians is considerable.[10,11,12,9]

PROFESSIONAL NURSING

The College of Nursing still exists as an academic entity at the University of Baghdad. While we have no specific information on numbers or gender of students, we can assume that life for both faculty and students is very difficult and that the economic situation brought about by the sanctions has made life extremely onerous. One Iraqi talking about visiting his former colleagues at the University of Baghdad, said, 'It is so sad to see them. Men who used to take such pride and care in the way they dressed...now they are shabby, their coats are frayed and their shoes have holes in them. They are very thin and hungry.'

In the 1990s, virtually all of the University's education budget went to pay minimal salaries; no regular budget exists for repairs or equipment.[8] Training for staff or professional development for faculty are no longer possible. The intellectual community is completely isolated as faculty are unable to travel; computers and the internet are not available, and the library holdings are antiquated. Per capita income has fallen and inflation has taken its toll on members of the faculty community. There has been a steady erosion of intellectual life.

Garfield estimates that from 2-4 million Iraqis have emigrated.[8] Many of the senior and most experienced faculty at the College of Nursing have left Iraq seeking a decent life in other countries. Not all of Iraq's neighbours welcome the fleeing Iraqis. Jordan has become the country of first choice for many nursing faculty, but those few who are allowed to stay there have experienced great difficulty finding employment. Even when individual nurses find positions, visas and other permits that would allow them to stay in a particular country on a permanent basis have been very difficult to obtain. Returning to Iraq is not always an option and we know of nursing faculty who have sought refuge in Libya, Oman and other nearby countries. A few have been able to settle in England or the United States. Still their lives have been disrupted, family and friends have been left behind and for professional nurses, the issues related to licensure and certification in other countries pose formidable barriers to work opportunities.

The departure of many of the senior faculty has obviously had a tremendous impact on the quality of the nursing programme at the University of Baghdad and on professional nursing in Iraq. A major strength of the college was the advanced educational level and expertise of the nursing faculty. Along with the loss of numerous faculty, the college has also suffered the loss of experienced administrators. This undoubtedly has led to leadership crises within the college. There are no longer adequate numbers of experienced administrators or well-prepared, senior faculty to teach the courses or to maintain the integrity of the curriculum. Funding for research and/ or technology is non-existent.

THE FUTURE OF NURSING

The easing of the sanctions as well as other political, social and economic changes has improved the quality of life for many Iraqis. Nevertheless, it is difficult to describe the devastation and destruction that the Gulf war and ensuing sanctions have had on the health care sector. Visits by patients to health centres, hospitalizations, diagnostic exams, including x-rays, lab tests, surgical procedures and prescriptions fell by half by the mid 1990s as there was literally nowhere to go for health care services or very little care available. In a country that once had an enviable programme for maternal and infant health services, at one time during the blockade only about one third of all women received prenatal care. Garfield[8] reported that there had been an increased demand for mental health services as the numbers of outpatient visits at mental health clinics and the number of hospital admissions for mental disorders have increased. The Oil for Food programme has improved living conditions for most Iraqis with the ensuing decrease in childhood malnutrition and the decreased numbers of communicable diseases, including gastrointestinal infections. Availability of medicines has improved; nevertheless, serious problems exist in access to education, food, employment and health care.

One can read between the lines about professional nursing. On a personal level, women have become increasing responsible for family income, often caring for extended family members as well as their own children. This increased responsibility has occurred in a terrible social situation including war and deprivation of basic requirements for existence. Nurses work in hospitals, clinics and health centres that were virtually destroyed during the bombing campaign.

Public employment (most nurses worked in the public sector) has drastically declined. The embargo has prohibited rebuilding the civilian intrastructure, including hospitals, but also extended to water purification plants, electrical supply, and pharmaceutical supplies. One can imagine that patients are sicker, more desperate, lacking clean water, decent food and medicine. Nursing care would be severely impacted as nurses struggled to provide anything other than the most fundamental measures of nursing care. One friend, a colleague living in Iraq, wrote to one of the authors: 'Living in Iraq is like living in a grave. I am waiting for the edges to slide in on me.'

In summary, the Gulf War and the economic sanctions have had devastating effects on women. Basic education, professional education and employment have all been effected. Deprofessionalization, declining public sector employment and rising unemployment have had serious effects on professional nursing. Women have had less flexibility in employment and their participation in the urban workforce has seriously declined. Similarly, the gender differential in education, nearly eliminated prior to 1990, has returned in basic education and grown in higher education. Socially, politically, and economically, sanctions have been associated with a marked decline in options for Iraqi women. As a women's profession, nursing has been extensively damaged; the leaders have gone, the numbers of nurses actually working in professional roles have decreased; nursing has become a menial professional. Nursing is not a professional career with a future in Iraq.

As Iraqi society struggles for survival, traditional views and ways of coping come to the forefront. The role of women becomes even more limited to marriage and family as educational opportunities become less available to women. The problems faced by professional nurses in Iraq—low status and a poor image of nursing, low pay, poor working conditions, lack of autonomy, and cultural constraints for women have all been confounded and worsened by the war and economic sanctions.

However, the situation is not totally bleak and without hope. Strong women and nursing leadership still exist in Iraq, albeit in different ways. This is the twenty-first century and there is beginning pressure on governments and countries across the world to address the cultural constraints that have traditionally oppressed women. Women throughout the world and in Iraq are pushing forward to make their lives and the lives of their family members better. We have recently learned that the College of Nursing at the University of Baghdad has established a collaborative doctoral programme with a university in Yemen. While we wonder about the quality of the programme, the academic preparation of the faculty and the level of funding for research, we cannot help but applaud the efforts of the faculty and students.

ACKNOWLEDGEMENTS

The authors are grateful for the help and support of our Iraqi friends and colleagues as well as faculty members at the University of Baghdad. We appreciate the assistance of Richard Garfield, RN, DrPH, Columbia University. We thank Khalid Al-Hitti, PhD, former Minister of Plenipotentiary and the former Ambassador of the Iraqi Mission to the United Nations, His Excellency, Nizar Hamdoon.

NOTES

1. N.H. Bryant, 'Progress and constraints of nursing and nursing education in Islamic societies,' in E.B. Gallagher and J. Subedi (eds.), *Global perspectives on health care*, pp. 45-72, Englewood Cliffs, NJ: Prentice Hall, 1995.
2. P. Abu Gharbich and W. Suliman, 'Changing the image of nursing in Jordan through effective role negotiation,' *International Nursing Review*, 39, 1992, pp. 149-52.
3. J.S. Boyle, 'Professional nursing in Iraq,' *IMAGE: Journal of Nursing Scholarship*, 21, 1989, pp. 168-171.
4. State Organization for Tourism, *IRAQ: A tourist guide*, Baghdad, Iraq: State Organization for Tourism, 1982.
5. *Curriculum 1962–1987*, Republic of Iraq, Ministry of Higher Education and Scientific Research, University of Baghdad, College of Nursing.
6. K. Salman, personal communication, December 2000.
7. T. Horowitz, *Baghdad without a map*, New York, NY: Dutton, 1991.
8. R. Garfield, personal communication, 10 November 2000.

9. J.S. Boyle and S.M. Bunting, 'Horsemen of the Apocalypse: Lessons from the Gulf War,' *Advances in Nursing Science*, 21, 1998, pp. 30-41.

10. J. Vickers, *Women and war*. Atlantic Highlands, NJ: Zed Books, 1993.

11. R. Garfield, 'The impact of economic embargoes on the health of women and children,' *Journal of American Medical Women's Association*, 52, 1997, pp. 181-184.

12. R. Garfield, S. Saidi and J. Lemmock, 'Medical care in Iraq after six years of sanctions,' *British Medical Journal*, 1997, pp. 315, 474.

14

Lebanon: An American Nurse Amidst Chaos, 1975–2002

The Story of the American University of Beirut Medical Centre during the Lebanese Civil War

Gladys Mouro

There once was a beautiful country on the Mediterranean. A country of Christians and Muslims living together and sharing a land of beauty and blessings.

Then came the war. Sixty thousand people died. Many lost their lives; others were left handicapped.

Lebanon, the peaceful country became a country of darkness and destruction. It became a country of people who suffered and cried for help.

- At the start of the civil war, the American University of Beirut (AUB) had 420 beds and was located 750 meters from the large hotels where the fiercest fighting took place. The American University of Beirut Medical Centre served during the civil strife as a referral centre for the whole of Lebanon. In addition, it acted as a field hospital because of its proximity to the area of struggle and the unavailability of other medical facilities in the region.
- It was my year to graduate, and I was so excited about wearing the cap and gown. But graduation was cancelled. I had joined AUB in 1973 to study nursing in Lebanon against my family's wishes. They were all in the States, but I fell in love with AUB the moment I stepped into it. I wanted to do my undergraduate studies there and return to the States to work, not knowing I would not do so for a very long time.
- The basic necessities of life slowly disappeared. Water was a rare commodity

- By February 1976 Beirut fell into total chaos.
- Students threatened faculty and administration.
- And on 17 February 1976, the Dean of Engineering and the Dean of Students were both assassinated by a student who was expelled for troubles he caused. He was caught and placed in prison for a few years but was released as he was well connected to a political party. Ironically, he returned to AUB to continue his studies and graduated before the war was over!
- For those who remained at the American University of Beirut, they had to cross-checkpoints when going home. It took them six hours walking that normally took ten minutes by car.
- I was a nursing student and a counselor at a girl's dormitory called Building No. 56.
- The first encounter of war at AUB was in May 1976. Two hundred and twenty casualties piled up in the ER. The dead were labeled as unknown I, II, III...
- On 8 June 1976, at 12 midnight, Building No. 56 was hit. Students had to move to a basement in another building with no facilities.
- On 18 June, the US Ambassador Francis Meloy was assassinated. The US State Department advised all Americans to leave. Convoys were arranged but I did not leave.
- Educational links with the outside world were cut. AUB was in the midst of a battlefield.
- Our Hospital became a military field hospital and all elective admissions were stopped.
- Physicians left, resident staff was reduced by 50 per cent and nursing by 30 per cent. Only eight of twenty-two surgeons remained and only two of our ten operating rooms functioned.
- Nurses and doctors worked long hours without breaks.
- From April 1975 to November 1976 the Emergency Unit received 8,326 casualties out of a total of 8,945 casualties in Lebanon and an additional 6,387 were killed during that period.
- Our admissions were limited only to patients with intracranial injuries, thoracic, cardiovascular, limb saving, and multiple injuries.
- In June 1976, I graduated but without a ceremony. My brother asked me to leave Lebanon. I did, but after some months in the States and many letters of encouragement from the Director of Nursing service in Beirut, I decided to return in 1977 as Head Nurse of a Ward Unit.

- From 1976 till 1981 the number of casualties and dead both in Lebanon and AUB rose to 148,724.

And the most difficult year of our lives was waiting for us in 1982.

- The Israeli invasion was the worst period during the entire war. Beirut once more was being destroyed and attacked severely.
- In 1981, I was promoted to a Nursing Supervisor.
- I was about to leave my patients to enter a world of management. This saddened me since I would drift away from bedside nursing.
- I learned to respond to emergencies, to stay calm, think, and act.
- I dealt with persistent shortages, repairing breakdowns in interpersonal relationships, replenishing supplies, and continuously arranging to cover staff shortage.
- There was an explosive conflict between East and West, Christians and Muslims, and I had to make sure not to take sides.
- When radio flashes reported the Israeli army invading South Lebanon a state of alert was declared. We were petrified.
- At the Hospital, a volunteer's office was established.
- Palestinians who lived in the camps in Beirut fled to our Hospital for safety, food, and sleep.
- The absentee rate for nursing staff rose to 70 per cent. Units closed, infection increased, open heart surgery stopped. And every time I closed a unit, there was an emotional strain.
- On 23 June 1982, the Israelis dropped leaflets from airplanes asking inhabitants of Beirut to leave. People began to leave and took whatever they could get hold of.
- We were all scared to death including myself. Staff came to my office requesting to go and join their loved ones. How could I tell them to stay?
- Casualties came to the ER burnt from the phosphorus bombs. Their flesh smelled and was on fire. The shouting, crying, and pain still exists in my ears and heart to this date.
- To ease the pain, we prepared a nursing show and called it 'Nursing Syndrome' with a part on the visit of the Joint Commission on Accreditation of Hospitals Organization (JCAHO) and how picky they are when they survey. There was also a scene about the war. It was in a way like a therapy for us. In spite of the sadness that existed we managed to enjoy some times of laughter. That was the

special thing about the Lebanese people. They were indeed survivors.

- At the hospital we had a special patient called Nisrine.
- Nisrine, was a favourite to us and to me particularly. She spent two years at our hospital treated for multiple injuries. She became our spoiled child and we all loved her.
- On 3 July, an Israeli blockade was enforced on West Beirut for ninety days. There were no fruits, vegetables, or other essentials. People waited in line for bread and had difficulty getting water.
- At the hospital, we ate rice and beans and beans and rice seven days a week waiting for our turn to eat due to the long queue in the dining room.

* * *

- There was no gas or oil for the power plant. The consumption was cut from 20,000 liters/day to 7,000. Oxygen was reduced as well. The Inhalation and Anesthesia Department had to decide which patients needed oxygen the most and give it to them.
- Air Raids began and we moved patients with their equipment and supplies to a safer place in the basement.
- We always had to be careful not to give medications to the wrong patients. It was a game of hide and seek to find the patients especially when the electricity went off.
- Medical staff continued to leave and we pleaded with them to stay. We needed them badly but who could keep them from leaving the country?
- We had ten operating rooms.
- The shortage of staff increased.
- Those who remained worked twenty-four hours a day.
- One of our surgeons operated on thirteen craniotomies in one day.
- Infections increased and physicians wore dresses because we ran out of scrub suits.
- Militia forced themselves into the OR thinking they had the right to be near their people. They would not listen.
- And the shortage of oxygen continued to horrify us.
- There was no air-conditioning, and the heat of the summer was terrible.
- Elective surgery stopped and people preferred not to be treated unless it was an emergency situation. The AUB emergency unit

received the majority of casualties in the country. From 1976–1991 the AUB treated 197,716 patients, which was 69 per cent of the total treated in Lebanon.

- Casualties rushed in hundreds at one time and were transported on top of the cars and not in them. Stretchers were always ready for transport outside the EU, but without mattresses because the militia would steal them.
- Armed militia guarded the doors of the EU.
- Explosions occurred in the emergency unit.
- There were attacks on staff by militia.
- Triaging was very important but unfortunately armed men interfered with the triage process.
- We set up trolleys to be prepared at all times with a contingency plan. A disaster team was on call. Our staff were well trained and they did an excellent job when mass casualties arrived.
- The militia improvised emergency sirens by firing their high powered rifles when rushing to the EU.
- In the tense work of sorting patients, physicians and nurses were attacked by militia while they were carrying on their duties.
- The emergency unit had three major surgery rooms and five cubicles. When mass casualties came in, complete chaos prevailed for 5-10 minutes. Patients and their families screamed. In twenty minutes all patients would be triaged and taken care of. I was always there the minute I knew of casualties coming.
- Usually, valuables of patients were taken from dead bodies by the Supervisor only and placed in a safe. Because there were no banks open, people kept huge amounts of money in their pockets and there was always a bystander waiting around to steal from the pockets of someone arriving at the EU.
- We had to serve both sides of the militia and many times we were caught in the middle.
- The militia had their own medical representative and press. However, they interfered constantly with our duties.
- Militia came with hand grenades in their pockets and often by mistake they would explode accidentally and hurt staff in the process.
- We closed the EU for a few hours once when an armed man hit the doctor who was caring for his friend because he thought he was not doing the right thing.

- I returned to the United States in 1983 to the University of Penn to complete my masters degree but could not attend the graduation ceremony. Again I did not get the chance to wear my cap and gown.
- In 1983 I was offered the position of Director of Nursing. Being an American was not popular at that time and being young also did not help, but I was still determined to succeed.
- Fortunately or unfortunately, I did not know that another decade of war was waiting for me.
- Shells continued to hit the AUB campus, and as for me, being an American did not help.
- Stray bullets entered patients' rooms. Nurses were injured while distributing medications. One day a big shrapnel went through the patient's room from his bathroom down to the lab and exploded there causing a lot of damage and injuring some staff.
- Doctors and staff continued to leave.
- Our hospital was sinking, with no leadership, no money, no staff, and no faculty. It fell under the control of one political faction after another.
- Families of patients threatened staff, and if patients asked for sedation and did not get it, they threatened them with guns that were kept hidden under their pillows.
- Families cooked food in bedpans.
- Housekeeping deteriorated and as a result infection continued to increase.
- On 23 May 1985, a dedicated employee called Hajji Omar, who was responsible for transportation, was killed by a sniper. He was one of these rare individuals who in the midst of the chaos of war would find supplies and get people safely to their destination and who performed these tasks with unfailing optimism, courage, and energy.
- The kidnappings of Americans started and my nightmares began as well. David Jacobson, Hospital Director, Peter Kilburn, Librarian, Tom Slade, Assistant VP, and finally Joe Ciccipio, who was my very close friend, were all taken and kept for years as hostages.
- Foreigners left and the fighting continued but AUB did not close. Had we quit, it would have meant a tremendous loss to the country in both medicine and education.
- If I had to choose the worse emotion, it was fear. It often leaves wounds too deep to heal.

- I was sinking into a depression, and I was afraid that I would be the next victim.
- The threats began and the pressure increased to employ unqualified people. Threats were continuously placed under my office door, and finally the car bomb threat. Someone had placed dynamite under my car. I was lucky they caught it in time. They did not want Americans around. I had been there too long and to them I had no place in Lebanon.
- I became more and more depressed but I was determined to survive and stay.
- My friends and support system continued to leave one by one.
- I was always afraid to start my car. I bought a gun and learned how to use it. My anxiety increased and nightmares haunted me. I was illegally in Lebanon for the Lebanese government and the US government.
- Then, it was my turn to receive a threat of kidnapping. The AUB President called from the US insisting I leave the country immediately or else I would be out of a job. Reluctantly, I left but my soul was at AUB. After four months, I was allowed to return, but with a bodyguard. The Dean of Medicine was well connected and took responsibility for my return. The hospital was in need of leadership, and Nursing needed it more than ever.
- Children suffered terribly. They drew pictures of guns, tanks and explosions, and incidents of psychosomatic ailments among children increased. They lost their homes and didn't know where to go. Some families moved to the hospital and started a home near the emergency unit. They cooked, washed their clothes using the facilities of the emergency and slept at night to the noises of casualties rushing in.
- As for adults, anxiety, depression, hysterical behavior and exaggerated emotional expressions increased. People no longer smiled. If violence happened only two blocks away, it went unnoticed.
- Water everywhere but not a drop to drink. We had to be creative. The water supply in our apartment was one hour/day. We connected a hose from the Kidney unit to provide soft water for babies' formula. Whisky was cheaper to drink.
- Fuel and oxygen continued to dwindle; we had to cook the patients' food using the steam supply from our own generators, which left us with hardly enough steam to sterilize equipment. Our faith in the

ability of AUB against all hardships continued. It stood as an enduring symbol of hope.

- Motivation was down and at work it was tough to keep people going. How could you motivate people and expect them to be loyal when their lives were constantly in danger and at risk?
- Imposing discipline, law and order was almost impossible.
- And personally, I refused to accept that we would be left behind while the whole world was advancing. I kept reading journals, books to keep up to date. I was afraid I would wake up one day after the war was over, and I would be far behind.
- My morale was going down slowly but surely. Suicide was on my mind. There were times when I hated myself for remaining, and yet I did not want to leave.
- I was emotionally on a roller coaster, out of control, not being able to predict my feelings from day to day. My support system was no longer there.
- On 8 November 1991, College Hall was hit. It was the last blow to AUB, and it was devastating. It took the next eight years to collect enough funds to rebuild College Hall. Students, staff, faculty, governments, friends of AUB all contributed to rebuild College Hall. And fortunately something very nice happened, Ceccipio, my good friend who had been a hostage, was released and the Hospital and AUB were on the road to recovery. It looked as if the war was over.

THE AFTERMATH OF WAR

- The economy was the key issue in 1992. The government failed to control inflation. The rich got richer and the poor got poorer.
- The Israelis had attacked again in the South in 1992. The Israeli attack forced 300,000 people to leave the South and come to Beirut.
- By 1993, the civil war in Lebanon was almost over. On 7 May 1992, I was awarded Lebanon's silver Order of Health for my services during the war, in addition to an award from the health sectors of the Arab Countries. I was surprised and gratified to have been recognized by the Lebanese Government. It was a day to remember. I only wish my family were there.
- The war was over but the aftermath of a war was just beginning. Resistance to change, drugs, loss of values, all prevailed.

- As for me, my mother still wanted me to return to the States. Why did I stay and still do? It was hard to make her understand what I myself did not understand. Is it the satisfaction of giving and knowing that by giving, I might make a difference? Is it because I gave so much and did not want to see my efforts go down the drain?
- In January 1998, a new President, Dr John Waterbury, who still remains, was appointed. For the first time in twelve years he assumed his responsibilities as the first resident president of AUB. During his first week, a car explosion occurred on campus. It was the first serious attack on AUB since the 1991 bombing of College Hall. Was it intended to scare Americans away, including Dr Waterbury? It did not, because it sent out a signal that AUB was determined to maintain stability and continue its mission against all odds. It was only those of us who remained in Lebanon throughout the entire war who could fully appreciate the significance of Dr Waterbury's decision to live on the AUB campus.
- As for the young generation, drugs became an escape mechanism. Post traumatic stress disorder was apparent in Lebanon after the war. Depression invaded the mental health of Lebanese men and women. The consequences of these disorders were and still are devastating on the individual, the family and on society at large.

CHALLENGE OF CHANGE

And now, after twenty-four years in Lebanon, from 1976–2000, I find myself facing a different struggle. A fight to change attitudes at the hospital. Promoting standards, improving quality of care, and regaining the credibility of AUB is a long and difficult road to embark upon.

It is so hard after so many disruptive years to rebuild an atmosphere of credibility and trust among patients, visitors, and medical staff. It is true that we kept the hospital surviving and saved so many lives, but at a high price. We were way behind in technology, health care advancements, and our last JCAHO survey was in 1982. We had so much to work on. When people in other countries were going on with their lives and keeping up with the new world of technology, we were figuring out how to survive and sustain our institution.

In the rest of the world there were changes going on in nursing that I kept up to date with through literature reviews. I wanted to compensate for our limited resources so I read every journal of management and nursing I could obtain. I listened to all the audiotapes of conferences to keep up with what was going on. I wanted to learn from the mistakes that happened in hospitals in the US and not make the same ones at AUB. I was more determined than ever.

This was a hospital that was comparable to the most prestigious medical centres in the world prior to the war and was suddenly faced with twenty years of merely meeting the basic needs for institutional survival. Nursing services had a critical but unsung importance in keeping the hospital alive. It was indeed a distinguished legacy. The health care system both in the US and the world has evolved tremendously, especially in nursing, with new methods and approaches to patient care. Computers have taken over. As the US stopped recruiting our nurses, we could breathe again. For the first time, we tried recruiting nurses from French speaking university graduates of nursing. It was not easy to approach a culture that disliked the American system. However, with a lot of effort and creativity we have been able to hire forty nurses from the East side. Today, the psychological dividing line between East and West has almost disappeared among our hospital staff.

Our Nursing Department had to be completely rebuilt. The staff, like the children of war still felt insecure. Many resented the influx of Lebanese academicians, doctors and others, returning to their country with new ideas. They feared being replaced.

In February of 1998, I was determined to set out a re-engineering process that would bring back our US accreditation. I reviewed the literature extensively, the staffing patterns, classification tools, and the different nursing approaches followed for patient care. It was like waking up from a Rip Van Winkle Sleep. I set out for a new dream.

The numbers of acute medical conditions in the hospital increased after the economy worsened once more. People could not afford to be treated. As a result, we received the most critical cases in the country. In the past, we followed the functional nursing approach due to the limited number of nurses. With planning, teamwork, and involvement of all, I successfully introduced a patient-centered care approach. The difficult part was to convince the staff, the administration, and the physicians of the need to change. Nurses were accustomed to shortcuts, shortages, and did not want to hear of any change. Moreover, those who had spent the majority of their professional life in a war situation were burnt out, tired, and could not cope with a change process.

Ironically, the new generation of nurses who did not experience this horrible war, were not interested in the challenge and could care less. The resources were few, nurses with expertise to assist in such a process were lacking both in nursing administration and the clinical areas. The administration was concerned with budget restrictions.

The nurses available were inexperienced. More than 75 per cent had less than two years of experience. I involved the nursing managers and empowered them with the decision making process. I knew if I could satisfy our patients and meet their needs, they would come back to our hospital. As a result, the image of nursing would significantly improve, an issue we have been working on for so many years. I introduced a new patient classification system, conducted time motion studies, introduced patient education, JCAHO standards, and based all interventions on outcome measurements. I worked closely with the staff and the nursing leaders. Fortunately, they trusted and believed in me. To do all this required a very strong passion and drive to make the change and achieve excellence.

I believed in the strength of every single staff member and did not give up on anyone. I tried to make them believe in themselves and in our ability to reach that vision. I believe that the University of Pennsylvania and the faculty who taught me, especially my adviser Dr Anne Keanne, helped me to soldier through these tough situations.

I missed out on continuing my education and joining a group of academicians in a profession I love so much. When I am asked why I stayed it is hard to answer because all I know is that I wanted to do what I did in spite of all the miseries I went through. I still am in pain and every time I think about those years, or talk about them, I want to cry. But, I am grateful to God that I had the opportunity to make a difference and still can. To survive a war of twenty-five years and start again and to re-build an institution, you must have courage, determination, a strong commitment, love, passion and a great deal of belief in the vision you want to achieve.

I am not sure I made the wisest decision by sacrificing the best years of my life. The future will tell me. I can only say that I have been privileged to serve the people of Lebanon, the AUB and as an American I am proud to follow the values and principles of the country and family in which I was brought up.

15

Nursing Education in Afghanistan: Yesterday and Today

Paula Herberg

Introduction

The education of young women as nurses in Afghanistan began in the 1930s and reached a peak in the mid to late 1970s before the advent of civil war and conflict, which has ravaged the country for the past twenty-three years. Today the Afghan Ministry of Public Health (MOPH) is in the process of 'reconstructing' the health care system, including the education of nurses, midwives, and allied health personnel. This chapter will explore the system of nursing education in place during the 1970s and the current plans for the future. It will try to shed some light on the transition period (1978-2001) in which the established educational system was abolished and new systems were put in place. Much of the information presented is based on the author's experiences while in Afghanistan from 1974 to 1976, 1978 through October 1979, and more recently from August to November 2002.

From 1932 to 1979: A Broad Overview of Nursing in Afghanistan

It was accepted in Afghan society that women were needed to care for the sick. However, the status of these women was low and few families envisioned their daughters becoming nurses. Therefore, young women chose nursing as a career for primarily financial reasons. A government job in nursing guaranteed a steady income. In addition the government provided a stipend for students while in nursing school. These were strong incentives for parents who were willing to let their daughters pursue a 'career' in any setting outside the home. In addition, nursing education did not require a 12th grade education and thus appealed to girls who did not complete high school. Finally, nursing skills were a salable commodity that could be used to supplement a government salary.

There were male nurses in Afghanistan. In fact they outnumbered the female nurses. In 1971, there were 280 male nurses and 141 females (Furnia, 1978). Male nurses were accepted by the public and often treated as medical doctors in the rural areas. It was not uncommon for villagers to address any male nurse wearing a lab coat as *daktar-sahib*. Male nurses were able to supplement their meager civil salary by practicing in such capacity or by offering their services as 'injectors/vaccinators.' This source of cash income helped to draw men into the nursing profession. Also, men often saw nursing as a stepping stone to a medical career. The MOPH and Ministry of Education (MOE) supported this through a policy of sponsoring the top male nursing school graduate for medical studies at Kabul Medical Institute of the University.

The first school of nursing in Afghanistan was connected to Kabul Hospital and began in 1932 with a class of sixty-nine students (Furnia, 1978). From the 1930s to the late 1960s, schools of nursing mushroomed throughout the country. Most were run by private organizations and connected to hospitals in which students were used for service. There were no standards to guide education or practice. In a 1970 study of nurses reported by Furnia, there were eight different categories of nurse listed. At that time a total of 694 'nurses' practiced in Afghanistan.

The MOPH slowly began to close the private schools of nursing and to set some standards of education. A Nursing Unit in the Curative Medicine Department of the MOPH was established in the late 1960s and by 1974, all the schools of nursing in Afghanistan were located in Kabul except for one in Nangarhar province (in Jalalabad). In 1976, a standardized curriculum was introduced.

In general, the responsibility for nursing in Afghanistan was given to the Nursing Unit. The unit was headed by a Director General and Directors of Nursing Education, Nursing Service, and Community Health Nursing. Under its control were all nurses working in MOPH hospitals, clinics, and schools of nursing (SON). The Nursing Unit was responsible for all continuing education in the country as well as standardizing the nursing school curricula. While this organizational structure helped to decrease the confusion of nursing categories, it did not solve the problem totally. The MOE also had authority over some nurses and nursing schools through the Kabul University Institute of Medicine and its affiliated hospital and clinics. The military had direct control over all nurses working in military hospitals.

The Nursing Unit, as a political entity, had several changes of administration during the 1970s. Due to the unstable nature of Afghan politics, many government leaders had short tours of office and nursing was no exception. Progress was difficult when leadership changed hands repeatedly but the women who held the position of Director General were all well educated (in the USA and England) and had real concern for and allegiance to nursing. Working within the male dominated world of the MOPH and medicine in general, these women made remarkable accomplishments in standardizing nursing education and contributing to community oriented nursing practice.

During the 1960s and 1970s, nursing had the official guidance of the World Health Organization through the assignment of a Nursing Advisor to the nursing schools and later to the Nursing Unit. Nursing also had the help and cooperation of international nurses who were in the community at any given time. This included British, French, Indian, Scandinavian, German and North American nurses from a variety of NGOs including USAID, CARE, Peace Corps and its international equivalents, and various missionary groups, the largest of which was the International Afghan Mission (IAM).

There were no nursing professional organizations or regulatory bodies in Afghanistan. A Board of Nursing was discussed in the early 1970s but not created. Afghans who graduated from an approved school of nursing were able to practice. There was no licensure exam or registration system, although new graduates were entered into the 'register' maintained in the Nursing Unit.

In order to recruit students for the nursing schools, the government made periodic trips into the provinces to visit local high schools and promote nursing. Village families weighed the benefits of increased family income, advanced education, and a working family member to the perils of sending a daughter to live in Kabul. If traditional values about women and work did not keep families from agreeing to nursing school, then the reputation and prospect of life in Kabul often did. The MOPH worked to assure parents that hostels were strictly monitored, secure, and maintained proper standards of decorum. In some cases, parents were known to visit the schools first to satisfy themselves that their daughters would be well chaperoned and cared for. Thus, in spite of the difficulties, these recruitment trips were often successful.

The entire situation was different for village boys. Should they decide to enter nursing school, they could usually find cheap lodging in the city. They were given much more independence than their sisters and were able to adjust to Kabul life more quickly. That is not to say the boys did not encounter difficulties or become homesick but that they had more social supports and coping mechanisms available to them.

NURSING EDUCATION IN THE 1970S

By 1970, all the nursing schools, except one, were located in Kabul. There were three types of training programmes: 1) professional nurse-midwives; 2) professional nurses: male and female; and 3) auxiliary nurse midwives (ANMs). Details about each school are shown in Table 1. Zaishgah School of Nursing (in Kabul) and Nangarhar School of Nursing (in Jalalabad) were the two professional nurse-midwifery programs available for women only. The two schools of professional nursing, both in Kabul, were Aliabad School of Male Nursing and Mastoorat School of Female Nursing. The ANM School was also in Kabul. Aliabad and Mastoorat were under the direction of the Ministry of Education. For many years, a French team of nurse educators worked at Mastoorat. The military recruited graduates from all the nursing schools but favoured Zaishgah.

The ANM Programme. The role of the auxiliary nurse midwife (ANM) was developed as part of a broader programme to provide basic heath care to rural families (Russell & Richter, 1981). ANMs functioned at the village level in basic health centres as female health workers for women and children. The one and a half year ANM training curriculum was conducted at the ANM School, in a new building provided by USAID funds and opened in 1971. Young women were recruited from the villages and returned home after training in order to live with their families and work in MCH clinics and/or basic health centres nearby.

The training programme emphasized preventive care such as family planning, nutrition, antenatal and postpartum care; basic midwifery and care of the newborn; infant-child growth monitoring and preventive

Table 1

Status of Nursing Schools in Afghanistan, March 1975

Name of School	Total student body	Number of Faculty including Director	Teacher/ Student Ratio	Teaching Experience of Faculty					Faculty Language Ability			Number of External Lectures[2]	Nursing Service Personnel (Teaching)
				< yrs	1-5 yrs	6-10 yrs	11-15 yrs	16+	Dari	Pashto	Eng French		
Aliabad School of Male Nursing	105	8	1:13	-	2	2	1	2	8	4	3	14	1
Mastoorat School of Female Nursing	71	8 + 3 French Nurse Educators	1:9	1	1	2	4	-	7	-	3	20	-
Zaishgah School of Nurse Midwifery	262	17	1:15	3	12	2	-	-	17	2	3	4	-
Nangarhar School of Nurse Midwifery	28	3	1:9	1	2	-	-	-	3	-	1	6	2
Auxiliary Nurse Midwives School	55	8 + 2 Peace Corps Nurse Teachers and 2 USAID/UCSC Nurse Educators	1:6	-	8	1			9	3	2	2	-
TOTALS:	521	39 Local		5	25	7	5	2			12	46	3

Adapted from Heber, 1975.

care; and health education. Students were also taught to do high risk assessments and make appropriate referrals. From 1974 to 1979, the ANM programme was assisted by the Division of International Programs of the University of California Extension at Santa Cruz, which provided two nurse midwife advisers to work on curricular, administrative and clinical training issues with the local faculty. The University was supported by a USAID contract. As part of the programme, ANM faculty were sent to UC Santa Cruz for one academic year to study in the family nurse practitioner programme. This training was tailored to their needs as nurse midwifery educators in a developing country. By early 1979, thirty-one teachers had participated in this training (Russell & Richter, 1981).

Schools of Nursing. The controlling authority appointed Nursing Directors for each school. The Ministry of Education schools were administered by the Faculty of Medicine, University of Kabul. Zaishgah SON was controlled by the President of the Zaishgah women's institutions: two hospitals, a community MCH clinic and the SON. It was the most prestigious school in the country. The President of Curative Medicine, MOPH, controlled the other SONs. All nursing directors had their appointments confirmed by the Prime Minister (Heber, 1975).

Application forms were used in all the SONs. At Aliabad School of Male Nursing, there were often more than 300 applicants for thirty spaces in the first year class. A competitive concourse examination was set by the Ministry of Education and announced in the press. Questions covered physics, chemistry, algebra and biology. The top applicants were selected according to a ranking system set by the Nursing Director and the teaching faculty. At Mastoorat School of Female Nursing the same procedure was followed if more than thirty applications were received. In practice, recruitment for Mastoorat was difficult and all seats were rarely filled. At Zaishgah, a Radio Afghanistan announcement was used to request letters of application from students. The nursing director, her assistant and five senior faculty made the final selection of students. Thirty to thirty-five students were admitted each year.

The SON in Jalalabad used recruitment visits to the neighbouring provinces of Laghman and Kunar to distribute application forms. Visits were made to local schools to talk to the 9th and 11th grade students and parental contacts were made to encourage them to visit the school in Jalalabad. Thirty students were typically admitted each year. The

ANM school used a similar recruitment campaign in the provinces to find suitable candidates. Selection of students was finalized by the Director of Nursing Education in the Nursing Unit according to a policy of geographic distribution and the needs of basic health units for ANMs (Heber, 1975).

Selection criteria differed according to the level of nursing education. Professional nursing candidates were required to complete the 9th grade; ANMs, at least the 6th grade. Stamped school 'certificates of completion' were required as proof at all nursing schools. At Mastoorat, girls had to be between the ages of 16 and 22 and be single. If they married once in school they were allowed to continue. At Zaishgah, girls had to be at least 16 years old to enter. Married students were allowed, but women who were pregnant and due to deliver within a school term were discouraged from applying. In reality, pregnant students were always present at the girls' schools. The minimum age for entry at the ANM school was 16, but often girls as young as 12 or 13 were admitted. ANM applicants were allowed to be married. There were no age requirements at Aliabad but candidates were usually between the ages of 16 and 20. All schools required character reports from head teachers at the applicant's secondary school (primary school for ANM students). A medical examination and inoculations were given to all successful candidates once they began school.

All students, regardless of programme, were issued two uniforms at the beginning of each school year. These uniforms were returned annually for re-issue. Each student received a food allowance in the form of free meals or cash/tickets. The University schools issued a stipend of 200 Afs ($4.00 USD) per month for the first year; 250 Afs/month in year two and 300 Afs/month in year three. MOPH professional school students received 150, 200, and 250 Afs/month for each respective year. Students in the ANM programme were promised a stipend of 100 Afs/month but were never paid. All the schools had difficulty issuing the stipends on a regular basis, but some cash was distributed at fairly regular intervals.

University students received thirty days of summer vacation and two months plus twenty days of winter vacation. Zaishgah students received fifteen days in the summer and thirty days in winter. Nangarhar had a two month summer holiday and the ANM school gave thirty days of vacation annually: fifteen days in summer; fifteen in winter. In practice the schools usually had longer winter breaks to conserve fuel and heating expenses.

In the professional schools, the Nursing Director in consultation with her faculty selected new teachers. The general rule was to take the top two or three graduates from the last examination period and offer them teaching positions if available. Since teachers did not have previous teaching experience or specialized education, they were assigned a light teaching load when they began. They were often teamed with a master teacher who had at least three years' experience. New teachers routinely sat and observed in the classroom for one semester before beginning to teach. SON teachers, not service personnel, supervised all clinical experiences. Teachers were allowed to specialize by expressing an interest in one area of nursing and being assigned to that area for clinical and classroom teaching. Over the years, teachers became experts in their field. There was very little attrition of teachers at the schools. All schools held routine meetings of the faculty to discuss student issues, curriculum implementation, and teacher promotions.

All nursing students attended classes, skills lab practice and clinical learning rotations. Students worked day and night shifts during their education and often came to class at 8 a.m. after working all night. Clinical placements included hospitals, outpatient clinics, MCH clinics, health centres, and specialized facilities such as clinical labs. All students were expected to receive the same amount of clinical experience but this did not always happen. Teachers were familiar with rotation plans, skills sheets, anecdotal notes and evaluation forms as part of the clinical assessment of students. Although most teachers were organized, they had little understanding of true clinical supervision of students or clinical teaching methods. Once students had been assigned to a patient care area, they were not supervised closely. On occasion, nursing service personnel took advantage of this to ask students to wash windows, mop floors, and carry out other household chores. But students were also allowed to be present during rounds and were sometimes questioned by the medical personnel in terms of their nursing knowledge.

Teaching in the classroom was conducted according to the traditional methods of the country: primarily through dictation, memorization and recitation of lessons. Thus the ebb and flow of the classroom was two-day cycles of dictation/recitation in endless repetition. Teachers who had command of English or French were able to use the library books available to them. Often huge passages were copied from texts then translated into Dari and dictated to students. Over the course of several years, English words began to take on a foreign flavor and were often incomprehensible as English. Efforts to correct the spelling or pronunciation of such terms were usually futile. Very few Dari/Farsi resources existed for teachers. Each teacher developed his or her course notes over time from library and other resources such as doctor's lectures, common experience, and the shared wisdom of other nurses. Those notes soon took on the form of short books. Gradually those books became the standard text for classes. New teachers copied the notes into their own books. And so the system was perpetuated. There was no quality control over content and little to no updating of materials.

The classroom is the central core of the Afghan educational system. Discipline is harsh and stylized. Students stand when the teacher enters the room. A tardy student stops at the door, says '*ejazas*'(with your permission), and waits to be recognized by the teacher, which might take up to ten minutes. When a student is called on to speak, she must leave her seat and walk to the front of the class. Posture and bearing are expected to be formal when addressing one's classmates. There is no talking, laughing, or playfulness allowed in the classroom (although some whispering and note passing does occur). Should the Director happen to pass by, all the students spring to attention. Teachers, who minutes before have been joking with their colleagues, become studies of sternness and decorum in front of their students. They do not smile. They stand erect and are quick to tell students to be quiet; they are generally hard taskmasters.

A student who is reciting a lesson is expected to remember the placement of every comma and to state every 'a, an and the' correctly while speaking quickly and assuredly. Students have exceptionally good memories and speaking skills. So do teachers. When teachers are not actually dictating, they give lessons from memory. No notes are used when speaking to the class. I have seen one hour lectures given without a break and with no use of prepared notes.

All SONs had a skills lab where students could practice procedures. Only at Zaishgah did the lab resemble a hospital environment in any way. All supplies and equipment were the responsibility of one person, the storekeeper or *tawildar*. Should anything get lost or broken, the *tawildar* had to pay. Therefore supplies and equipment were routinely inventoried and kept behind locked cupboards. Rarely were supplies used freely. Often, teachers who needed equipment could not find the *tawildar*, so were forced to change their plans. Skills labs were used most often to practice bedmaking, vital signs, dressings, isolation techniques, and preparation of injections.

Afghan nursing students were kept very busy. Before the standardized curriculum was implemented in 1976, it was not uncommon for students to study eighteen subjects in one semester. All students were required to study Dari, Pashtu, Islamic Studies and English or French. The curriculum included chemistry, math, biology, anatomy and physiology, pharmacology, medical terminology, growth and development, psychology, sociology, nutrition, microbiology and all the traditional nursing subjects from fundamentals to critical care.

All the professional nursing school programmes were three years in length. The professional curriculum focused on curative medicine. Graduates were expected to work in hospitals and staff polyclinics. Only a few worked in health centres. The first year of the curriculum was spent in the classroom and skills lab with minimal clinical experience. The second and third years were usually divided 50 per cent in class and 50 per cent in clinical practice. At Zaishgah students spent a 4th year in midwifery. Classes were in session from Sunday to Thursday at noon. The 'weekend' was Thursday afternoon and Friday. Girls in residential schools were not allowed to leave the school grounds on weekends without an escort.

All students were required to pass a final examination to progress to the next semester. Although in-class tests were used, only the final exam was official. Final examinations were written. The security system in effect at exam time was rigidly enforced. The rules and procedures for the preparation of exams, conduct of exams and grading of exams were explicitly stated. There were always those who managed to subvert the rules, but they had to be very familiar with the system or in a position of high authority to do so. The responsibility for typing and security of the test items was given to the Nursing Unit.

Except at Mastoorat, the written exam used a combination of essay and objective type questions. At Mastoorat students were given five essay questions for each subject and chose one per subject to answer. All the schools, except Aliabad required a practical examination as well. If a student failed one or two subjects of the final exam, a re-sit exam was allowed one week later. If more than two subjects were failed, the student was required to repeat the semester. The third time the same subject was failed, the student was expelled from school.

Likewise, if a student failed more than four subjects in one exam, training was discontinued.

The procedures for the practical examinations were just as stringent. All procedures were written on pieces of paper and placed in a bowl. Students selected one procedure and demonstrated complete mastery of the skills involved. That included setting up supplies, technique, understanding of the procedure, and final clean up. The teacher of the subject and one external nurse from a local hospital graded each student.

Although all nursing students were generally serious about their studies, there were differences between the male and female students. The difference was most apparent in the clinical area. Female students were usually willing to try most procedures and to give bedside care. The male students tended to perform only the most technical of skills and rarely showed enthusiasm for routine nursing procedures. Neither group of students were required to assist patients with bedpans and urinals (the work of the *nanas* and *bachas*—housekeeping/nursing aids), but only female students seemed willing to do so when the need arose.

Discipline tended to be higher among the female students as observed in the classrooms. For example, when I visited Zaishgah the students were rarely aware of my presence after a few smiles and giggles. This was due to the nature of the classroom and the authoritarian rule of the environment by the teacher. By contrast, when I visited Aliabad, I found that the teacher, a male, was able to exert little to no control over the students. Talking, staring, turning around to look at me instead of the teacher, and not standing when called on to answer questions were common. Although the teacher attempted to maintain discipline, the boys ignored him. This was often mentioned as a problem at Aliabad where physical violence against teachers was not unheard of.

All Afghan students looked very professional while in the clinical area. Students took pride in their appearance. Student uniforms at Zaishgah were blue and white checked dresses with a white bib. ANM students wore pink and white uniforms. The Aliabad students wore all white shirts and pants of western style. Students at Mastoorat wore a blue shirtdress. All female students wore caps. Female nursing instructors wore white uniforms except at Zaishgah where they wore blue. Male instructors usually wore a lab coat. All the teachers at the ANM school, Mastoorat and Zaishgah were women. Of the five

Aliabad teachers, one was a woman. The directors of all the schools were women.

Generally then, nursing schools were places of serious study in Afghanistan. Students were expected to master a great deal of content in short periods of time. They put in long hours of study and clinical work. Many had family obligations to fulfill while in school. After graduation, most found work and continued in the nursing profession.

In 1976, a new level of nursing education was created: the Post Basic School of Nursing. With the help of CARE, WHO and IAM nurse educators (including the author), the Nursing Unit was able to plan and obtain approval for a school for graduate nurses to further their education. The school was designed to prepare nurse teachers, administrators, and clinicians who could help upgrade nursing from within. The school opened in 1978. The first class was devoted entirely to teacher training and twenty-six students were admitted. A faculty of eight Afghan nurses was recruited from the existing schools and four international nurse educators worked in counterpart with them. The program of studies was two years in length and twenty-four students were due to graduate in 1979.

THE LOST YEARS

By the beginning of 1979, it was obvious that the routine existence of most Afghans had come to an end. Due to increasing Soviet influence, tensions were high throughout Kabul. Forced patriotic marches and demonstrations disrupted normal classroom activities. The noise of helicopter gunships flying overhead interrupted the best efforts of teachers to keep their students' attention. All teachers were aware that there were political 'spies' in place at the schools and that their behavior was being monitored. Interactions with foreigners became impossible if not dangerous. Families were being disrupted by nocturnal visits in which, at best their sleep was disturbed, and at worst, family members were taken away never to be seen again. Fighting broke out in the city; bombing of buildings became commonplace; tanks appeared on the streets.

At this time I was working at the Post Basic School of Nursing. By June 1979, it was clear that we could not continue our programmes there. I left Kabul in October 1979 when the CARE team was flown to New Delhi, India. I left behind many friends and colleagues and shattered hopes for the burgeoning nursing profession. I watched while the wealthier and educated health/medical professionals I knew made plans to leave the country. I understood that many of my nursing colleagues would not be able to leave and faced the horrors of war. I assumed our new Post Basic School of Nursing would close its doors, but had no way of knowing what would happen.[1]

In fact, it is hard to put together a coherent picture of what transpired during the years from 1979 when the Soviets invaded Afghanistan to the time when the Taliban took over control of the country in the 1990s. I have been told that all the schools of nursing I knew were closed by 1981. Soviet systems of education were initiated throughout the country and basic nursing and midwifery education was transferred to the Intermediate Medical Education Institutes (IMEI) established in the mid-1960s to train mid level public health workers for underserved and underdeveloped areas. The ANM programme was not restarted. The Nursing Unit in the MOPH was closed.

The Soviet system remained in place during the years of war and internal conflict until the Taliban seized control. A new curriculum for nurses was established and given to the IMEIs in Kabul and at other regional sites throughout the country. Male nursing students continued to be trained. Reports are conflicting as to whether female students continued to study nursing during the Taliban years. It appears that nursing schools in Kandahar and Herat were operational. Certainly there were pockets of training going on throughout the country that were considered 'underground' efforts to provide women health care workers. In effect, nursing education went full circle again as various private NGOs proliferated different cadres of 'nurses' with little to no standardization of training or outcomes.

2002: DOORWAY TO THE FUTURE

In December 2001, the Interim Afghan Authority was formed to begin the work of reconstructing the Afghan civil sector. A Minister of Health, Dr Suhaila Seddiq was appointed and given the charge of revitalizing the MOPH and its regional centres in Kandahar, Jalalabad, Faizabad, Mazar-e-Sharif, Herat, Ghazni, and Kunduz. Following twenty-three years of conflict, the country's health human resources were severely depleted due to the loss of qualified health professionals (both migration and lack of proper educational preparation in the country). The MOPH, in collaboration with WHO and other international agencies, has begun the task of reorganization and identification of policies and procedures. Eighty per cent of the MOPH resources come from aid agencies, the UN and NGOs. Sixty-six international and local NGOs are currently supporting the health sector in Afghanistan. All civil service salaries are being paid through a UN trust fund (MOPH National Health Sector Planning Workshop, 16-19 March 2002). The salary is set at $5.00/month plus food allowance. The range of monthly payments is from $35.00 to $50.00 USD (Dr Malang, HRD/MOPH, 2002).

A final draft of a National Health Policy (February 2002) has been approved and a Health Services Package (May 2002) plan prepared. An MOPH organogram was approved at the beginning of the year (WHO, *Afghanistan Bulletin* February 2002). The new organizational structure, unfortunately, does not recreate a nursing unit in the MOPH or even make clear who will be responsible for monitoring nurses and nursing education in the country.

INTERMEDIATE MEDICAL EDUCATION INSTITUTE

The Intermediate Medical Education Institutes (IMEI) are responsible for nursing, midwifery and allied health education in Afghanistan. No other individual schools of nursing exist. The IMEI in Kabul provides training programmes at two levels. Institute level programmes require 12th grade education and offer a three-year course of studies for Radiologists (a technical programme), Dental Technicians, Lab Technicians, Pharmacy Technicians, and Physical Therapists. School level programs require 9th grade education and offer two to three year training for general nursing, nurse-midwifery, x-ray technicians, and ophthalmology technicians.

The auxiliary nurse midwife is being reconceptualized as a 'community nurse midwife' who will serve at the basic health unit/ village level. A model programme has been developed by a Dutch NGO, Health Net International, with financing from USAID, and with support from UNICEF through the Johns Hopkins Program for International Education in Obstetrics and Gynecology (JHPIEGO). This two-year training programme (one year of theory and practice; one year field experience) will begin at the Jalalabad University Hospital in the near future.

There are seven regional IMEIs throughout the country in Kandahar, Herat, Helmand/Farah, Mazar, Faizabad, Kunduz and Jalalabad. The Kabul IMEI is the central coordinating body for curricula, policies and procedures, but in reality little communication takes place between the institutes. Not all are functioning adequately due to damages sustained during the war years. The IMEI in Mazar is operating from tents as the building was destroyed. Nursing and midwifery are taught in Herat, Kandahar, Jalalabad, and Mazar. Nursing but not midwifery is taught in Faizabad, Farah, and Kunduz. Only the IMEIs in Kabul and Jalalabad offer programmes in allied health.

The Kabul IMEI, like other educational facilities, faces acute operational constraints. There is not a guaranteed steady source of electricity. Running water and plumbing are inadequate. Classrooms are stark and labs in poor condition. Equipment and supplies are nonexistent (except for NGO provided necessities). There is no transportation for students going to clinical facilities. No hostels exist and the male students are currently housed in tents on the barren land near the school. They contend with heat, dust, snakes, scorpions, and totally inadequate sanitation on a daily basis.

The Kabul IMEI has received technical assistance and infrastructure support from the International Medical Corps (IMC). In July 2002, the Aga Khan Development Network (representing the Aga Khan University), WHO and the Government of Afghanistan signed an agreement to strengthen the IMEIs in general and to enhance the nursing and midwifery programmes specifically. One faculty member from the Aga Khan University School of Nursing (AKUSON) is stationed at IMEI and a nursing education consultant is working to develop a five-year technical assistance plan. WHO will provide a nursing adviser and other technical assistance for IMEI. A WHO Educationist/Training Coordinator is working with the HRD unit of the MOPH. The HRD unit represents the MOPH in collaborating with AKDN and WHO on this project.

The Kabul IMEI has a large nursing programme, with over 350 students. Of those students, however, only thirty-two are women. The Institute and the MOPH have committed to increasing the numbers of female students admitted and set a target of 70 per cent female intake for the 2002 admissions cycle. Results are not yet known. The nurse midwifery programme admits a class of thirty-five women each year. A consultant from UNICEF/JHPIEGO has recently revised the 3rd year curriculum and will work with faculty on clinical supervision of students during a six-month residency programme.

The three-year nursing curriculum has recently been reviewed and modified slightly from the Taliban proscribed version. The number of hours of religious training has decreased significantly. However, the curriculum continues to focus on the medical model and is woefully outdated. A major curriculum revision is needed.

The IMEI faculty is organized into departments, which do not represent the programmes taught. Thus, faculty from all programmes are spread out among the departments. The faculty teaching the 'discipline specific nursing content' can be found in several departments. For example, the faculty teaching Fundamentals of Nursing and Fundamentals of Midwifery (including related skills lab training) are in the Principles of Medicine Department. Other nursing faculty are in the Diseases Department. Support courses, such as sciences, languages and social studies have separate departments. To coordinate the programmes, managers are appointed.

Among the nursing faculty are two teachers who once worked at Mastoorat School of Nursing. One of the midwifery faculty was once the Director of the Post Basic School of Nursing. All faculty need to be educated in current teaching methodologies and to be exposed to current trends in curricular and course development. Content upgrading is urgently required. The issues of clinical expertise and clinical supervision of students will require much time and attention.

SUMMARY

Afghanistan continues to educate nurses for its health workforce. Whereas in the 1970s, all the schools were located in Kabul, more provincial schools exist today. Young women are able to remain at home and study nursing. Young men are still attracted to a career in nursing. The number of female students remains inadequate to meet the needs for access to health care by the majority of Afghan women. The caliber of training offered does not meet international standards and requires major upgrading. The training facilities need renovations and an infusion of physical and educational resources. The service sector requires major infusions of material and human resources. Faculty need to be exposed to new ideas about teaching methodologies and brought up to date about all things related to nursing and health care delivery in the new millennium. This will take time and patience, but the opportunity is now at hand.

BIBLIOGRAPHY

Furnia, A.H. (1978). *Syncrisis: The dynamics of health. XXIV: Afghanistan.* Washington, DC: US Department of Health, Education and Welfare Public Health Service (DHEW 78-50056).

Heber, B. (1975). *Report on a study of nursing schools in Afghanistan.* Kabul, Afghanistan: WHO Nursing Advisory Services (afg/68/015/g/01/14/UNDP).

MOPH. (May 2002). *A Basic Package of Health Services for Afghanistan Second Draft.* Kabul, Afghanistan: author.

MOPH. (February 2002). *National Health Policy. Policy Statement Document Final Draft.* Kabul, Afghanistan: author.

MOPH. (March 2002). *Report of the National Health Sector Planning Workshop.* Kabul, Afghanistan: author.

Russel, L., and Richter, A. (1981). The training of auxiliary nurse midwives in Afghanistan. *Journal of Nurse-Midwifery, 26* (6). 23-25.

WHO Afghanistan. (January/February 2002). *Afghanistan Bulletin,* 1(1), 1-4.

NOTES

1. I learned in September 2002 from a former teacher at the Post Basic School that the first class of students was able to graduate in 1980 and then the school was closed. Several of the graduates are still working as nurse teachers in Kabul. Of the faculty, one has died, one has gone to North America, one teaches at the Intermediate Medical Education Institute; and, one, at least, is working in a health clinic in Kabul.

2. This refers to non-nursing faculty including physicians.

16

Reflections and Future Directions
Nancy H. Bryant

The struggles that have faced the nursing profession since early times have also been the struggles faced by all women in male-dominated societies. Over the years, nurses' work has been looked down upon, thought to be demeaning, needing few educational qualifications, subservient to physicians and meagerly rewarded. At the same time, the concept of the truly caring person who takes care of the sick, comforts the family and works selflessly for long hours is glorified and ennobled as the perfect nurse. But a paradox occurs: people want that kind of person to take care of themselves and their family members when they are ill, but they are reluctant to permit their daughters, sisters or wives to choose nursing as a career.

Throughout the years in the West, women from all social backgrounds have entered nursing. Early leaders in nursing were often women from refined backgrounds, with advanced education for their times, often with strong religious convictions and a mission to help society and the poor. At the same time, nursing has long provided the mobility for women from low-income families to move up economically, socially and professionally.

Nursing has reached the level of an accepted and well-paid profession in many western countries such as the US, UK and Scandinavia, as well as in Australia and New Zealand. Several European countries, however, are still working on recognizing the modern nurse as a full member of the health team. In contrast, countries of the Middle East and South Asia have a long way to go in their recognition of nursing as a true profession comparable to medicine, dentistry and pharmacy. The reasons for this situation are many and have been ably discussed in the preceding chapters.

The situation is not static, and examples of progress can be found in even the most conservative societies. In addition, the International

Council of Nurses is conducting a final review of its 'ICN Framework of Competencies for the Generalist Nurse: Report of the Development Process and Consultation' and 'ICN Framework of Competencies for the Generalist Nurse and an Implementation Model.' When finalized these guidelines will greatly help individual countries establish norms for registered nurses.[1] By having an internationally accepted framework of nurse competencies, many countries will be able to establish one set of competencies for the 'nurse.' To illustrate the importance of these advances, in the Eastern Mediterranean Region of the World Health Organization, there are currently twenty-two different categories of nurses prepared by countries in this region.

This change will not be easy to accomplish for several reasons. First, ministries of health must be convinced that nurses educated to these competencies are necessary to provide quality health care to their populations. Nurses currently prepared at lower levels of education and with fewer competencies cannot perform adequately in institutions of increasing high technology or as managers in community health settings. A plan must be developed to bring them up to basic competency levels.

Second, any programme requiring major changes to reach increased competency levels will also require sufficient funding, and this is where problems will develop. Presently, many ministries of health (except perhaps in the Gulf States) are being forced to cut back budgetary expenditures in all areas and nurses (and nurses associations) do not often have the clout (as compared with medical associations) to demand a greater share of the health budget. Nevertheless, the ICN competencies are a valuable beginning for supporting the upgrading of nursing worldwide, and governments, national nurses associations, private health providers, educational institutions, foundations the corporate sector and donor agencies should be encouraged to begin the effort to promote and require these competencies.

There are many other hopeful signs for the future of nursing in Islamic societies. There are also some stubborn problems that will not be resolved easily. The promotion of education for girls and women by governments, parents and society as a whole is a positive sign for nursings' future. Without general primary and secondary education for both girls and boys, students will not be prepared to enter the post-secondary professional nursing programmes which are considered the minimum for a practicing nurse. Unfortunately, as described by El-Sanabary, many Middle Eastern and South Asian countries still have low literacy rates, and their high population growth rates and poor economies make it impossible for them to provide even basic education for all children. Countries such as Egypt, Pakistan and Bangladesh have female literacy rates from 28 to 44 per cent while at the same time their growth rates are from 1.6 to 2.5 per cent.[2]

We can, however, be encouraged by the overall increase of employment of women in the regions, especially in the health sector. The 1998 ILO study by Richard Anker on gender and jobs (as reported by Sarfati) found that the female share of non-agricultural employment in the MENA region averaged 14.8 per cent. Although their share of employment has increased over the past few decades, women in this region generally have not entered the work force in large numbers. The nursing profession, however, appears to be a genuinely 'female' occupation worldwide and provides an opportunity for women in Islamic countries to enter the labour market.[3] Although the numbers appear small, it is a first step toward making full use of the human resource potential of half the population.

It must be noted that increased employment in nursing will depend on a number of factors. First, MOE and MOH must work together to establish educational institutions and appropriate clinical work settings for educating modern nurses and compensating them in accordance with other health professionals. Adequate compensation, which provides a living wage, is essential to attract both women and men into nursing. It can not be assumed that because most nurses are women that their salaries can be low because they are living free in the homes of their parents, in-laws or husbands. It was our experience at the Aga Khan University Medical Centre (AKUMC), Karachi, that a livable salary, with benefits, pensions, opportunities for continuing and higher education, planned promotions and day care for pre school children, were important factors in attracting young women into nursing and retaining them in the work force.

At the same time that educational qualifications, salaries and benefits are being upgraded, MOH and private health providers need to maintain ongoing public relations programmes that educate the public, parents, brothers and spouses about the value of nurses to society, the nobility of the profession and the economic opportunities it offers young women and their families. It is well known that families play an important part in the career choices girls make and their approval is crucial in recruiting and retaining young women into nursing.

Sarfati and Biscoe discuss the important role that governments must play if they are to recruit enough nurses for their health care systems. Unlike the US, the governments in countries of the Middle East and South Asia are the major employers of doctors, nurses, pharmacists, etc. They are also responsible for providing health care to nearly the entire population. A serious fault of these systems is that a severe shortage of female nurses and doctors leaves many women without health care because of cultural taboos against their being seen by male health workers. In addition, the shortage of nurses in hospitals means that most patients receive inadequate care, or they depend on relatives or attendants for care.

We recognize that most countries under discussion are experiencing cost constraints in their health budgets. However, the previous trends to over-emphasize the education of doctors and not recognize the wide range of services that nurses can provide, have resulted in serious neglect of the nursing profession.

Fortunately, these conditions are changing—even if slowly. Affara and Biscoe note that improvements in basic and post-basic nursing programmes, development of regulations and standards, and preparation of nursing leaders and managers in the WHO EMR have served to elevate and strengthen the profession. Many of these changes and improvements are dependent on or initiated by national nurses associations. As noted by Sarfati and Affara, these organizations vary considerably in their influence and effectiveness within the region. The ICN has played a substantial role in upgrading and supporting the national associations in their efforts to improve educational standards and working conditions of nurses and to provide a strong voice in policy matters related to health.

STATUS OF WOMEN

An important issue that holds a dominant place in future trends for nursing in Islamic societies is the role of women and their place in society. The natural progression for all women in Islam after education is marriage and family. It is still against the established norm to consider working and supporting oneself. Although many women in Middle Eastern countries do prepare themselves for a profession and do hold jobs outside the home, it is still done by only a small proportion of the population, who are mostly urban, and usually within the traditional context of marriage and children. Conditions for most Muslim women do not differ greatly today from the 1930s when Woodsmall reported: 'Eastern society as a whole, not only the Islamic system, has assigned to women a position of economic dependence as regards their earning a livelihood. The Eastern man has always assumed the responsibility for the support of all the women in his family, and guarded this responsibility as a matter of personal honour and pride. Hence, the idea of having a woman earn her own living has been considered a direct reflection on the husband or father or brother, whoever may be responsible for her support...A woman under the established social order of the East, therefore, has never been regarded as an independent member of society, but always as a part of a home group.'[4]

Minai and other authors note the contradictions existing in this situation when from 50 to 70 per cent of rural workers in agriculture are women and most of them receive no wages for their arduous work.[5] We do know, however, that the single professional woman in the West, who previously made up a large part of the teaching and nursing professions, is not yet an acceptable alternative in Muslim society.

In examining the roles of men and women in society, Khan notes that usually the reproductive role is assigned to women and the productive role is assigned to men. When this occurs, the activities assigned to women are those of 'caring' for family members (unpaid) while men are primarily involved in productive work (paid). Unfortunately, this concept has become imbedded in the thinking of health care policy makers. It leads to the generally low wages, low status and poor working conditions that nurses have endured from early times and are still facing today in numerous societies worldwide.

STATUS AND IMAGE OF NURSING

The greatest factor affecting the progress of nursing is its generally low image and status in many countries in South Asia and the Middle East. This has been mentioned again and again by each author who discussed issues relating to women and nursing.

From the time of Florence Nightingale and her efforts to establish nursing as a profession—and up to the present time—it has been an uphill battle to raise both the image and the status of nursing. To a large extent, nursing has achieved professional status in the West. But, as most of the authors note, nursing still suffers from a low image and is not held in high esteem in many Islamic cultures. The caring and nurturing aspects of nursing are highly appreciated and congruent with Islamic values, but the interacting with male physicians and patients, and the necessity to work night and evening shifts are still not accepted by most members of those societies. This paradox presents a major constraint to the development of nursing within Islamic countries.

The violent treatment of women and nurses as described by both Khan and Kingma is a disturbing condition that does not bode well for the future of nursing in these regions or elsewhere. These incidents, documented and publicized, are holding back potential nursing candidates from entering the profession. The climate for change, however, is present in many countries. It will be up to country nursing leaders, national nursing associations and organizations like ICN and WHO, along with the help of enlightened government officials in ministries of health and education as well as health care administrators, to take positive steps to eliminate the injustices, violence and subjugation of women and nurses.

Another issue that greatly affects the status and image of nursing is that of control. It is felt that until nurses, rather than government officials, health planners and physicians, gain control over their profession, nursing will continue to be viewed as a paraprofession and will not attract the bright, committed females who are seeking careers and have the potential to make significant contributions to the profession of nursing.

It is worth mentioning one factor—demand for services—that helps immensely to raise the image and status of nursing. In each of the countries under consideration, the need for nurses far exceeds the numbers available. This situation was true in the 1920s and it is still true now, at the beginning of the twenty-first century. But unless governments, national nurses associations and educational institutions act quickly, the relatively few qualified nurses they are producing will be gobbled up by the United States and other developed countries. A recent article in the *New York Times* by Gail Collins points out that the impending nursing shortage in the US is projected at 400,000 nurses in twenty years. Collins writes about a situation that is all too familiar to the authors of this book:

'It was only in the 19th century that respectable American women were allowed to work for pay, and their natural fields were deemed to be teaching and nursing. Women, the authority figures decreed, had an innate capacity for nurturing—low-cost nurturing....

'We know, in theory, that our hospitals and schools have always been staffed by cheap female labor. But we haven't really grappled with what happens to the health care and education systems when the captive pool of future teachers and nurses dries up....

'Nursing is being reshaped by market forces, in a society that still doesn't quite believe that the old days are over. The average [annual] salary for a nurse right now [in the US] is somewhere between $40,000 and $45,000. The hospitals, in an age of tight budgets and managed care, think that's fair. From now on, a fair salary is going to be whatever it costs to get qualified people in the profession... Management has a right to be efficient and demand results, as long as everybody remembers that the nurses of the future have a right to sign up for dentistry or accounting.'[7]

This situation has already occurred in the oil-rich Gulf States where young women are provided with education up through doctorates if they want them. But, as El-Sanabary and others point out, young women in those countries have opted not to select nursing as a career. Instead, they choose medicine, law or a career in the humanities. It is essential for countries in the Middle East and South Asia to make nursing a desirable and well paid profession in order to slow down migration of future nurses to the US, Europe and other wealthy countries.

There can be no doubt that more and better educated nurses are urgently required to serve present as well as future needs of increasing populations in Islamic societies. Our contributing authors have spoken out courageously on the subject, providing compelling evidence of the dire need to attract, train and nurture a new cadre of intelligent, committed women nurses to supplement the present dedicated nurses who most often carry far too heavy loads under far less than satisfactory conditions. It is true that leaders in many countries in these early years of the twenty-first century are beginning to recognize and respond to the impetus to provide adequate nursing care to their people—whether that impetus be demands of war, rapidly advancing medical technology or global reforms in health service delivery. The hope is that these countries will formulate, fund and implement appropriate nursing reforms—using their nursing leadership as valuable advisery resources—and that these actions will take place soon.

NOTES

1. International Council of Nurses, 'ICN Framework of Competencies for the Generalist Nurse: Report of the Development Process and Consultation' and 'ICN Framework of Competencies for the Generalist Nurse and an Implementation Model.' In preparation.
2. World Bank, *World Development Report 2000/2001: Attacking Poverty*, New York: Oxford University Press, 2001, pp. 276-279.
3. Ricahrd Anker, *Gender and Jobs—Sex segregation of occupations in the world*, Geneva: ILO, 1998, pp. 145-147.
4. Ruth F. Woodsmall, *Women in the Changing Islamic System*, New York: The Round Table Press, 1936, pp. 239-240.
5. Naila Minai, *Women in Islam*, New York: Seaview Books, 1981.
6. Gail Collins, 'Nursing a Shortage,' New York: *New York Times*, 13 April 2001, p. A19.

Contributors

1. **Fadwa A. Affara**, RGN, SCM, MA, MSc, practised as a nurse and midwife for ten years in the UK and abroad. She then spent twelve years in nursing education, in Scotland and Bahrain, where as chairperson of the Division of Nursing at the College of Health Sciences she oversaw the reform of nursing education to an articulated system ranging from the practical nurse level to post-basic specialities and a post-registration BSc. She joined the International Council of Nurses in 1987, initially as director on an international nursing regulation project which involved over eighty countries before taking up the position in 1991 as one of ICN's consultants for nursing and health policy. Among her special responsibilities at ICN were regulation and education. She has been World Health Organization consultant on several occasions, and a member of various WHO working groups. Now retired from ICN she is undertaking consultancy work for ICN and WHO particularly in the field of regulation.

2. **Rahima Jamal Akhtar**, SRN, BScN, MPH(HE), MEd(PHC), obtained her higher nursing education from NIPSOM, Dhaka and from Manchester University, UK. She is presently working as a teacher at the College of Nursing, Dhaka and also works as an editor of the quarterly Nursing Newsletter. She previously worked as Senior Registered Nurse in different hospitals of Bangladesh and also served as a National Nurse Consultant to the Strengthening Nursing Education and Services (SNES) Project, Dhaka, Bangladesh.

3. **Yasmin Amarsi**, RN, BScN, MSN, PhD is Professor and Associate Dean at the Aga Khan University School of Nursing, Karachi, Pakistan. She received her MSN from the University of Arizona and her BScN and PhD from McMaster University, Canada. Her areas of interest are community health and nursing human resources. She has served on numerous committees and held senior offices in the Pakistan Nurses Federation and has taken part in several major donor nursing programmes in Pakistan and East Africa. As the first Pakistani nurse to earn a doctoral degree, she is widely sought after as a speaker and consultant.

4. **Gillian Biscoe**, RN, PhD, is an international nurse consultant who has worked extensively in areas of health system reform, poverty and health, health financing, strategic planning, technical and organizational reviews, and a wide variety of human resource issues. She has facilitated global,

regional and national strategic plans for nursing and midwifery development, is adviser to WHO's SEAR Regional Committee on strengthening management of nursing and midwifery workforce, and works with ICN on their Leadership for Change programme. She is the first nurse and the first woman to be Permanent Secretary for Health and for Human Services in Australia (1991-1996) and was formerly Chief Executive of the Royal Canberra Hospital, a Deputy Director-General in the New Zealand Ministry of Health, and Assistant Secretary in Australia's Commonwealth Department of Health. Her clinical specialty when a practising nurse was intensive care (general and open heart surgery).

5. **Joyceen S. Boyle**, RN, PhD, FAAN, is Chair and Professor, Department of Community and Mental Health Nursing, School of Nursing, Medical College of Georgia. She obtained her PhD in nursing from the University of Utah in 1982. Her masters' degree (MPH) is in public health nursing from the University of California at Berkeley. Her interest is in ethnographic research with diverse cultural groups, especially high risk populations. She is an Associate Editor for the Journal of Transcultural Nursing and is active in teaching and research.

6. **Nancy H. Bryant**, RN, MPH, most recently worked for nine years in various administrative and teaching positions and as Assistant Professor at The Aga Khan University School of Nursing, Karachi, Pakistan. She obtained her bachelor's and masters' degrees from Columbia University, New York City and worked for the Grenfell Association in Newfoundland, Canada and as a school nurse at the International School, Bangkok, Thailand. She was Director of the Office of Consumer Health Education, University of Medicine and Dentistry of New Jersey before moving to Washington, DC where she worked in the advertising department of the Health and Education section at the Washington Post. She is the author of Progress and Constraints of Nursing and Nursing Education in Islamic Societies' in *Global Perspective on Health Care*.

7. **Fariba Al-Darazi**, RN, MSc, PhD, is the Regional Adviser for Nursing and Allied Health Personnel, Eastern Mediterranean Region, WHO, Cairo, Egypt. She was previously Director of Training, Ministry of Health, State of Bahrain, Arabian Gulf. She obtained her PhD from the College of Nursing, University of Illinois at Chicago.

8. **Ira Dibra**, SRN, DPHN, BSc in PHN, Dip in PHC, Med (PHC), is presently working as a Nursing Officer to the Nursing Directorate. She received her higher nursing education from Manchester University, UK. She served as National Nurse Consultant to the SNES Project, Dhaka, Bangladesh and as an assistant editor for the Nursing Newsletter. Prior to that she worked as a District Public Health Nurse at Mymenshing, Bangladesh.

9. **Paula Herberg**, RN, PhD, is Associate Professor, California State University, Fullerton, California. She previously worked for ten years at The Aga Khan University where she was a Professor and Director of the School of Nursing; and Associate Dean, Nursing in the Faculty of Health Sciences. She obtained her masters' degree from the University of Maryland and her PhD from the University of Utah. She is a Family Nurse Practitioner. Her major areas of interest are transcultural/ international nursing and nursing systems/nursing educational programme development worldwide. She has been involved in several major donor funded nursing development projects in Pakistan and East Africa and has lived and worked in Afghanistan, Nepal, Thailand and Pakistan. She has done short term consultation work in Kenya, Uganda, Tanzania/ Zanzibar and Tajikistan.

10. **Kausar S. Khan**, BS, MA, is a sociologist and Associate Professor, Community Health Sciences Department at the Aga Khan University, Karachi, Pakistan. She has been active in the human rights movement in Pakistan, especially as it relates to women's issues. She is also the author of numerous articles.

11. **Mireille Kingma**, RN, PhD, is a Consultant, Nursing and Health Policy with the International Council of Nurses, a federation of over 120 national nurses' associations. She obtained a Bachelor Degree in Nursing and post-basic qualifications in Human Resources Development and Health Policy. Her doctoral thesis was on Economic Policy: Incentive or disincentive for community nurses? During the past eighteen years she has been responsible for international consultations and workshop programmes in more than sixty countries. Her major job portfolios include socio-economic welfare of nurses, human resources development, occupational health and safety, care of the older person, refugees, nursing students, and international trade in health services. Her main interests are human resources development, violence reduction, impact of health and economic policy on the delivery of care, negotiation, and process of policy formulation.

12. **Gladys Mouro**, RN, MSN, is Assistant Hospital Director, American University of Beirut Medical Centre, Beirut, Lebanon. She received a BS in Nursing from the American University of Beirut and her MS in Nursing from the University of Pennsylvania. Her entire professional career has been spent at AUB where she began as a staff nurse in 1976 and rose to Director of Nursing Services in 1983, and to her present position in 1995. She was awarded the Silver Order of Health by the Lebanese Government in 1994. She is the author of *An American Nurse Amidst Chaos (1975-1998), The story of the American University Medical Centre during the Lebanese Civil War.*

13. **Khlood Salman**, RN, DrPH, completed her doctoral work from the University of Pittsburgh in 2001. Her masters' degree in nursing (MSN)

is from the University of Pittsburgh also. She is a pulmonary nurse specialist. She taught for approximately nine years at the College of Nursing, University of Baghdad. Her research has focused on chronic diseases and diabetic related complications in Middle Eastern populations.

14. **Nagat El-Sanabary**, MA, PhD, is a gender and education development specialist with extensive academic and practical field experiences. She is currently a senior visiting scholar at the Centre for Middle Eastern Studies, University of California at Berkeley (UCB). She received her undergraduate education at Cairo University in Egypt and her MA and PhD degrees from UCB. She began her career in Egypt as a secondary school teacher and radio broadcaster. In the USA she has held teaching and academic administrative positions at UCB, Holy Name College in Oakland, California, and at King Abdelaziz University in Jeddah, Saudi Arabia. An internationally recognized expert on women's education in the Arab and Islamic countries, she has written and published extensively on the subject. She is the author of a book on Education in the Arab Gulf States and the Arab World and has also contributed numerous journal articles and book chapters. She has been a consultant to the World Bank, USAID, UNDP, UNESCO and several Arab universities and international consulting firms and NGOs. She has done extensive fieldwork on education and gender and development in most of the Arab countries and in several Asian and African countries.

15. **Hedva Sarfati**, a political scientist, analyst of comparative employment, social protection and labour relations policies, is the former Director of the Industrial Relations and Labour Administration Department, ILO, Geneva, Switzerland. At present she is a consultant to the Geneva-based International Social Security Association (ISSA) and director of the ISSA project on the Interactions between labour market and social protection reforms. As Chief of the Salaried Employees and Professional Workers Branch, ILO (1987-1997), she launched and was responsible for the implementation of a broad research programme and publications on the remuneration and career development of nursing personnel in various world regions. Her most recent publication is *Labour market and social protection reforms in international perspective:Parallel or converging tracks*? (with Giuliano Bonoli).

Index

North Africa, 6, 8, 10, 67, 90, 93, 96-
99, 115, 122
Norway, 102
Nursing
– education, 11, 176-179, 181,
182, 185, 186, 215, 216, 285
– image, 4, 5, 53, 79, 183, 217,
234, 267, 269, 274, 275, 282,
307, 320, 342
– leadership, 5, 6, 19, 24, 26, 27,
29, 31, 32, 34-36, 37, 38, 123,
302
– status, 4, 5, 10, 12, 25, 46, 61,
62, 75, 90, 104, 107, 115, 117,
118, 123, 161, 171, 188, 191,
205, 206, 208, 209, 217-219,
234, 260, 281, 282, 290, 293,
301, 304, 307, 342, 343
Nursing and Midwifery, 4, 6, 14, 15,
18-20, 23-29, 31, 32, 34-39, 49,
92, 100, 120, 176, 186, 289, 333,
335
– health system
reform and development
(HSRD), 5, 19, 20-22, 37
Nursing Shortage, 90, 115, 116, 123,
129, 178, 196, 219, 223, 256, 257,
270, 272, 289, 290, 296, 302, 343

O

OECD, 22, 93, 107
Oman, 26, 27, 47-49, 97, 99-101,
103, 104, 122, 306
Ortin, E., 121

P

Pakistan, 1, 7, 9-11, 47, 49, 57, 58,
60, 65-69, 71, 73-75, 77, 80-82,
85, 86, 94, 100-104, 120, 122,
141-143, 159-162, 164, 169-173,
180, 188-197, 200-212, 214-216,

218, 220, 221, 223-225, 232, 281,
284, 286, 289, 340
– Karachi, 1, 143, 170, 195, 281,
286, 289, 340
– Nursing   Health   Human
Resource
cultural trends and status of
women, 192
current health, 194
demographics, 192
health   human   resources
development (HRD), 195
implications, 224
Overview, 188
perceptions of how it works
management, 217
planning, 201
production, 210
similarities and differences,
219
planning, 221
study, 197
– Pakistan Nursing Council, 210,
215, 284
– Punjab, 81, 160, 172, 188
– Sindh, 81, 160, 188, 197, 205,
208, 211-213, 215, 216, 220,
223
– Women
critical periods in history, 171
hard facts, 161
trapped but struggling, 10, 159,
169
Palestine, 76
Philippines, 15, 17, 18, 102-104, 120-
122, 125, 190
Poland, 102
Primary Education, 65, 67, 69-71, 75,
81, 259, 261, 292, 296
Primary Health Care (PHC), 92, 101,
107, 130, 131, 178, 233, 255, 260,
271-273, 276, 286
Productive Roles, 168, 169
Public Health Nurses, 118